S0-ARN-819

DATE DUE

Diagnosis and Therapy
of Fetal Anomalies

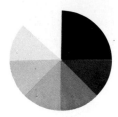

CLINICS IN DIAGNOSTIC ULTRASOUND
VOLUME 25

EDITORIAL BOARD

Kenneth J.W. Taylor, M.D., Ph.D., F.A.C.P., *Chairman*
Diane Babcock, M.D.
James P. Crane, M.D.
Barry B. Goldberg, M.D.
John C. Hobbins, M.D.
Joseph A. Kisslo, M.D.
George R. Leopold, M.D.
Wesley L. Nyborg, Ph.D.
P.N.T. Wells, D.Sc.
Marvin C. Ziskin, M.D.

Diagnosis and Therapy of Fetal Anomalies

Edited by

John C. Hobbins, M.D.

Professor
Department of Obstetrics and Gynecology
(Perinatal Medicine)
Yale University School of Medicine
Director
Department of Obstetrics and Gynecology
Yale-New Haven Hospital
New Haven, Connecticut

Beryl R. Benacerraf, M.D.

Clinical Associate Professor
Department of Obstetrics and Gynecology
Clinical Assistant Professor
Department of Radiology
Harvard Medical School
Consultant
Departments of Obstetrics and Gynecology,
and Radiology
Brigham and Women's Hospital
Boston, Massachusetts

CHURCHILL LIVINGSTONE
NEW YORK, EDINBURGH, LONDON, MELBOURNE
1989

Library of Congress Cataloging in Publication Data

Diagnosis and therapy of fetal anomalies / edited by John C. Hobbins,
    Beryl R. Benacerraf.
        p.   cm.—(Clinics in diagnostic ultrasound; v. 25)
    Includes bibliographies and index.
    ISBN 0–443–08609–5
    1. Fetus—Abnormalities.   2. Fetus—Diseases.   3. Prenatal
diagnosis.   4. Diagnosis, Ultrasonic.   I. Hobbins, John C., date.
II. Benacerraf, Beryl R.   III. Series.
    [DNLM: 1. Abnormalities—diagnosis.   2. Fetal Diseases—
diagnosis.   3. Fetal Diseases—therapy.   4. Prenatal Diagnosis.
5. Ultrasonic
Diagnosis.   W1 CL831BC v. 25 / WQ 211 D536]
RG626.D53 1989
618.3′2—dc19
DNLM/DLC
for Library of Congress   88–25658
                                                                        CIP

© **Churchill Livingstone Inc. 1989**

All rights reserved. No part of this publication may be reproduced, stored in a retrieval
system, or transmitted in any form or by any means, electronic, mechanical,
photocopying, recording, or otherwise, without prior permission of the publisher
(Churchill Livingstone Inc., 1560 Broadway, New York, NY 10036).

Distributed in the United Kingdom by Churchill Livingstone, Robert Stevenson House,
1–3 Baxter's Place, Leith Walk, Edinburgh EH1 3AF, and by associated companies,
branches, and representatives throughout the world.

Accurate indications, adverse reactions, and dosage schedules for drugs are provided in
this book, but it is possible that they may change. The reader is urged to review the
package information data of the manufacturers of the medications mentioned.

The Publishers have made every effort to trace the copyright holders for borrowed
material. If they have inadvertently overlooked any, they will be pleased to make the
necessary arrangements at the first opportunity.   ·

Acquisitions Editor: *Linda Panzarella*
Copy Editor: *Kathleen M. Carroll*
Production Designer: *Melanie Haber*
Production Supervisor: *Christina Hippeli*

Printed in the United States of America

First published in 1989

Contributors

Beryl R. Benacerraf, M.D.
Clinical Associate Professor, Department of Obstetrics and Gynecology,
Clinical Assistant Professor, Department of Radiology, Harvard Medical School;
Consultant, Departments of Obstetrics and Gynecology, and Radiology,
Brigham and Women's Hospital, Boston, Massachusetts

Richard L. Berkowitz, M.D.
Professor and Chairman, Department of Obstetrics—Gynecology and
Reproductive Science, Mount Sinai School of Medicine of the City University
of New York, New York, New York

Jason C. Birnholz, M.D., F.A.C.R., F.A.C.O.G.
Professor, Department of Radiology, Rush Medical College of Rush University,
Chicago, Illinois

Frank A. Boehm, M.D.
Professor, Department of Obstetrics and Gynecology; Associate Professor,
Department of Radiology, Vanderbilt University School of Medicine; Director
of Maternal-Fetal Medicine, Vanderbilt University Medical Center, Nashville,
Tennessee

Luciano Bovicelli, M.D.
Professor, Cattedra di Fisiopatologia Prenatale, Instituto di Clinica Ostetrica e
Ginecologica, School of Medicine, Bologna, Italy

James Campbell, M.R.C.O.G.
Professor, Department of Obstetrics and Gynaecology, King's College School of
Medicine and Dentistry; Department of Obstetrics and Gynaecology, Harris
Birthright Research Centre for Fetal Medicine, London, England

Joshua A. Copel, M.D.
Assistant Professor and Director of Resident Education, Department of
Obstetrics and Gynecology, Yale University School of Medicine; Attending
Physician, Yale–New Haven Hospital, New Haven, Connecticut

Terri L. Daniel, M.D.
Diagnostic Radiologist, Department of Radiology, Baptist Regional Medical Center, Corbin, Kentucky

Arthur C. Fleisher, M.D.
Professor of Radiology and Associate Professor in Obstetrics and Gynecology, Vanderbilt University School of Medicine; Chief, Ultrasound Section, Department of Radiology, Vanderbilt University Medical Center, Nashville, Tennessee

Peter A. T. Grannum, M.D.
Associate Professor, Department of Obstetrics and Gynecology (Maternal-Fetal Medicine), Director of Medical Studies and of High Risk Obstetrics, Yale University School of Medicine, New Haven, Connecticut

Philippe Jeanty, Ph.D., M.D.
Associate Professor and Director of Perinatal Research, Vanderbilt University School of Medicine, Nashville, Tennessee

Charles S. Kleinman, M.D.
Professor of Pediatrics, Diagnostic Imaging, and Obstetrics and Gynecology, Department of Pediatric Cardiology, Yale University School of Medicine, New Haven, Connecticut

Alfred B. Kurtz, M.D.
Professor, Departments of Radiology and Obstetrics and Gynecology, Jefferson Medical College of Thomas Jefferson University; Associate Director, Division of Diagnostic Ultrasound, Department of Radiology, Thomas Jefferson University Hospital, Philadelphia, Pennsylvania

Lauren Lynch, M.D.
Assistant Professor, Division of Maternal-Fetal Medicine, Department of Obstetrics–Gynecology and Reproductive Science, Mount Sinai School of Medicine of the City University of New York, New York, New York

Frank A. Manning, M.D.
Professor and Head, Department of Obstetrics, Gynecology, and Reproductive Sciences, Division of Maternal-Fetal Medicine, University of Manitoba Faculty of Medicine; Chairman, Department of Obstetrics, Gynecology, and Reproductive Sciences, Women's Hospital, Winnipeg, Manitoba, Canada

Karen E. Mehalek, M.D.
Fellow, Division of Maternal-Fetal Medicine, Department of Obstetrics—Gynecology and Reproductive Science, Mount Sinai School of Medicine of the City University of New York, New York, New York

Kypros Nicholaides, M.R.C.O.G.
Deputy Director, Department of Obstetrics and Gynaecology, Kings College
School of Medicine and Dentistry; Department of Obstetrics and Gynaecology,
Harris Birthright Centre for Fetal Medicine, London, England

Rebecca G. Pennell, M.D.
Assistant Professor, Department of Radiology, Jefferson Medical College of
Thomas Jefferson University; Division of Diagnostic Ultrasound, Thomas
Jefferson University Hospital, Philadelphia, Pennsylvania

Gianluigi Pilu, M.D.
Attending Physician, Section of Prenatal Pathophysiology, Second Department
of Obstetrics and Gynecology, University of Bologna School of Medicine,
Bologna, Italy

Roberto Romero, M.D.
Associate Professor and Director of Perinatal Research, Department of
Obstetrics and Gynecology, Yale University School of Medicine, New Haven,
Connecticut

Glynis A. Sacks, M.D.
Clinical Assistant, Ultrasound Section, Department of Radiology, Vanderbilt
University Medical Center; Consultant, West Side Medical Plaza Diagnostic
Center, Nashville, Tennessee

Dinesh M. Shah, M.D.
Associate Professor, Department of Obstetrics and Gynecology (Maternal-Fetal
Medicine), Vanderbilt University School of Medicine; Director, Obstetric
Diabetic Unit, Vanderbilt University Medical Center, Nashville, Tennessee

Marina Sirtori, M.D.
Post-doctoral Fellow, Department of Obstetrics and Gynecology (Perinatal
Medicine), Yale University School of Medicine, New Haven, Connecticut

Contents

Preface

Many obstetric ultrasound texts have either a predominately obstetric or radiologic slant because the authors tend to represent one discipline. Although the co-editors, a radiologist and obstetrician, have attempted to attain an even mix in the authorship, it will become apparent to the reader that there is now very little difference between radiologists and obstetricians in their approach taken to the diagnosis of fetal anomalies.

This volume of the Clinics has been designed for the experienced sonographer or sonologist who is confronted with obstetric patients having developmentally abnormal fetuses. The chapters comprehensively address prenatal diagnosis according to fetal body system and are written by authors who were chosen because of their experience and expertise in their assigned topics.

The concepts and the data incorporated in this text represent the most up-to-date information in the literature because the authors are in the forefront of current investigation and the "turn around" time for these volumes is remarkably short. Even though we tailor-made this book for the busy ultrasound practitioner, we sincerely hope that medical students, residents, and sonographers-in-training will find this an invaluable reference resource.

John C. Hobbins, M.D.
Beryl R. Benacerraf, M.D.

1 Fetal Syndromes

Jason C. Birnholz

The term *syndrome* is taken from two Greek roots meaning "running together." The term appears to have been introduced in English usage around the mid-sixteenth century conveying, as in the works of Sydenham, a combination of symptoms pertaining to a particular disease. In recent times, the term has received several technical definitions, each tending to imply a combination of findings or observations concerning individual patients. If the combination recurs, the syndrome becomes legitimized, and when a mechanism is found explaining a syndrome, we refer to it as a *disease*. Syndromes are named eponymically (e.g., Potter syndrome, Robert syndrome) descriptively by some of their major features (e.g., bird-headed dwarf, CHARGE association), by outcome (e.g., thanatophoric dwarf), or by cause (e.g., trisomy 21).

Whenever any fetal abnormality is found, we must try to determine whether it is an isolated problem or one that represents a systemic process, the latter implying a syndrome and generally conveying a poor prognosis. The same rationale underlies our obtaining amniotic fluid or fetal blood for chromosomal analysis with apparently isolated anomalies. One recent study found an unexpectedly high incidence of aneuploidy in cases of umbilical hernia or abdominal wall defects.[1]

There are no definitive guidelines for a "routine" examination suitable for a referral center. However, we perform an exhaustive survey when there are abnormal image findings or when a past, family, or current history indicates further attention. We use minor morphologic signs for classification, and we compensate for the difficulties of achieving total visualization under all conditions by performing serial restudies.

DEFINITIONS

Categorical terms concerning fetal anomalies have been used loosely in ultrasound practice, although they are defined stringently by international convention[2,3] and in textbooks.[4] We use the term *malformation* to refer to a

1

primary defect in morphogenesis, and *malformation syndrome* when there are developmental abnormalities in two or more organs or physiologic systems. An *embryopathy* is an acquired abnormality; this group is subdivided into *deformations*, usually compression or restriction associated with oligohydramnios or myometrial tumor, and *disruptions*, usually the result of an amniotic band. An *association* is a combination of presumably unrelated findings, whereas a *complex* or *sequence* constitutes several findings with a common cause. This scheme emphasizes anatomic findings, as sought by ultrasonic imaging and recognizes that additional terms will be required for metabolic or biochemical disorders and for dyshistogenic processes without grossly visible morphologic abnormalities.

External insults operating around the time of conception will be expected to have an all-or-none effect. Malformations are usually dated to the mid-first to mid-second trimester, although a variety of atresias and hypoplasias can be caused by vascular insults later in pregnancy. Abnormalities of remodeling, especially of the face, may not appear until later in development (Fig. 1.1). The embryopathies tend to be concerns of the second half of pregnancy,

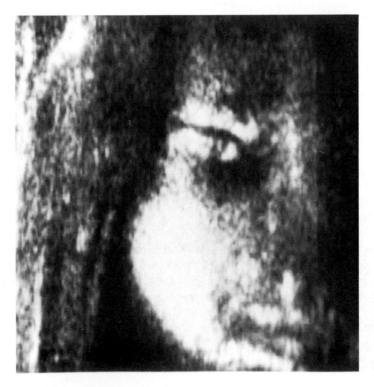

FIG. 1.1.   Trisomy 21. Right coronal face view showing the characteristic epicanthal fold and lax cheek. These third-trimester features are absent even by visual inspection of afflicted abortuses less than 20 weeks old.

although we have seen amniotic band disruptions in the early second trimester.[5]

SYNDROMES WITH LUNG HYPOPLASIA

One of the most important assets of the ultrasonic study, and one infrequently discussed, is confirmation of adequate lung volume. This is accomplished easily[7] in transverse thoracic sections through the crux of the heart, expecting that the heart itself will only occupy about one-third of the total area. Fetal myocardium is stiff and has little tendency for volume loading. A relatively large heart in ultrasound images is usually due to lung hypoplasia with reduction in the bulk of thoracic contents. Also, the diameters of the chest will be considerably less than those of the adjacent upper abdomen, reconfirming the impression (Fig. 1.2). Lung hypoplasia encompasses a range of severity. Those forms obvious in ultrasound images are key to syndrome evaluation because, no matter what other findings may be present, neonatal mortality can be expected.

Lung hypoplasia is an invariant component of Potter syndrome,[6] in which the primary malformation is (bilateral) renal agenesis. It is possible, but unlikely, that there is some component of fetal urine that contributes to lung development, given the potential for amniotic fluid entry into the respiratory tract when the larynx is open during diaphragm descent. Rather, it would appear that chest wall restriction due to oligohydramnios is causative.[7] Lung

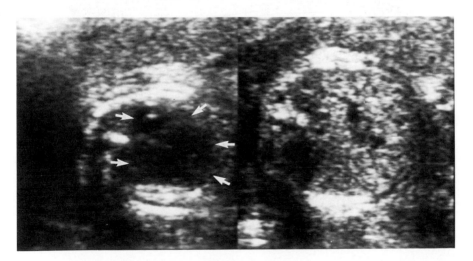

FIG. 1.2.   Oligohydramnios. Split-screen views comparing transverse sections of the chest and upper abdomen. The heart (arrows) fills the thorax. Note severe lung hypoplasia.

hypoplasia complicates longstanding oliogohydramnios from any cause, including bilateral obstructive uropathy and prolonged rupture of membranes. Lung hypoplasia is also a feature of skeletal dysplasias with thoracic involvement such as osteogenesis imperfecta with multiple rib fractures (Fig. 1.3), thanatophoric dwarfism, asphyxiating thoracic dystrophy, and spondylocostal dysostosis.

The time course of lung compression is likely a major determinant of its clinical severity. We presume that each organ has critical or vulnerable phases during which otherwise minor insults can arrest or seriously impair development.[8] For the lung, 15 to 19 weeks gestational age (during the cannicular phase of development) is a particularly critical phase. Primary renal agenesis is always associated with an irreversible pulmonary growth deficit, whereas mild lung hypoplasia acquired in the early third trimester as a result of prolonged rupture of membranes may be recovered postnatally, if satisfactory respiratory support can be achieved throughout the neonatal period. Severely compromised lung growth occurs with large diaphragmatic hernias (which accompany various malformation syndromes), with cystic adenomatoid lung malformation, and with large pleural effusions (which generally have a mid-second trimester occurrence and may be related to delayed lymphatic development) or persistent diaphragmatic elevation with ascites.

Lung hypoplasia has also been created in experimental animals by cervical

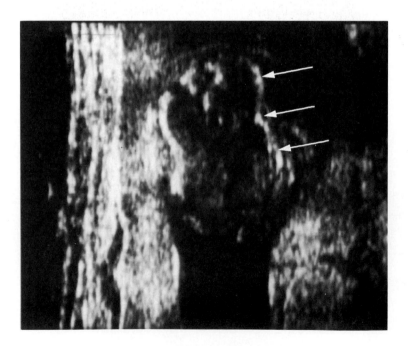

FIG. 1.3. Central rib fractures result in an hourglass deformity (spine 12 o'clock, arrows along left eighth rib). Mid-second-trimester thoracic wall injury stunts lung growth.

cord injury, which abolishes diaphragm (and costal) movement.[9] Spontaneous diaphragm movements are normally present during the critical phase of lung development, decreasing in incidence to the start of the third trimester (as central inhibition develops), and then increasing progressively until the later third trimester, when sleep states differentiate. Inasmuch as diaphragm movements are initiated at the brain stem level,[10] lung hypoplasia does not tend to be a complication of most cortical brain malformations in which subcortical development is unaffected. Diaphragm movements are present in Potter syndrome.

SYNDROMES WITH CENTRAL NERVOUS SYSTEM COMPONENTS

The brain is involved in malformation syndromes by grossly dysmorphic development, by delayed growth, or by depressed function (these last two categories with macroscopically normal anatomy). Dysmorphic changes are usually obvious ultrasonically (Figs. 1.4 and 1.5), while the image findings

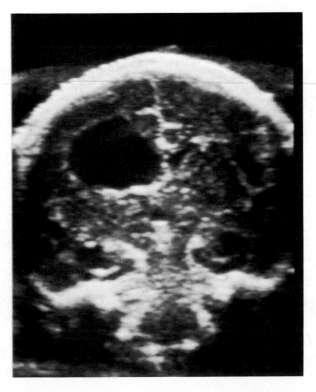

FIG. 1.4.   There is an obvious disparity in lateral ventricular size and shape in this coronal section (34.8 weeks). The left ventricle is normal and the right is expanded (porencephaly), because of vascular injury with hypoplasia of the overlying cortex.

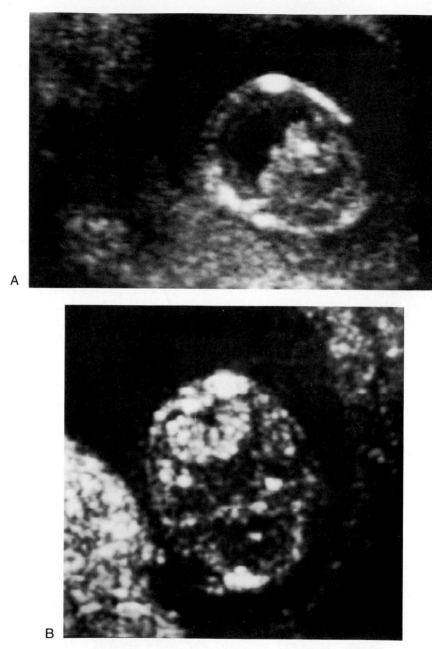

FIG. 1.5. (A) Holoprosencephaly at 12 weeks gestational age. There is a single central ventricle. Compare with the normal condition (B), in which choroid glomi fill the upper cranium.

in delayed growth are typically subtle. Examples of dysmorphic development include the single U-shaped ventricle of alobar holoprosencephaly (which can occur sporadically, with trisomy-13, with partially swallowed amniotic bands, and, possibly, with maternal cocaine use[11]), cerebellar agenesis with Dandy-Walker cyst formation (which occurs sporadically and with first trimester maternal coumadin exposure[12]), and absence of the cerebellar vermis with occipital flattening (frequently accompanying lumbar or sacral neural tube defects[13]).

The eye is an embryologic derivative of the forebrain that is uniquely suited to ultrasound examination[14] (Fig. 1.6), including recognition of coloboma, micropthalmia, or delayed hyaloid artery regression, which has a frequent association with aneuploidy.[15]

Partial or complete agenesis of the corpus callosum is frequently associated with other anomalies and is particularly easily sought (or excluded) with ultrasonic imaging (Fig. 1.7). It has been suggested that callosal agenesis is a forme fruste of holoprosencephaly,[16,17] and it is frequent with trisomy 13[18] and with various types of facial or palatal clefts.[19] Agenesis of the corpus callosum often occurs with, or induces, a characteristic ventricular configuration of dilated occipital horns narrowing to rudimentary frontal horns, referred to as colpocephaly.[20] We have seen four cases of ambiguous genitalia with absence of the corpus callosum (one also with a Dandy-Walker cyst), and an association with hypospadias has been reported.[21] The Aicardi syndrome[22] associates agenesis of the corpus callosum in females with choreoretinal abnormalities, infantile spasms, and mental retardation. It is important to distinguish the absence of the corpus callosum from the innocuous typically isolated occurrence of absence of the septum pellucidum.

In the early ultrasound experience, fetal brain growth was inferred from the size and shape of the cranium, whereas today we evaluate some brain features directly. The mantle becomes measurable, ultrasonically, at about 12 weeks gestational age. We have observed an abrupt increase in cortical thickness between about 14 and 16½ weeks gestational age (GA), a relative plateau for about 10 days, followed by a later surge in thickness. These phases appear to correspond to neuronal proliferation, neuronal migration (with selective cell death), and glial proliferation.[23] In the second trimester, ventricles are passive, their configuration dependent on regional brain growth (Figs. 1.4 and 1.8). There is some fluid accumulation in the anterior portions of the frontal horns at 14 to 16 weeks, and there is some mild fullness of the occipital horns until the start of the third trimester. The ventricular atria are filled with choroid glomi and have little free fluid (Fig. 1.5B). Ventricular dilation in the second trimester is always significant clinically, because its presence implies a primary deficiency in brain growth. Delayed brain growth is a feature of Down syndrome, wherein the entire triphasic sequence is delayed 2 to 3 weeks. These cases also show delay in sulcation in the third trimester in our own experience and in isolated case reports.[24]

The Miller-Dieker syndrome[25] is a rare condition that illustrates potential associations of temporally disordered cortical growth. Neuronal migration

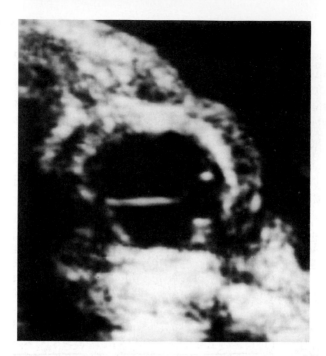

FIG. 1.6. Sagittal section through the eye at 17 weeks gestational age. The hyaloid artery bridges the retina (9 o'clock) with the cup-shaped lens (9 o'clock).

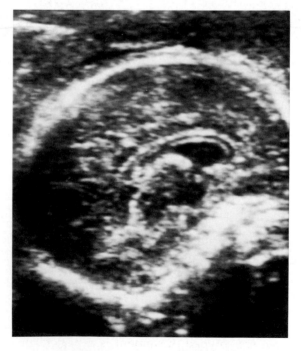

FIG. 1.7. The corpus callosum is an obvious landmark in the midline sagittal view. It is outlined interiorly by fluid in the cavum septi pellucidi.

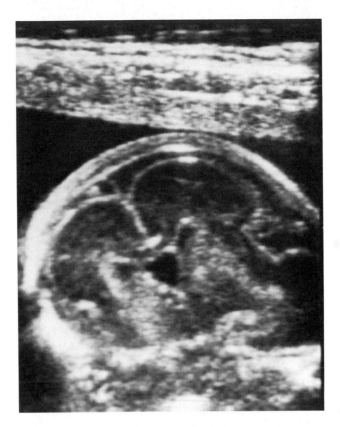

FIG. 1.8.   Coronal views after 16 weeks should show small symmetric lateral ventricles surrounded by a thick cortical mantle. At this stage, the brain surface is smooth, and there is a fluid rim over the convexities outlining the falx.

leading to sulcation fails, and the brain surface is smooth (lissencephaly), the cortex is thick (decreased selective cell death) but there is an atrophy-like ventriculomegaly, and there is severe mental retardation. There appears to be an underlying short-arm chromosome 17 abnormality and there are associated renal (unilateral agenesis to bilateral cystic dysplasia) and occasionally cardiac anomalies. It is essential to evaluate lung volume, whenever a maldevelopment syndrome is found. The Miller-Dieker association illustrates an extension of that hierarchial structure, namely, that with any visceral anomaly, brain anatomy should also be studied in detail.

Functional information about the brain is inferred through observing motor activity. Some observations will concern the quality of movements. Seizure activity is uncommon but of obvious importance. Second-trimester movements tend to be abrupt. These are distinguished from tonic-clonic seizures, in which the same stereotyped movement is repeated for at least 10 to 20 seconds, followed by postictal depression of further motor activity for at least a short time. Seizures tend to be asymmetric. A related concern is consistent absence of movements on one side. Major seizures are dramatic, unlikely to be confused with normal activity. Repetitive series of hiccups are a normal occurrence that lack obligatory limb movements or postictal phases.

Another potentially misleading situation is a slender anxious mother in whom aortic or iliac artery pulsations are transmitted to the posterior wall of the uterus with pulsatile bobbing of a dependent second-trimester fetus. A general paucity and rapid fatigue for simple movements are characteristic, dynamic features of some of the muscle development problems, including Werdnig-Hoffmann syndrome and central nuclear palsy. A milder form of fatigue occurs with maternal myasthenia gravis, in which antimuscle antibodies cross the placental barrier. Motor activity is suppressed centrally as an energy-conserving mechanism with hypoxemia, and it is depressed extrinsically with maternal sedative or narcotic use.

There are few options for assessing fetal sensory competence, although auditory stimulation is practical in the third trimester.[26] We assess hearing by observing a motor response to a startling sound, which requires not only function of the sensor, but perception and completion of circuits to motor effectors. Failure to elicit auditory responsiveness prompts consideration of primary deafness and of a depressed central nervous system (CNS) as with trisomies 13 and 18, fetal alcohol and marijuana syndromes, and hypoxia.

SYNDROMES INVOLVING GROWTH DISTURBANCE

Most systemic malformation syndromes involve an abnormality of growth. The growth deficit may be regional or general, absolute or relative (i.e., involving some disproportion). An isolated structural abnormality associated with generalized growth deficit implies a systemic process. Likewise, growth retardation of such severity as to be recognized before 28 weeks prompts a search for any evidence of a developmental syndrome including blood sampling or amniocentesis for aneuploidy, TORCH infection, or some dysmetabolic state. Triploidy is a common chromosomal disorder, but it is not encountered with great frequency in ultrasound practice because of the high incidence of death and spontaneous abortion in the first and early second trimesters.[27] The condition involves hypoplastic development of many organs, including soft tissues compositely. Growth delay is demonstrable from crown-rump length increments in the first trimester, as well as from any somatic measurements obtained later. In this case, and in some other chromosomal problems, growth rates at the cellular level are below average. This is a completely different mechanism of growth restriction from the energy-conserving compensation for placental insufficiency that accounts for most clinical cases of growth retardation. There are also syndromes involving fetal overgrowth, not discussed further herein.

Developing bone and cartilage are depicted with unique clarity with ultrasound imaging. Consequently, a fundamental diagnostic capability for ultrasound is the antenatal detection of skeletal disorders, including many forms

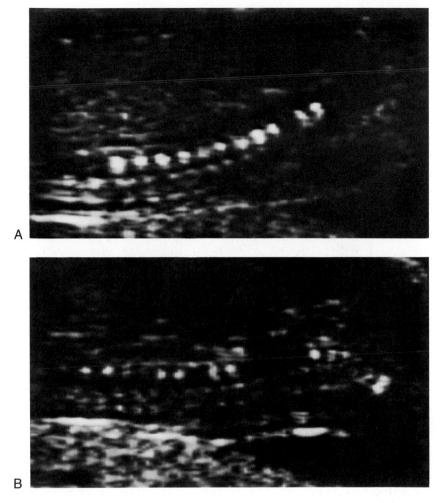

FIG. 1.9. Hypophosphatasia at 15 weeks. View through the lateral processes of the spine (A) shows a focal absence. Section through the centra (B) demonstrates a gross deficiency in ossification.

of dwarfism. The primary disorders that we encounter range from defective ossification as in hypophosphatasia (Fig. 1.9); the production of thin, weak, and readily fractured bone (osteogenesis imperfecta and the rare Needles-Melnick syndrome); and those conditions in which limb length is foreshortened but with structurally sound bone and joint formation (Fig. 1.10).

Limb reductions are subclassified as distal (acromelic), middle (mesomelic), and proximal (rhizomelic). It is now reasonably standard practice to assess GA from femur-shaft length. This measurement will fortuitously disclose rhizomelic dwarfism; however, other portions of the limbs should also be surveyed, particularly when any type of general growth disturbance is suspected.

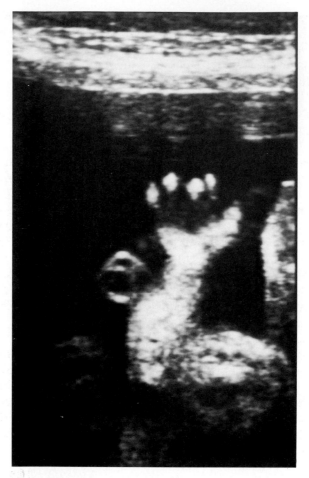

FIG. 1.10. Note the obvious disproportion between the size of the hand and the length of the forearm in this case of dwarfism.

Inspection demonstrates gross limb-reduction problems; recognition of more subtle forms requires measurements. We tend to think in terms of absolute measurement discrepancies when we compare individual values with tables, although proportional discrepancies requiring comparisons of separate parts may be more revealing in syndrome identification.[28] For example, conventional skeletal staging measurements include one or more diameters of the head and femur length. In the normal fetus, there is very little variation in growth patterns through at least 20 weeks, with cranial measurements becoming a progressively poor measurement in the third trimester; this is because they are insensitive to changes in surface area of the brain that account for the principal component of growth then.[29] In any case, a very small head, in comparison with long-bone growth implies microcephaly, while an appropriately sized head and short femurs suggest other forms of regional growth disturbance, including Down syndrome. We tend to concentrate on the "standard" measurements. In the case of Down syndrome, the growth disturbance is more general, affecting other parts of the skeleton and body for which we will have to develop or retrieve additional "standards."[30]

We try to distinguish, conceptually, "delayed" and "retarded" growth patterns. A delayed pattern resembles the normal pattern but is shifted in time, while, with the retarded pattern, growth velocity (i.e., the slope of the growth curve) declines progressively. For the delayed pattern, there are diagnostic "windows of opportunity" after which the part in question will appear normal. This occurs, for example, with Down syndrome. Brain growth is slow in the mid-second trimester and the ventricles are relatively large, but after the fifth month they appear normal; sulcation is delayed in the early third trimester but appears normal by term. Two additional considerations with retarded patterns are their times of onset and severity. For example, some forms of microcephaly involve failure of glial proliferation, which begins around 18 or 19 weeks. Consequently, earlier diagnosis is not possible. Similar considerations pertain with milder forms of achondroplasia, in which limb appearance may be normal initially.

Cases of dwarfism have tended to be classified diagnostically on the basis of classic radiographic findings, that is, by other skeletal features, such as vertebral body shape. Vertebral bodies are square with thanatophoric dwarfism (Fig. 1.11), although practically, chest configuration and lung volume are the important features. In any case, in terms of antenatal syndrome identification, our range of applications goes far beyond traditional radiographic possibilities, and our antenatal assessment will include observations from a variety of body systems (Fig. 1.12).

"SMALL" MORPHOLOGIC FEATURES

When a major malformation is detected or there is high clinical suspicion that a particular syndrome may occur or recur, ancillary morphologic features may be very helpful. These are typically small structures that are not usually a part of the routine examination. For example, a single artery umbilical cord occurs with a variety of syndromes. There is little point in seeking the number of cord vessels in a routine examination, because the sensitivity and specificity of that finding are so low. However, in conjunction with other findings, its presence may help define a specific syndrome. It must be remembered that with ultrasound imaging we need not rely on indirect signs, as we can visualize the principal organs directly. Low-set ears suggest renal malformations that are occult by newborn physical examination; however, in the ultrasound case, we look at the kidneys themselves.

Small morphologic findings are not the same as minor malformations. We consider the face a region to be studied thoroughly in each examination

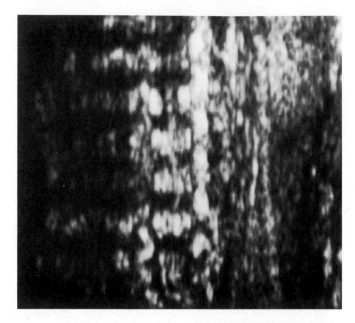

FIG. 1.11. Thanatophoric dwarfism. The vertebral bodies are short and square.

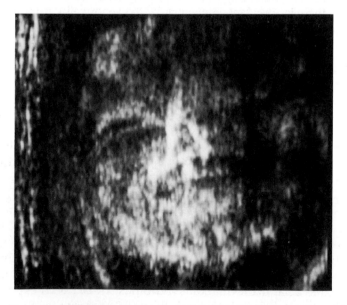

FIG. 1.12. Turner syndrome at 14 weeks. This facies is due to diffuse skin edema. The right eyelids are accentuated. A portion of a large cystic hygroma descends below the chin as a crescent.

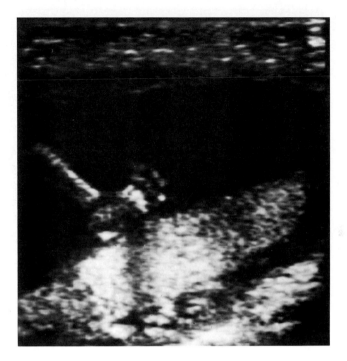

FIG. 1.13.   Clubfoot deformity with altered position of the foot relative to the ankle. In this case, there is abundant amniotic fluid; the abnormality is primary.

with lateral coronal views, because of the psychological impact, on unprepared parents, of cleft lips and cleft palates. Micrognathia, on the other hand, is best appreciated as a receding chin in sagittal views and by configuration in frontal base plane views, which often must be sought specifically. Areas that are particularly helpful in syndrome classification are the appearance of the hands and feet with specific clues from the number of digits, rocker-bottom feet, clubfeet, clinodactyly, shortening of individual metacarpals or metatarsals, or relative positions of individual parts (Fig. 1.13).

We rely greatly on the appearance of the external ear[31] (Fig. 1.14). The growth rate of pinna length is normal under a variety of conditions. It is increased with macrosomic growth acceleration. It is normal with growth retardation due to placental vascular insufficiency. Ear length normally increases from about 9 mm at 16 weeks to 33 mm at term. Grossly, short ears are a characteristic finding with aneuploidy; they can occur as well with regional craniofacial malformation syndromes. In our own experience, short ears imply an extremely high probability of a chromosomal abnormality, while, in a case with multiple malformations, normal ear length mitigates strongly against that possibility.

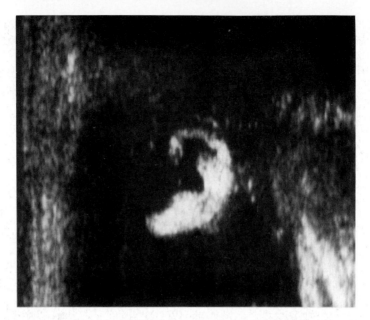

FIG. 1.14. The external ear (length: 28.8 mm).

PHYSIOLOGIC SYNDROMES

Ultrasonic definition of syndromes in fetuses tends to focus on dysmorphology. In routine practice, however, combinations of findings implying disordered physiology are of equal importance. In Rh factor isoimmunization, there is red cell hemolysis counterbalanced by fetal erythropoiesis. When the degree of hemolysis is slight and erythropoiesis is satisfactory, the fetus is essentially normal. When extramedullary hematopoiesis is excessive, liver replacement results in progressive hypoalbuminemia. The signs are hepatomegaly, gallbladder wall edema, and fluid transudation into the peritoneum, pleural, and pericardial spaces. Finally, when hemolysis is not compensated, there is progressive anemia with high output congestive failure. The signs in this case will be systolic pulse broadening of the thoracic aortic Doppler wave form (Fig. 1.15) dilation of the right atrium, and hydrops (including skin edema and increased subdural fluid). Each of these combinations of signs defines a pathophysiologic syndrome. The severity will govern the particular signs that appear. This is analogous to variable penetrance with genetic syndromes.

A particular physiologic syndrome we are now trying to define is one that includes growth retardation. We refer to this entity as placental dysfunction syndrome with individual grades. As fibrin deposits about the small vessels within the placenta, vascular resistance increases, and diastolic flow components in the umbilical artery Doppler signal decline. Several fetal compensatory mechanisms are invoked for failing placental function, which we

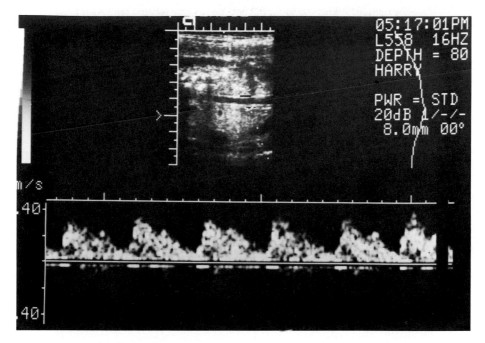

FIG. 1.15.   Aortic Doppler tracing shows a broad, double-humped systolic pattern associated with anemia (decreased blood viscosity).

simplify to a primary emphasis on oxygen transport. First, there is an attempt to increase venous return to the heart. We have observed dilation of the normally closed ductus venosus as an early sign (Fig. 1.16). When ductal flow is prolonged, there is stealing of blood flow from the right portal vein, which results in the small right lobe of the liver typical of so-called asymmetric growth retardation. Opening of the ductus probably also alters blood flood streaming through the atria. The blood flow redistribution preferentially maintains cerebral, myocardial, and probably adrenal blood flow. Decreased renal blood flow and decreased urine output eventuate in oligohydramnios. Anterior and middle cerebral artery Doppler waveforms have increasing diastolic flow components. Energy is conserved by decreasing body movements, by decreasing heart rate 8 to 12 beats per minute, and, later in development, by decreasing the time spent in rapid eye movement (REM) sleep.[32] These activity changes are due to central inhibition. Over a long time, the growth rate itself declines, possibly mediated by a change in growth factor secretion from the gut. With acute hypoxemia, there is clamping of the larynx,[33] decline in diaphragm and rapid eye movements, depression of cortical function, and eventually, a preterminal, comalike state, usually associated with bradycardia. The signs we seek in defining and grading this syndrome are largely dynamic.

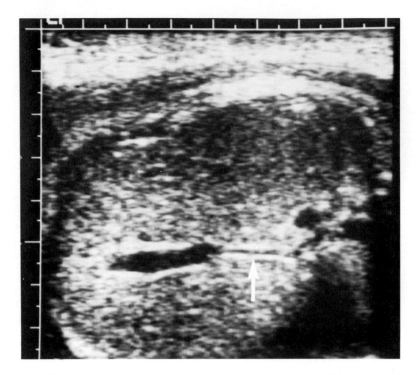

FIG. 1.16.   The ductus venosus (arrow) is the small thick-walled channel bridging the umbilical vein (left) and IVC. This vessel is usually closed by a sphincter at its origin.

CONCLUSION

The fetal ultrasound examination can now be pursued at a finely detailed level. When preliminary imaging or historical clinical findings pertain, global perusal provides great opportunities for specific syndrome identification, essential for prognosis and management planning, including the route, timing, and site of delivery. Each study is individualized; consequently, its thoroughness and accuracy are entirely dependent on the interest, knowledge, experience, and technique of the operator.[34]

In addition to antenatal detection of the range of abnormalities, precise ultrasound observations reviewed in retrospect, when problems are unmasked in infancy or later, will aid in identifying unknown environmental prenatal insults, the elimination of which will further optimize human development.

ACKNOWLEDGMENTS

This chapter is dedicated to my friends Beryl Benacerraf and Fredric Frigoletto, Brigham and Women's Hospital, Boston, with whom it was my privilege to work and learn during critical phases in the development of ultrasonic imaging and fetal medicine.

REFERENCES

1. Gilbert WM, Nicolaides KH: Fetal omphalocele: associated malformations and chromosomal defects. Obstet Gynecol 70:633, 1987
2. Smith DW: Classification, nomenclature, and naming of morphologic defects. J Pediatr 87:162, 1975
3. Spranger J, Benirschke K, Hall JG, et al: Errors in morphogenesis: Concepts and terms. Recommendation of an international working group. J Pediatr 100:160, 1982
4. Cohen MM: The Child with Multiple Birth Defects. Raven Press, New York, 1982
5. Bieber FR, Moustoufi-Zadeh M, Birnholz JC, Driscoll SG: Amniotic band sequence associated with ectopia cordis in one twin. J Pediatr 105:817, 1984
6. Potter EI: Bilateral renal agenesis. J Pediatr 29:68, 1946
7. Moessinger AC, Bassi GA, Ballantyne G, et al: Experimental production of pulmonary hypoplasia following amniocentesis and oligohydramnios. Early Hum Dev 8:343, 1983
8. Dobbing J: Later development of the brain and its vulnerability. p. 565. In Davis JA, Dobbing J, (eds): Scientific Foundations of Paediatrics. WB Saunders, Philadelphia, 1974
9. Wigglesworth JS: Fetal lung growth and lung hypoplasia in animals and man. p. 242. In Van Assche F, Robertson WB, (eds): Fetal Growth Retardation. Churchill Livingstone, New York, 1981
10. Bystrzycka E, Nait BS, Purves MJ: Central and peripheral neural respiratory activity in the mature sleep foetus and newborn lamb. Respir Physiol 25:199, 1975
11. DeMeyer W: Classification of cerebral malformations. Birth Defects 7:78, 1971
12. Warkany J: Warfarin embryopathy. Teratology 14:205, 1976
13. Nicolaides KH, Gabbe SG, Guidetti R, et al: Ultrasound screening for spina bifida: cranial and cerebellar signs. Lancet 1:72, 1986
14. Birnholz JC: Fetal ophthalmology. Early Hum Dev 12:199, 1985
15. Birnholz JC: Fetal hyaloid artery regression. Radiology 166:781, 1988
16. Loeser JD, Alford EC Jr: Agenesis of the corpus callosum. Brain 91:553, 1968
17. Marburg O: So-called agenesis of the corpus callosum (callosal defect). anterior cerebral dysraphism. Arch Neurol Psychiat 61:295, 1949
18. Warkany J, Passarge E, Smith CB: Congenital malformations in autosomal trisomy syndromes. Am J Dis Child 112:502, 1966
19. Belle W, Van Allen MS: Agenesis of the corpus callosum with associated facial anomalies. Neurology 9:694, 1959
20. Herskowitz J, Roseman P, Wheeler CB: Colpocephaly: clinical, radiologic, and pathogenetic aspects. Neurology 35:1594, 1985
21. Butler IJ, Beal S, Simpson DA: Agenesis of the corpus callosum in infancy. J Aust Clin 3:137, 1968
22. Aicardi J, Chevrie J-J, Pouselle F: Le syndrome spasmes en flexion, agenèse calleuse, anomalies chorio-rétinienes. Arch Fr Pediatr 28:1103, 1969
23. Sidman SL, Rakic P: Neuronal migration with special reference to developing human brain. Brain Res 62:1, 1973
24. Trounce JY, Fagan DG, Young ID, Levene, MI: Disorders of neuronal migration: Sonographic features. Dev Med Child Neurol 28:467, 1986
25. Dobyns W, Stratton R, Parke J, et al: Miller-Dieker syndrome: lissencephaly and monosomy 17p. J Pediatr 102:552, 1983
26. Birnholz JC, Benacerraf BR: The development of fetal hearing. Science 222:516, 1983
27. Wertelecki W, Graham JM, Sergovich FR: The clinical syndrome of triploidy. Obstet Gynecol 47:69, 1976

28. Robinow M, Chumlea WC: Standards for limb bone length ratios in children. Radiology 143:433, 1982

29. Birnholz JC: Biological foundations for fetal growth studies. p. 49. In Deter RL, Harrist RB, Birnholz JC, Hadlock F (eds): Quantitative Obstetrical Ultrasonography. Wiley, New York, 1986

30. Scammon RE, Calkins LA: The Development and Growth of the External Dimensions of the Human Body in the Fetal Period. University of Minnesota Press, Minneapolis, 1929

31. Birnholz JC: Fetal ear length. Pediatrics 81:555, 1988

32. Koos BJ, Sameshima M, Power GC: Fetal breathing, sleep state, and cardiovascular responses to graded hypoxia in sheep. J Appl Physiol 62:1033, 1987

33. Harding R: Perinatal development of laryngeal function. J Dev Physiol 6:249, 1984

34. Birnholz JC, Hayes T: The effect of instrumentation and examination. p. 143. In McGraham JP (ed): Controversies in Ultrasound. Churchill Livingstone, New York, 1987

2 The Use of Sonography for the Antenatal Detection of Aneuploidy

BERYL R. BENACERRAF

Ultrasound technology has progressed over the past several years and now permits identification and detailed delineation of fetal abnormalities. Increasing expertise among ultrasound personnel has also contributed dramatically to our ability to diagnose fetal abnormalities, in particular those associated with an abnormal chromosome complement. Although many fetal abnormalities—such as anencephaly, hydrocephalus, and anterior abdominal wall abnormalities—can now be diagnosed sonographically even in the second trimester,[1-4] more refined diagnoses involve examination of the face and extremities. It is not sufficient, however, to diagnose isolated cleft lip and palate or a clubfoot. Rather, the presence of these lesions should stimulate the ultrasonographer to seek a pattern and fit the pieces of the puzzles together in order to recognize the syndromes associated with chromosomal anomalies.

Fetuses with trisomy 13, trisomy 18, triploidy, and so forth are known to develop intrauterine growth retardation (IUGR).[5-7] Clearly, the ultrasonographer must recognize the structural abnormalities associated with these trisomies in order to institute appropriate obstetric management. Many fetuses who have severe IUGR may be subject to premature delivery by cesarean section for fetal distress.[8] If the diagnosis of a lethal trisomy can be made antenatally, the parents can be prepared for the poor outcome and the patient can be saved lengthy antenatal monitoring and operative delivery.

Only small numbers of the pregnant women are candidates for amniocentesis or chorionic villous sampling; however, an increasing portion of pregnant women are undergoing ultrasound for a variety of indications. The ultrasonographer must therefore be aware of the signs and pattern of abnormalities associated with chromosomal anomalies so that cytogenetic studies can be done when these findings are present.

TRISOMY 13

Trisomy 13 is a rare disorder resulting from the presence of three chromosome 13. Trisomy 13 was first described in 1960 by Patau; it has an incidence of 1 in 5,000 births.[9,10] Reports of the sonographic diagnosis of fetuses with trisomy 13 have been described and require a careful search for multiple congenital abnormalities that fit a pattern. Morphologic features include anomalies of the brain, such as holoprosencephaly, congenital heart defects, ventral wall defects, polydactyly, and cystic kidneys.[9,11–14] The exceedingly poor outcome of neonates with this syndrome makes identification of fetuses with trisomy 13 particularly helpful for obstetric management. The mean survival for an infant with trisomy 13 is 130 days; only 18 percent of infants survive the first year, and they are severely handicapped.[9,15]

Cranium

The fetal cranium can be identified as early as 8 weeks, and the intracranial structures are visible by 11 to 12 weeks gestation. At that time, the choroid plexus, lateral ventricles, and falx can be well defined. By 16 weeks, the entire outline of the lateral ventricles, shape of the choroid plexus, and sometimes the third ventricle can be identified.

Holoprosencephaly is a severe intracranial abnormality that arises from failure of normal cleavage of the prosencephalon, often accompanied by abnormal midfacial development. As early as 12 weeks, the diagnosis of alobar holoprosencephaly can be made by noting the absence of the falx and the presence of a single ventricle crossing the midline (Fig. 2.1). Sonographically, none of the usual midline structures is visible, and the large central ventricle can be seen with a mantle around it (Figs. 2.2 and 2.3). The thalami and brain stem have an abnormal fused sonographic appearance, which is characteristic (Fig. 2.4). Holoprosencephaly is often associated with trisomy 13 and alobar holoprosencephaly is the most severe form.[11,13]

In a series of 10 consecutive cases of holoprosencephaly, 4 (40 percent) of the fetuses had trisomy 13, showing a high association between trisomy 13 and this intracranial abnormality.[13] Associated midline facial anomalies commonly include severe cleft lip and palate (Fig. 2.5), hypotelorism, occasional cyclopia (Figs. 2.6 and 2.7), nasal abnormalities, and abnormal positioning of the ears.[11–13] In cases of cyclopia, the proboscis (nose) can be positioned above the eye (Fig. 2.8). Because of this association, careful assessment of the fetal face is an extremely important part of the structural survey when looking for chromosomal abnormalities, in particular, trisomy 13.

Imaging the fetal face is best accomplished using a coronal view through the soft tissues of the face and the maxilla.[11,12,16–23] The ultrasound beam can then be angled cephalad to view the upper lip and nostrils, which is the most helpful manuver for detecting midline clefts (Fig. 2.9). The longitudi-

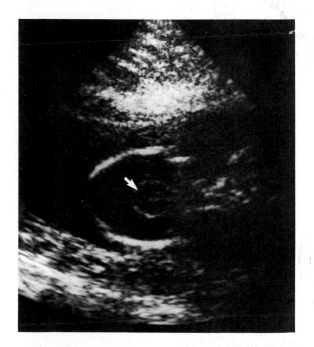

FIG. 2.1. A 12-week fetus with holoprosencephaly. Note the large central ventricle with no falx and the abnormal-appearing thalami (arrow). The karyotype was trisomy 13.

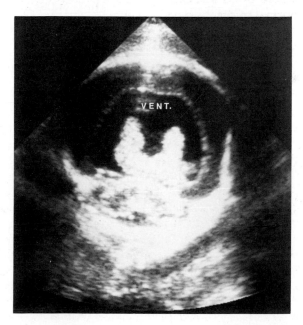

FIG. 2.2. Coronal view showing holoprosencephaly with a central ventricle (VENT) and lack of midline structures. A mantle of brain is present, and the choroid plexus is prominent.

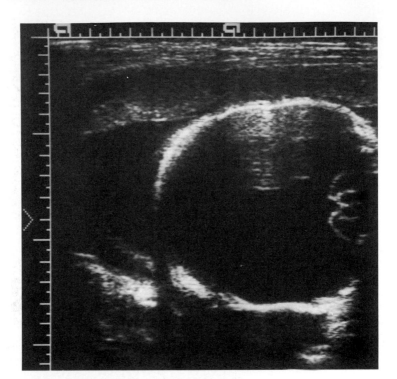

FIG. 2.3. Markedly expanded head of a fetus near term, showing almost no visible brain mantle and a large amount of fluid in the single ventricle. No falx is identified.

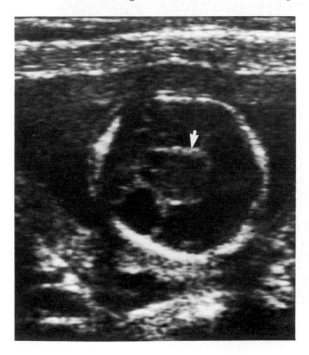

FIG. 2.4. A 19-week fetus with trisomy 13, showing typical features of alobar holoprosencephaly. Note the abnormal appearance of the thalami (arrow) and lack of falx.

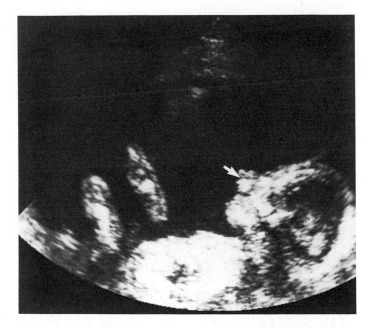

FIG. 2.5. A 16-week fetus with severe midline cleft involving the nose (arrow). The entire midline facial structures were disrupted.

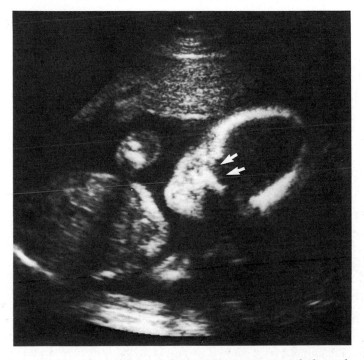

FIG. 2.6. Frontal view of a 19-week fetus with holoprosencephaly and a cyclopic deformity. The single orbit is shown by arrows.

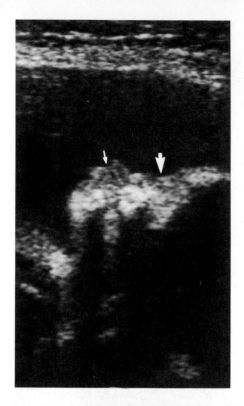

FIG. 2.7. Same fetus in profile showing complete absence of the nose. The region of the central orbit is shown by the large arrow, and the mouth by the small arrow.

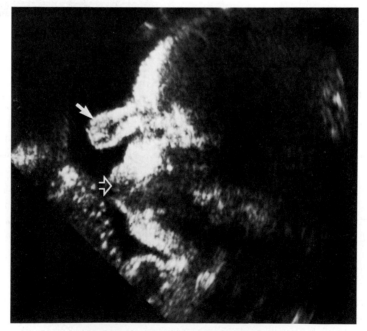

FIG. 2.8. Trisomy 13 fetus shown in profile at 25 weeks. A large proboscis (thin arrow) is present above the single orbit. The region of the mouth is protuberant (open arrow).

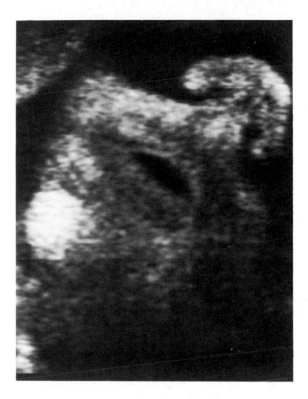

FIG. 2.9.   Magnified view of the lower face of a normal fetus showing the mouth and nose. This view is commonly used to look for clefts.

nal view of the fetal profile is also necessary for complete evaluation of the face (Fig. 2.10), as some facial defects will be visible only in this projection.

In a study by Saltzman et al.[12] 12 fetuses with facial clefts were reviewed, showing that 3 (25%) of the fetuses with facial clefts had trisomy 13 and 1 (8.75%) had trisomy 18. These findings demonstrate that amniocentesis is indicated in patients in whom a facial cleft is identified antenatally, particularly when other anomalies are also present. Facial abnormalities of all types have been well described sonographically as early as 16 weeks; in fact, our earliest case of trisomy 13 with holoprosencephaly and cyclopia was seen at 12 weeks (see Fig. 2.1). Dysmorphic features of the face may also occur in fetuses with trisomy 13 without accompanying holoprosencephaly, usually characterized by micrognathia.

To determine the rate of identification of fetuses with trisomy 13 in an ultrasound laboratory, all cases diagnosed by cytogenetics and also having undergone an ultrasound were reviewed, and 9 such cases were found. Abnormal facial features had been identified prospectively in all 9 cases, 6 of which also had holoprosencephaly.[24] The cranial and facial abnormalities are therefore crucial findings for detecting fetuses with trisomy 13 and should prompt cytogenetic studies.

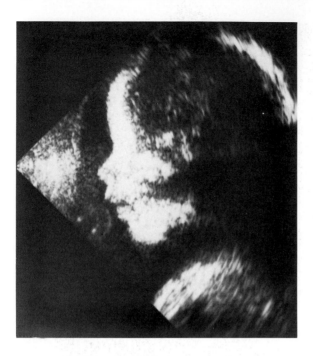

FIG. 2.10. Longitudinal view of the fetal profile showing a normal fetal face at 28 weeks.

Extracranial Abnormalities Associated with Trisomy 13

Trisomy 13 is associated with abnormalities of both hands and feet, most commonly seen sonographically as postaxial polydactyly[9,24] (Fig. 2.11). Abnormalities of the hands and feet are identifiable ultrasonographically as early as 15 or 16 weeks, although perseverence is often necessary when fetal position is not optimal.[11,25] When polydactyly is discovered, other anomalies associated with trisomy 13 should be sought, such as cardiac, renal, and cranial malformations.[9,11,14,24]

Congenital heart disease is present in 90 percent of fetuses with trisomy 13; the most common lesion is a ventriculoseptal defect (VSD)[14] (Fig. 2.12). Given the presence of a congenital heart lesion in a fetus, the risk of coexistent chromosomal abnormalities can be as high as 5 percent, indicating that cytogenetic studies may be helpful in these patients. Despite the high frequency of congenital heart disease in this syndrome, sonography has been disappointing for the detection of minor heart defects such as VSD.[26-28] Major heart lesions, such as hypoplastic ventricle, tetralogy of Fallot, and transposition of the great arteries, are reliably detected by fetal echocardiography, but more minor heart defects are easily overlooked, particularly in the second trimester.[26]

Fetuses with trisomy 13 also commonly exhibit anormalities of the kidneys, in particular polycystic kidneys (31%) and horseshoe kidney[9] (Fig. 2.13). Midline defects of the anterior abdominal wall, such as omphalocele, can also be present (Fig. 2.14). Because trisomy 13 can be associated with polycys-

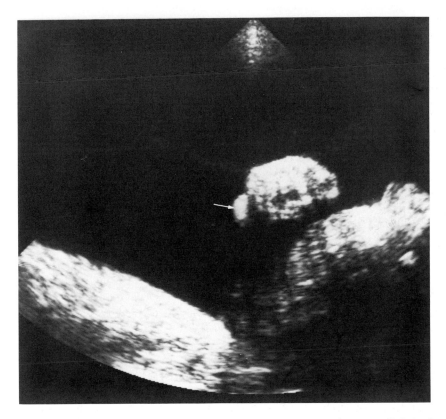

FIG. 2.11.   Postaxial polydactyly in a fetus with trisomy 13. The extra digit is shown by the arrow.

tic kidneys, polydactyly, and occasionally posterior encephaloceles, it can easily be confused with Meckel-Gruber syndrome, which has similar findings. Cytogenetic studies would be necessary to make this differentiation.

TRISOMY 18

Trisomy 18 (Edwards syndrome) is characterized by three chromosome 18 with an incidence of 0.3 in 1,000 births and a 3:1 female preponderance.[9] Along with trisomy 13, it is one of the most common chromosomal defects associated with multiple malformations. Abnormalities most commonly associated with trisomy 18 include growth deficiency with polyhydramnios, clenched hand with overlapping index finger, clubfeet or rockerbottom feet, forearm abnormalities, congenital heart disease, umbilical, diaphragmatic or inguinal hernias, and renal anomalies such as horseshoe kidney.[6,7,9,11,25,29–31] The ability to identify the specific pattern of malformations that would suggest trisomy 18 is crucial, since fetuses with trisomy 18 have a very poor prognosis.[32] The mean survival for an infant with trisomy 18 is 48 days,

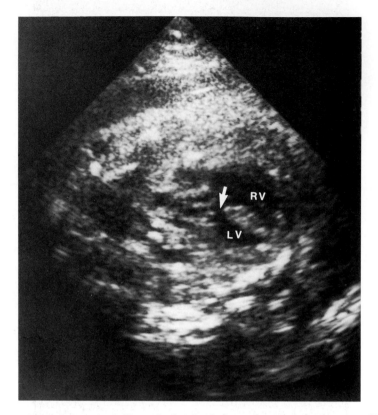

FIG. 2.12. Transverse view through the fetal chest showing the heart at 30 weeks. This fetus with trisomy 13 had a VSD (arrow). RV, right ventricle; LV, left ventricle.

but most of them die within the first few hours or days.[32] Because trisomy 18 fetuses are associated with severe IUGR, many of these fetuses are delivered by emergency cesarean section for fetal distress when, in fact, an operative delivery does not improve the dismal outcome.[6–8] Knowledge of trisomy 18 therefore is important for planning intrapartum management.

Extremities

The most common sonographically identifiable abnormalities associated with trisomy 18 involve the fetal hands and feet. Many fetuses with trisomy 18 have clubfeet or rockerbottom feet[24] (Fig. 2.15). In a series of 18 consecutive cases of clubfoot identified sonographically, 22 percent had trisomies, a percentage in agreement with Jeanty's series on the same subject.[25,29,33] When congenital clubfoot is noted sonographically, particularly in a fetus who has polyhydramnios and IUGR, trisomy 18 should be suspected, and cytogenetic studies are indicated.[25]

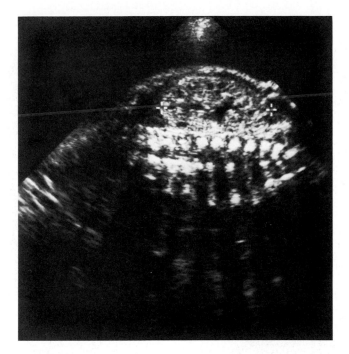

FIG. 2.13. Longitudinal view of a cystic kidney in a 36-week fetus with trisomy 13. Note the increased echogenicity and large size of the kidney.

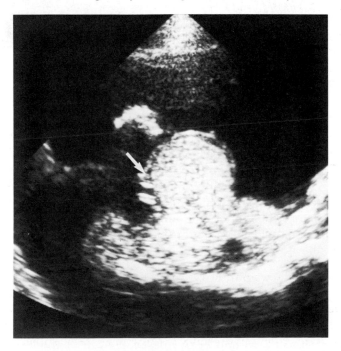

FIG. 2.14. Longitudinal view of the fetal body at 16 weeks, showing a large omphalo-cele involving the fetal liver. Note the insertion of the umbilical cord (arrow) in the region of the defect.

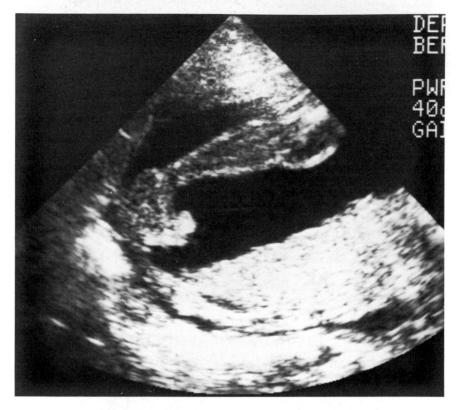

FIG. 2.15.   Longitudinal view of the fetal lower extremity showing a clubfoot at 20 weeks, associated with trisomy 18.

Abnormalities of the upper extremities can be quite characteristic of trisomy 18, in particular, fixed clenching of the hands with an overlapping index finger[9,24] (Fig. 2.16). Occasionally polydactyly is also present. Marked limb reduction of the forearm is occasionally encountered, although less frequent than the clawhand with overlapping finger[31] (Fig. 2.17). Examination of fetal hands can be accomplished on almost all fetuses 16 weeks and older. In many cases, the normal fetal hands are clenched; however, prodding on the maternal abdomen can often elicit enough fetal hand movement to rule out a fixed deformity.

We evaluated 15 cases of trisomy 18 identified cytogenetically and scanned in our ultrasound laboratory and found that in 12 of these 15 cases, obvious malformations of the fetus had been identified, suggesting the diagnosis.[24] Three cases of trisomy 18 had been missed. Eleven of the 12 fetuses who had sonographic structural abnormalities had anomalies of the hands or feet. Unlike trisomy 13, however, only one fetus had sonographic facial abnormalities, in particular micrognathia and prominence of the nose (Fig. 2.18).

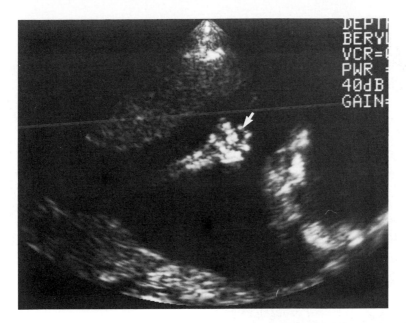

FIG. 2.16.   This 17-week fetus with trisomy 18 demonstrates the typical hand deformity, with an overlapping index finger and clenched fist.

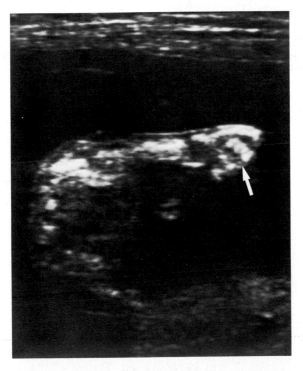

FIG. 2.17.   An unusual deformity occasionally associated with trisomy 18 is the abnormality of the forearm, short radial ray, and clubhand shown here (hand indicated by the arrow).

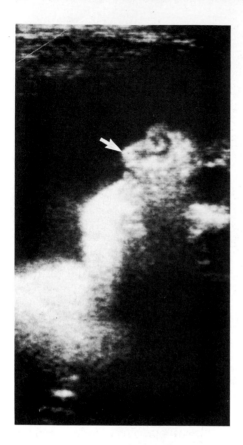

FIG. 2.18. Abnormal profile in a fetus with trisomy 18. Note the severe micrognathia and the protuberant upper lip (arrow).

Other Structural Abnormalities Associated with Trisomy 18

An estimated 99 percent of fetuses with trisomy 18 have congenital heart disease.[14] Of the typical lesions occurring in association with trisomy 18, VSD, complete arteriovenous canal, and double-outlet right ventricle are the most common, although other complex cardiac anomalies also occur.[14] Although major congenital heart lesions are easily detectable, such as double-outlet right ventricle and complete atrioventricular canal and tetralogy of Fallot, identifying a VSD in second-trimester fetuses can be difficult.[26–28] The presence of congenital heart disease, in particular VSD, in fetuses with trisomy 18 may not be as useful for detecting these fetuses as abnormalities of the extremities, which may be more readily visible.

Diaphragmatic hernia and omphalocele can be associated with trisomy 18; of our 12 fetuses with sonographic findings suggestive of trisomy 18, 3 had diaphragmatic hernia[24] (Fig. 2.19). One of these fetuses had diaphragmatic hernia as the only visible sonographic abnormality that prompted cytogenetic studies. In a recent study on 19 consecutive fetuses with sonographically diagnosed diaphragmatic hernia, 2 (11%) had trisomy 18, suggesting

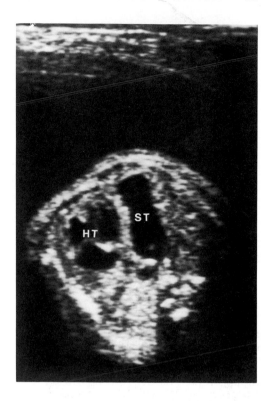

FIG. 2.19. A 25-week fetus with a large diaphragmatic hernia, a feature of trisomy 18. Note that the stomach (ST) is adjacent to the heart (HT) and pushing the heart and mediastinum to the right.

that cytogenetic studies are indicated when this diagnosis is made, particularly when accompanied by deficient growth.[30]

Other dysmorphic features such as low-set ears, prominent occiput, high-arched palate, short sternum, small pelvis, and adducted hips, are unfortunately not abnormalities that can be identified sonographically to date.[6] We have based our surveillance for trisomy 18 mostly on abnormalities of the hands and feet, facial profile, diaphragmatic hernia, omphalocele and congenital heart defects.[24]

DOWN SYNDROME

The antenatal diagnosis of Down syndrome (trisomy 21) has depended on cytogenetic evaluation; screening programs have included almost exclusively women 35 years or older or those with an abnormal serum α-fetoprotein (AFP). Although the rate of fetuses with Down syndrome is 1 in 385 to 1 in 250 for a 35-year-old woman, it is known that only 20 percent of Down syndrome fetuses are born to mothers 35 or older.[34–35] Thus, as many as 80 percent of fetuses with Down syndrome are born to mothers who are not candidates for cytogenetic evaluation. In 1981, it was estimated that less than one-half of women 35 years or older even elect amniocentesis.[35–37] It is possible that 90 percent of fetuses with Down syndrome still remain undetected antenatally. Most of the structural fetal abnormalities associated with Down syndrome are too subtle to be relied on for second trimester antenatal diagnosis, such as epicanthic eye fold, flat nasal profile, simian crease of the palm, dysplastic pelvis (iliac crest), hyperflexibility of joints, hypotonia, dysplastic ear, and brachycephaly.[9,38] However, several sonographic signs for the detection of Down syndrome can be used to detect fetuses at high risk of having the syndrome and prompt further testing by cytogenetic evaluation. These include an abnormally thick nuchal skin fold at the back of the fetal neck,[39–41] slightly short femurs,[42–43] dysplastic middle phalanx of the fifth digit with incurving finger,[44] congenital heart disease, and duodenal obstruction[45] (Fig. 2.20).

Thickened Nuchal Fold

Excess skin at the back of the fetal neck is present in 80 percent of newborns with Down syndrome, a finding well established in the pediatric literature.[9,38] We have studied this finding in 3,825 consecutive second-trimester fetuses undergoing genetic amniocentesis between 15 and 20 weeks.[41] The region of the back of the neck was evaluated prospectively in each case. The view used to obtain a biparietal diameter is modified and the beam angled posteriorly to include the cerebellum and occipital bone. The nuchal fold measurement is then made from the outer surface of the occipital bone to the outer skin edge (Figs. 2.21 and 2.22). A measurement of 6 mm or more was considered abnormal.[46] Of the 3,825 consecutive fetuses undergoing genetic amniocentesis, 21 had a positive karyotype for Down syndrome, and 9 of these 21 fetuses with trisomy 21 had an abnormal nuchal fold. In six of these nine fetuses, the abnormal skinfold was the only abnormality seen sonographically. The remaining three fetuses had generalized hydrops with a cardiac abnormality, multiple congenital abnormalities, and hydrocephalus, respectively. An additional four of the remaining 3,804 control fetuses had an abnormal skin thickening at the back of the neck (6 mm or greater) and did not have Down syndrome. Three had normal karyotypes and one had a 5P+ karyotype and multiple congenital abnormalities.

It is of note that three patients chose to have amniocentesis based only on the abnormal sonographic finding of the thickened nuchal fold and would otherwise not have undergone cytogenetic testing.[41] The sensitivity for the detection of Down syndrome in our series, therefore, was 9 of 21 (42.9%). The four false-positive cases represented a false-positive of 0.1 percent (4 of 3,804), and our sign was therefore 99.9 percent specific for Down syndrome. The positive predictive value of our sign for the diagnosis of Down syndrome in the second trimester was 9 of 13 (69%). Twenty-three percent (3 of 13) had a positive nuchal fold but a normal karyotype, and 8 percent (1 of 13) had a positive nuchal fold and an abnormal karyotype other than Down syndrome. It is clear that not as many fetuses with Down syndrome have the abnormal skinfold in the second trimester as they do in the neonatal

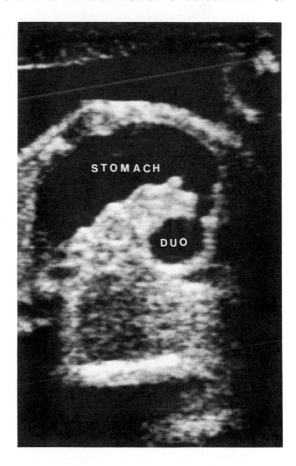

FIG. 2.20. Transverse view through the fetal abdomen at 30 weeks, showing dilation of the stomach and duodenum. This fetus had Down syndrome and associated duodenal atresia. DUO, duodenum.

period (80%). It appears, however, that this finding is reliable and quite specific for the diagnosis of Down syndrome. A quick evaluation of the back of the neck is easy to perform as an adjunct to measuring the biparietal diameter, and the appearance of the nuchal soft tissues can be assessed. With the increasing number of women undergoing ultrasound examination for a variety of different indications in the second trimester, a simple evaluation of the nuchal fold may be extremely helpful for women who are not otherwise candidates for cytogenetic evaluation and who may be carrying a fetus with Down syndrome.

For the thickened nuchal skinfold to be helpful, the measurement must be done accurately. Angling the beam too far posteriorly beyond the point where the occipital bone is visible will yield false-positive results. Care must also be taken not to include the occipital bone itself in the measurement.[47] The largest number of controls in whom we evaluated the normal nuchal fold was between 15 to 19 weeks, with fewer fetuses at 19 to 20.5 weeks.[46] We recommend the use of the nuchal fold thickness as described here for fetuses at 15 to 19 weeks, since normal measurements are not established conclusively for the older age groups.

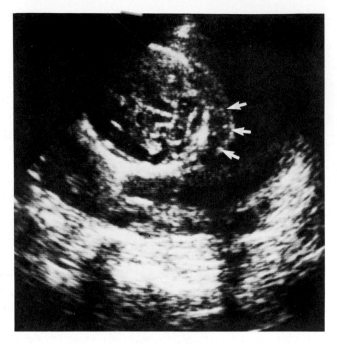

FIG. 2.21. Transverse view through the head of a fetus with Down syndrome at 16 weeks. Note the thickened nuchal skinfold (arrow).

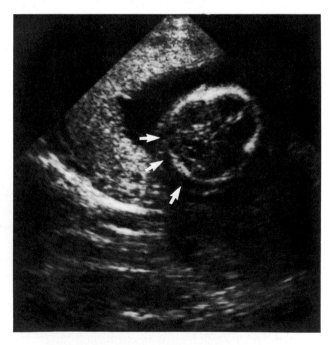

FIG. 2.22. Transverse view through a 17-week fetal head showing the thickened nuchal fold associated with Down syndrome. The mother would not have undergone amniocentesis were it not for this sonographic finding. She was 22 years old.

Abnormal Femur Length

During our study of fetuses with Down syndrome, it appeared that affected fetuses had slightly shorter femurs.[42-43] We evaluated 28 consecutive fetuses with Down syndrome out of more than 5,000 fetuses who were scanned at the time of amniocentesis (15 to 20 weeks) before knowledge of the abnormal karyotype.[42] Femur lengths of the 28 fetuses with Down syndrome were compared with those of 192 controls between 15 and 21 weeks to establish the normal femur lengths for gestational age in our laboratory. A simple linear regression model of the normal femur length based on biparietal diameter (BPD) was developed:

$$\text{Expected femur length} = -9.645 + 0.9338 \times \text{BPD}.$$

This equation accounted for 94 percent of variations in normal femur lengths ($P < 10^{-7}$) and was used to plot actual femur length versus expected femur length based on the BPD.[42] If the ratio (actual/expected femur length) of 0.91 is used as a limit for normal, specificity and sensitivity for a shorter femur is 98 percent and 69 percent, respectively (this would identify 2% of normal fetuses and 69% of fetuses with Down syndrome as needing amniocentesis). If a higher ratio is selected (i.e., 0.97), as many as 93 percent of fetuses with Down syndrome would be identified, but the specificity would fall to 72 percent, possibility subjecting 28 percent of normal fetuses to amniocentesis, an unacceptable number. It is also possible to choose a ratio of 0.89 percent, which would select 50 percent of fetuses with Down syndrome and only 0.4 percent of normal fetuses for cytogenetic studies. The cutoff point can therefore be chosen, depending on the specificity and sensitivity desired. For a ratio of 0.91, which we have selected, the positive predictive value for the use of a slightly shortened femur would be 12 percent for the population at risk for Down syndrome (1 of 250), that is, offspring of women 35 years or older.

Care must be taken to measure the femur in its entirety without foreshortening it, since this would result in false-positive results. Some variation exists among different ultrasound laboratories in the technique of femur measurements; it is crucial to obtain the longest measurement even if several tries are necessary.[43] This technique eliminates potential false-positive results.

We evaluated the same 28 consecutive fetuses with Down syndrome for the presence of an abnormal nuchal fold.[42] Twelve of 28 (42%) had an abnormal nuchal fold of 6 mm or more. Because two fetuses had generalized hydrops, and a thickened nuchal fold may have been secondary to the hydrops, these two were removed and 10 of 26 (38%) had a thickened nuchal fold as the only area of skin thickening. It is of note that six of the 28 fetuses had other abnormalities in addition to the abnormal femur and nuchal fold. In particular, two had generalized hydrops and an AV canal, one each had clubfeet, hydrocephalus (Fig. 2.23), meconium peritonitis, and cystic hygroma. We combined the morphologic abnormalities seen in these fetuses

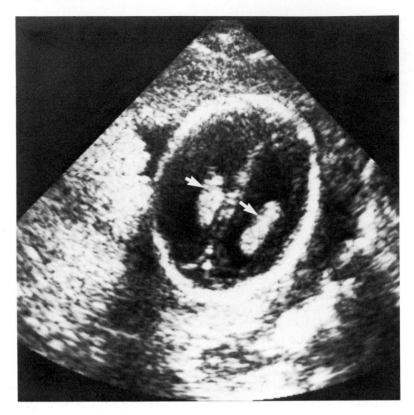

FIG. 2.23. Fetus with Down syndrome at 20 weeks who also had hydrocephalus. Note the asymmetry of the choroid plexuses (arrows), consistent with early ventricular dilation.

with the abnormal measurement of the femur length over the expected femur length of less than 0.91 and a nuchal skin fold of 6 mm or more. The sensitivity of these signs for the diagnosis of Down syndrome was 82 percent. This would mean that by using the combination of abnormal femur length, nuchal fold, and other congenital abnormalities, 82 percent of fetuses with Down syndrome could be identified with a false-positive rate of 2 percent.[42]

Abnormal Fifth Digit

Hypoplasia of the middle phalanx of the fifth finger is present in 60 percent of neonates with Down syndrome.[9,38] Identifying the phalanges of the fingers is possible with regularity as early as 15 or 16 weeks (Fig. 2.24). Some expertise is required to obtain a good image of the fifth digit at that gestational age, particularly when fetal position is not optimal. Perseverence, changing the maternal position, and prodding on the abdomen can often facilitate obtaining an adequate image of the hand. We evaluated five fetuses with Down syndrome for the presence of an abnormal fifth digit.[44] Four fetuses were known to have Down syndrome at the time of sonography, and the diagnosis was strongly suspected in the fifth due to generalized hydrops and an AV canal. Four of these five fetuses clearly had an abnormal configuration of the fifth digit with ulna deviation (inward curving) and a smaller than expected middle phalanx of the fifth digit (Fig. 2.25). The positive predictive value and use of this sign have not yet been established, and it is therefore premature to speculate its use for the detection of Down syndrome in a large population. More work is necessary to establish the efficacy of this additional and promising sign for antenatal detection of Down syndrome.

Congenital Heart Disease

Fifty percent of fetuses with trisomy 21 have congenital heart disease, most commonly ventriculoseptal defect or complete AV canal.[14] In our main series of 28 consecutive fetuses with Down syndrome, two were noted sonographically to have a complete AV canal with hydrops[42] (Fig. 2.26). How many of the other fetuses had a complete AV canal or a VSD is not known. It is likely that several fetuses with more minor congenital heart disease were missed in our series, since 2 of 28 is a far smaller percentage than anticipated for the presence of congenital heart disease in fetuses with Down syndrome.

We have evaluated the accuracy of sonographic detection of congenital heart disease in 49 non-Down syndrome fetuses who had 66 cardiac lesions.[26] Our study showed that the major heart lesions, such as hypoplastic ventricle, transposition of the great vessels, tetralogy of Fallot, and complete AV canal, were accurately identified. The identification of VSD and ASD was much more disappointing, since only half of fetuses with VSD were diagnosed antenatally and well under half of ASD were detected. Other investigators also report false-negative results when dealing with VSD.[27,28] It follows that second-trimester sonography cannot be relied on to detect Down syndrome by echocardiography, since VSD, typical lesions in fetuses with Down syndrome, are not always reliably detectable, particularly in the second trimester.

Identifying Down Syndrome by Morphological Features

Amniocentesis is done when the risk of giving birth to a fetus with Down syndrome is 1 of 250 (0.4%), because of either advanced maternal age or a low AFP.[34,48–50] The positive predictive value for using the combination of abnormal nuchal fold and short femur length for those at a 1 in 250 risk of Down syndrome is 13 percent, far superior than simply advanced maternal age or low AFP alone.[42] It may eventually be possible to combine the sonographic findings with the screening programs such as AFP testing to better identify women at risk for carrying a fetus with Down syndrome. However, since only 20 percent of fetuses with Down syndrome are born to women

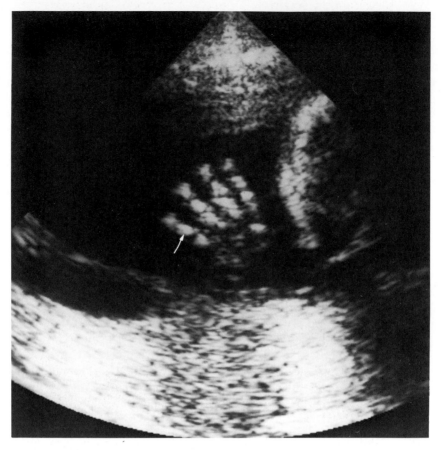

FIG. 2.24. Normal fetal hand at 17 weeks showing that the phalanges can be well seen. An arrow indicates the middle phalanx of the fifth digit, which is abnormal in 60 percent of patients with Down syndrome.

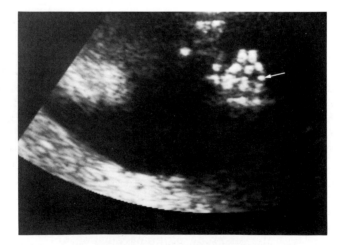

FIG. 2.25. An 18-week fetus with Down syndrome showing evidence of the hypoplasia of the middle phalanx of the fifth digit (arrow) with inward deformity of the digit, known to be associated with Down syndrome.

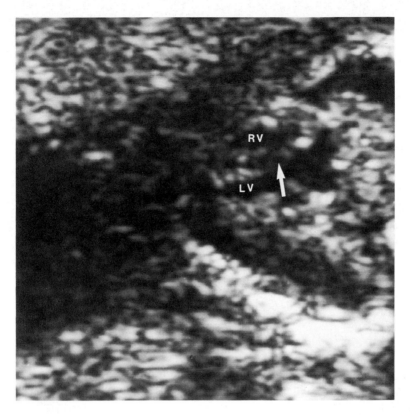

FIG. 2.26.   Transverse view through the fetal chest at 16 weeks, showing an endocardial cushion defect (AV canal) of the heart (arrow). Note the bilateral pleural effusions in this hydropic fetus. RV, right ventricle; LV, left ventricle.

35 years or more and less than half of these women elect to undergo antenatal diagnosis, 90 percent of fetuses with Down syndrome remain undetected by the advanced maternal age method.[35-37] A low serum AFP may detect 20 to 30 percent of fetuses with Down syndrome, but as many as 5 to 11 percent of women with normal fetuses are offered amniocentesis, a positive predictive value of 0.7 to 1 percent for a 1 in 250 risk of Down syndrome.[48,49] Even when low serum AFP and advanced maternal age are combined, no more than 40 percent of fetuses with Down syndrome can thus be identified.[48]

As more pregnancies are scanned in the second trimester for all indications, sonologists must be aware of the morphologic signs that might suggest a fetus with Down syndrome. If these signs are generally known and looked for, a large increase in the detection of Down syndrome is possible and, if cytogenetic evaluation were to follow each case in which an abnormality such as an abnormal nuchal fold, shortened femur, or congenital anomaly were discovered, potentially 82 percent of fetuses with Down syndrome would be identified, with 2 percent of normal fetuses being offered amniocentesis.[42]

TURNER SYNDROME

Turner syndrome (XO) was described in 1938 by Turner as a syndrome of sexual infantilism, small stature, web neck, and cubitus valgus. Most XO conceptuses result in miscarriage, and the incidence of XO newborns is approximately 1 per 5,000 births (excluding mosaics, partial deletions of an X chromosome, etc.).[9,51] Many variations of the XO syndrome exist, including mosaics with varying degrees of abnormalities and varying amounts of an X chromosome missing. These fetuses are less severely malformed than those with the full-blown XO syndrome. Abnormalities include short stature, ovarian dysgenesis (streak ovaries), congenital lymphedema of varying amounts, abnormal nipples that may be hypoplastic, prominent oracles, abnormalities of the facies with a relatively small mandible, low hairline, short or web neck, cubitus valgus, short fourth metacarpal, occasional renal abnormalities such as horseshoe kidney, and cardiac anomalies (20%), most of which involve the left side of the heart, such as coarctation of the aorta or abnormal aortic valve.[9,14]

Sonographic Findings

Fetal cystic hygroma colli are large cystic masses originating from the back of the fetal neck, which can be present very early in pregnancy; we have seen this at 9.5 weeks[52] and others have reported it from 12 weeks on.[53–60] Fetal cystic hygromas are thought to represent congenital lymphatic malformations arising from obstruction of the lymphatic system or failure to communicate with the venous system in the neck.[60] They are often associated with generalized hydrops and severe skin and scalp edema, often to a disproportionate degree to the ascites and pleural effusions. Sonographically, these cystic hygromas are fluid-filled thin-walled cysts, often with septations, occurring at the back of the fetal neck (Figs. 2.27 and 2.28). They can be very large, even larger than the fetal cranium. Marked scalp edema is usually present with varying degrees of generalized hydrops (Fig. 2.29). Cystic hygromas should not be confused with cervical encephaloceles, since disruption of the posterior aspect of the skull or cervical spine is present in the latter.

Many cases of fetal cystic hygroma are associated with Turner syndrome (XO)[59,60]; however, several other congenital malformation syndromes with normal karyotype have been reported in association with cystic hygromas, including Noonan syndrome, fetal alcohol syndrome, and nuchal bleb syndrome.[61,62] In Chervanak's series, 73 percent of fetuses with cystic hygroma had cytogenetic findings consistent with Turner syndrome. When hydrops occurs in association with cystic hygromas, the outcome is extremely poor; none of the fetuses with hydrops in Chervanak's series survived.[60] Even when hydrops is not present, the outcome of fetuses with cystic hygroma colli is disappointing.

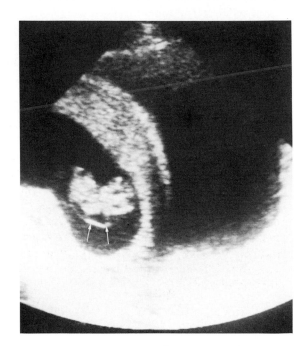

FIG. 2.27. Longitudinal view of 9½-week fetus with cystic hygroma (arrows). Subsequent scan at 15 weeks confirmed a large bilobed cystic hygroma, also seen at pregnancy termination.

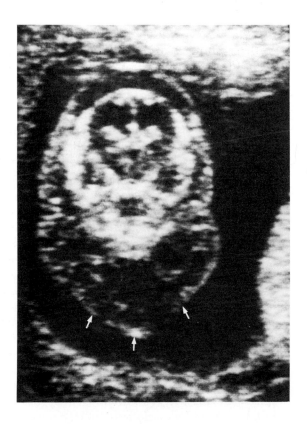

FIG. 2.28. Transverse view through the head at 13 weeks in a fetus with Turner syndrome, showing large cystic hygromas (arrows) behind the fetal head.

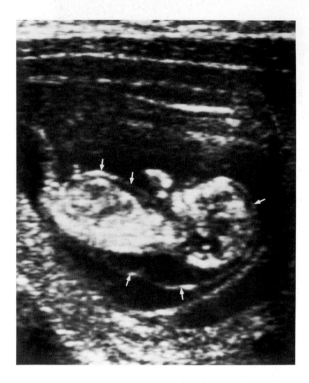

FIG. 2.29. A 12-week fetus with cystic hygromas and overall body edema (arrows).

Cystic hygromas are not always present at the back of the neck and occasionally, large lymphangiomas (cystic hygromas) can occur in the abdomen, abdominal wall, chest, or anterior aspect of the neck. These are not usually associated with chromosomal abnormalities, nor are they associated with generalized hydrops unless they mechanically compress venous return. We described four such fetuses, three of which survived after surgery.[63]

More than 20 percent of fetuses with Turner syndrome have a cardiac defect, 70 percent of which are coarctation of the aorta.[9] Antenatal detection of left heart lesions has been reported and abnormalities of the aortic valve can be demonstrated sonographically (Fig. 2.30). In our series evaluating the antenatal detection of congenital heart disease, three fetuses had coarctation of the aorta, two of which were correctly identified antenatally by echocardiography[26] (Fig. 2.31).

TRIPLOIDY

Triploidy occurs in approximately 1 percent of conceptions, but most of these end in spontaneous abortion before the end of the first trimester. Survival of a fetus beyond 20 weeks is rare.[64] Fetuses with triploidy can have a variety of structural malformations that are nonspecific and include abnormal shape of the head, cleft lip and palate, neural tube defects, congenital heart disease (ASD and VSD), hydrocephalus, holoprosencephaly, renal abnormalities including cystic dysplasia and hydronephrosis, and clubfoot.[9,65-70] The most

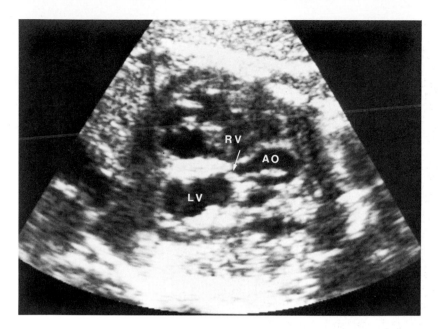

FIG. 2.30.   A 30-week fetus with critical aortic stenosis. Note the dilation of the ventricles and the very small region of the aortic valve (arrow). This fetus was hydropic due to congestive heart failure and died shortly after birth due to critical aortic stenosis. LV, left ventricle; RV, right ventricle; AO, aorta.

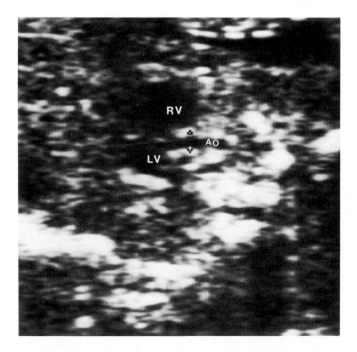

FIG. 2.31.   Magnified view of the fetal heart in a fetus that had a severe coarctation of the aorta. At 20 weeks in this image, the aortic outflow tract, indicated by the small cursors, is more narrow than expected for this gestational age. LV, left ventricle; RV, right ventricle; AO, aorta.

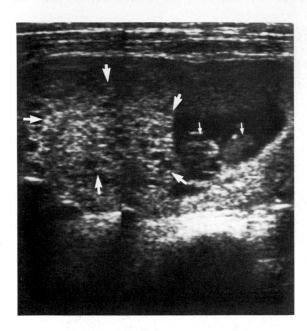

FIG. 2.32. Transverse view of the uterus at 11 weeks, showing the fetus on one side (small arrows) and a markedly enlarged placenta on the other (large arrows). Note that the placenta consists of multiple small echolucencies, consistent with a partial mole.

common abnormality involves severe IUGR, which is asymmetric, affecting the skeleton and body more severely, with some sparing of the head.[65–71] The placenta can either be very large with hydatidiform changes or may be very small and prematurely aged (Fig. 2.32).

Characteristically, IUGR can occur early, and growth deficiency in the first trimester has been detected sonographically.[71] Growth retardation in the second trimester is normally extremely rare and, when encountered, triploidy should be strongly suspected. The malformations that occur in triploidy are sufficiently nonspecific that a pattern is difficult to establish. In this particular chromosomal abnormality, therefore, the growth deficiency is by far more useful than a particular constellation of malformations. The appearance of the placenta may also be helpful, particularly when it has the configurations of a partial mole or hydatidiform.[72] Infants with triploidy, when born alive, die within the first few days of life, with the longest survivor being 10½ months. It is therefore extremely helpful to make this positive diagnosis, particularly when a fetus with severe IUGR is encountered in the late second or third trimester. The fetus is otherwise likely to be delivered by cesarean section for fetal distress and growth deficiency unless the presence of a lethal chromosomal abnormality is known.

CONFIRMING THE DIAGNOSIS OF ANEUPLOIDY

Sonographic identification of morphologic signs suggesting a fetal trisomy or triploidy is extremely helpful, since the fetus may not otherwise be a candidate for cytogenetic studies; however, cytogenetic analysis of amniotic

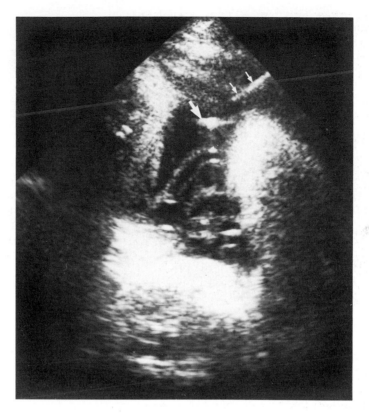

FIG. 2.33.   Amniocentesis performed under continuous ultrasound guidance. The needle shaft is shown by the small arrows and the large arrow indicates the tip of the needle in the amniotic fluid. Note several loops of umbilical cord directly underneath the needle.

fluid, blood, or tissue is necessary to make the definitive diagnosis. We are often faced with a fetus with abnormalities suggesting a possible chromosomal aberration, either just prior to 24 weeks or later in pregnancy, when the fetus may be at risk of fetal distress associated with IUGR. A rapid karyotype is crucial in these cases, in order to obtain the definitive diagnosis as quickly as possible. The percutaneous umbilical blood-sampling procedure has been used to obtain fetal blood for karyotyping.[73–76] A karyotype on fetal blood can be done in 48 hours, a much shorter time than needed to process amniotic fluid.

The technique used to obtain fetal blood is similar to our amniocentesis method, whereby the needle is visualized throughout the procedure[77] (Fig. 2.33). An appropriate location is chosen on the maternal abdomen and, after prepping, a 22-gauge needle is advanced toward the insertion of the umbilical vein on the placenta. The transducer is located 3 to 5 cm from the needle, and the needle angle can be altered during its path to reach the umbilical

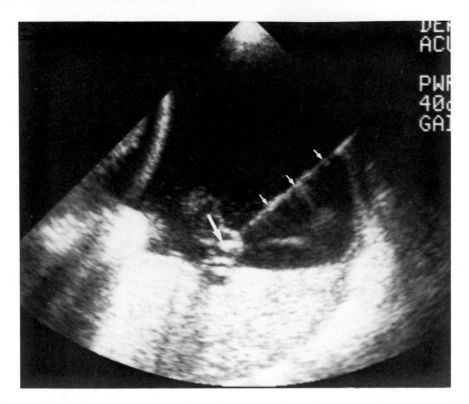

FIG. 2.34. Percutaneous umbilical blood sampling. The needle shaft is indicated by small arrows, and the tip of the needle in the umbilical vein is shown by the larger arrow. Because the placenta was posterior in this case, the amniotic cavity had to be traversed to gain access to the umbilical vein at its insertion on the placenta.

vein (Fig. 2.34); 3 cc of fetal blood is obtained with a procedure time of 5 to 15 minutes. In our first 100 cases of percutaneous umbilical blood sampling, 21 were done for the purpose of karyotyping with results available between 2 and 4 days.[73] This procedure has become an important adjunct to the sonographic detection of fetuses with chromosomal abnormalities, since confirmation by cytogenetics is necessary before obstetric management can be altered definitively.

CONCLUSIONS

Until recently, the diagnosis of chromosomal abnormalities had been left to the cytogeneticist. We are now able to identify subtle morphologic abnormalities that fit into a pattern suggesting a particular chromosomal anomaly. In our experience, we have been able to identify morphologic abnormalities suggesting trisomy 13 in nine of nine (100%) consecutive fetuses with trisomy 13 in our laboratory and in 12 of 15 (80%) fetuses with trisomy 18.[24] We also have developed morphologic signs for the detection of fetuses with trisomy 21 that can potentially identify 82 percent of fetuses with Down syndrome, subjecting only 2 percent of normal fetuses to amniocentesis.[42] Fetuses with triploidy are identified by combining severe IUGR with congenital abnormalities that may not fit a pattern but, when associated with the early onset of growth retardation and placental abnormalities, should suggest the diagnosis of triploidy. The rate of identification of fetuses with Turner syndrome has not been established, but severe nuchal cystic hygromas with associated body edema is an indication for a cytogenetic evaluation.

It is no longer enough to diagnose isolated fetal anomalies without looking for patterns of a recognizable syndrome or chromosomal abnormality. Increasing numbers of pregnant women are undergoing sonography for many different indications, but very few are candidates for cytogenetic studies. An important role for the sonologist is fetal surveillance for signs that would prompt the need for cytogenetic evaluation. The vast majority of patients carrying fetuses with chromosomal anomalies are not undergoing amniocentesis or chorionic villus sampling, and the only opportunity for detection may rest on the sonologist's ability to recognize a pattern of malformations. We have found percutaneous umbilical blood sampling an excellent method for further evaluation of fetuses with abnormal morphologic findings by ultrasonography to establish the abnormal karyotype both definitively and rapidly.

REFERENCES

1. Chervenak FA, Isaacson G, Mahoney MJ: Advances in the diagnosis of fetal defects. N Engl J Med 315:305, 1986
2. Horger EO, Pai GS: Ultrasound in the diagnosis of fetal malformations: implications for obstetrical management. Am J Obstet Gynecol 147:163, 1983
3. Vintzileos AM, Campbell WA, Nochimson DJ, et al: Antenatal evaluation and management of ultrasonically detected fetal anomalies. Obstet Gynecol 69:640, 1987
4. Sabbagha RE, Sheikh Z, Tamura RK, et al: Predictive value, sensitivity, and specificity of ultrasonic targeted imaging for fetal anomalies in gravid women at high risk for birth defects. Am J Obstet Gynecol 152:822, 1985
5. Kurjak A, Kirkinen P: Ultrasonic growth pattern of fetuses with chromosomal aberrations. Acta Obstet Gynecol Scand 61:223, 1982
6. Bundy AL, Saltzman DH, Pober B, et al: Antenatal sonographic findings in trisomy 18. J Ultrasound Med 5:361, 1986
7. Johnson TR, Corson VL, Payne PA, et al: Late prenatal diagnosis of fetal trisomy 18 associated with severe intrauterine growth retardation. Johns Hopkins Med J 151:242, 1982
8. Schneider AS, Mennuti MT, Zackai EH: High cesarean section rate in trisomy 18 births: a potential indication for late prenatal diagnosis. Am J Obstet Gynecol 140:367, 1981
9. Smith DW: Recognizable Patterns of Human Malformation. Vol. VII. Major Problems in Clinical Pediatrics. WB Saunders, Philadelphia, 1982
10. Patau K, Smith DW, Therman E, et al: Multiple congenital anomaly caused by an extra chromosome. Lancet 1:790, 1960
11. Benacerraf BR, Frigoletto FD, Greene MF: Abnormal facial features and extremities in human trisomy syndromes: prenatal ultrasound appearance. Radiology 159:243, 1986

12. Saltzman DH, Benacerraf BR, Frigoletto FD: Diagnosis and management of fetal facial clefts. Am J Obstet Gynecol 155:377, 1986

13. Greene MF, Benacerraf BR, Frigoletto FD: Reliable criteria for the prenatal sonographic diagnosis of alobar holoprosencephaly. Am J Obstet Gynecol 156:687, 1987

14. Copel JA, Pilu G, Kleinman CS: Congenital heart disease and extracardiac anomalies: associations and indications for fetal echocardiography. Am J Obstet Gynecol 154:1121, 1986

15. Redheendran R, Neu RL, Bannerman RM: Long survival in trisomy 13 syndrome: 21 cases including prolonged survival in two patients 11 and 19 years old. Am J Med Genet 8:167, 1981

16. Benacerraf BR, Frigoletto FD, Bieber FR: The fetal face ultrasound examination. Radiology 153:495, 1984

17. Seeds JW, Cefalo RC: Technique for early sonographic diagnosis of bilateral cleft lip and palate. Obstet Gynecol 62:2(S), 1983

18. Chervenak FA, Taortaora M, Mayden K, et al: Antenatal diagnosis of median cleft face syndrome: Sonographic demonstration of cleft lip and hypotelorism. Am J Obstet Gynecol 149:94, 1984

19. Savoldelli G, Schmid W, Schinzel A: Prenatal diagnosis of cleft lip and palate by ultrasound. Prenat Diagn 2:313, 1982

20. Christ JE, Meinigner MG: Ultrasound diagnosis of cleft lip and cleft palate before birth. Plast Reconstr Surg 68:854, 1981

21. Jeanty P, Romero R, Staudach A, et al: Facial anatomy of the fetus. J Ultrasound Med 5:607, 1986

22. Hegge FN, Prescott GH, Watson PT: Fetal facial abnormalities identified during obstetric sonography. J Ultrasound Med 5:679, 1986

23. Pilu G, Reece EA, Romero R, et al: Prenatal diagnosis of craniofacial malformations with ultrasonography. Am J Obstet Gynecol 155:45, 1986

24. Benacerraf BR, Miller WA, Frigoletto FD: Sonographic detection of fetuses with trisomy 13 and 18: accuracy and limitations. Am J Obstet Gynecol 158:404, 1988

25. Benacerraf BR: Antenatal sonographic diagnosis of congenital clubfoot: a possible indication for amniocentesis. JCU 14:703, 1986

26. Benacerraf BR, Pober BR, Sanders SP: The accuracy of fetal echocardiography. Radiology 165:847, 1987

27. Sandor GGS, Farquarson D, Wittmann B, et al: Fetal echocardiography: Results in high-risk patients. Obstet Gynecol 67:358, 1986

28. Allan LD, Crawford DC, Anderson RH, et al: Echocardiographic and anatomical correlations in fetal congenital heart disease. Br Heart J 52:542, 1984

29. Benacerraf BR, Frigoletto FD: Prenatal ultrasound diagnosis of clubfoot. Radiology 155:211, 1985

30. Benacerraf BR, Adzick NS: Fetal diaphragmatic hernia: ultrasound diagnosis and clinical outcome in 19 cases. Am J Obstet Gynecol 156:573, 1987

31. Christianson AL, Nelson MN: Four cases of trisomy 18 syndrome with limb reduction malformation. J Med Genet 21:293, 1984

32. Carter PE, Pearn JH, Bell J, et al: Survival in trisomy 13: Life tables for use in genetic counseling and clinical pediatrics. Clin Genet 27:59, 1985

33. Jeanty P, Romero R, D'Alton M, et al: In utero sonographic detection of hand and foot deformities. J Ultrasound Med 4:595, 1985

34. Hook EB, Cross PK, Schreinemachers DM: Chromosomal abnormality rates at amniocentesis and in live-born infants. JAMA 249:2034, 1983

35. Adams MM, Erickson JD, Layde PM, et al: Down's syndrome: recent trends in the United States. JAMA 247:758, 1981

36. Lippman-Hand A, Piper M: Prenatal diagnosis for the detection of Down syndrome: why are so few eligible women tested? Prenat Diagn 1:249, 1981

37. Hook EB, Schreinemachers DM, Cross PK: Use of prenatal cytogenetic diagnosis in New York State. N Engl J Med, 305:1410, 1981

38. Hall B: Mongolism in newborn infants. Clin Pediatr 5:4, 1966

39. Benacerraf BR, Barss VA, Laboda LA: A sonographic sign for the detection in the second trimester of the fetus with Down syndrome. Am J Obstet Gynecol 151:1078, 1985

40. Benacacerraf BR, Frigoletto FD, Laboda LA: Sonographic diagnosis of Down syndrome in the second trimester. Am J Obstet Gynecol 153:49, 1985

41. Benacerraf BR, Frigoletto FD, Cramer DW: Down syndrome: sonographic sign for diagnosis in the second-trimester fetus. Radiology 163:811, 1987

42. Benacerraf BR, Gelman R, Frigoletto FD: Sonographic prediction of the second trimester fetus with Down syndrome. N Engl J Med 317:1371, 1987

43. Lockwood C, Benacerraf B, Krinsky A, et al: A sonographic screening method for Down syndrome. Am J Obstet Gynecol 157:803, 1987

44. Benacerraf BR, Osathanondh R, Frigoletto FD: Sonographic demonstration of hypoplasia of the middle phalanx of the fifth digit: a finding associated with Down syndrome. Am J Obstet Gynecol (In press)

45. Balcar I, Grant DC, Miller WA, et al: Antenatal detection of Down syndrome by sonography. AJR 143:29, 1984

46. Benacerraf BR, Frigoletto FD: Soft tissue nuchal fold in the second trimester fetus: standards for normal measurements compared to the fetus with Down syndrome. Am J Obstet Gynecol 157:1146, 1987

47. Toi A, Simpson GF, Filly RA: Ultrasonically evident fetal nuchal skin thickening: is it specific for Down syndrome? Am J Obstet Gynecol 156:150, 1987

48. Palomaki GE, Haddow JE: Maternal serum α fetoprotein, age, and Down syndrome risk. Am J Obstet Gynecol 156:460, 1987

49. Spencer K, Carpenter P: Screening for Down's syndrome using serum α fetoprotein: a retrospective study indicating caution. Br Med J 290:1940, 1985

50. Merkatz IR, Nitowsky HM, Macri JN: An association between low maternal serum α fetoprotein and fetal chromosomal abnormalities. Am J Obstet Gynecol 148:886, 1984

51. Turner HH: A syndrome of infantilism, congenital web neck and cubitus valgus. Endocrinology 23:566, 1938

52. Benacerraf BR, Lister JE, Duponte B: First trimester diagnosis of fetal anomalies. J Reprod Med (In press)

53. Exalto N, Van Zalen RM, Van Brandenburg WJA: Early prenatal diagnosis of cystic hygroma by real time ultrasound. JCU 13:655, 1985

54. Rahmani MR, Fong KW, Connor TP: The varied sonographic appearance of cystic hygromas in utero. J Ultrasound Med 5:165, 1986

55. O'Brien WF, Cefalo RC, Bair DG: Ultrasonographic diagnosis of fetal cystic hygroma. Am J Obstet Gynecol 138:464, 1980

56. Phillips HE, McGahan JP: Intrauterine fetal cystic hygromas: sonographic detection. AJR 136:799, 1981

57. Garden AS, Benzie RJ, Miskin M, et al: Fetal cystic hygroma colli: antenatal diagnosis, significance, and management. Am J Obstet Gynecol 154:221, 1986

58. Miller JM, McCarter L, Pai GS, et al: Hygroma cervicis: antepartum ultrasonic findings. J Reprod Med 26:567, 1981

59. Robinow M, Spisso K, Buschi AJ, et al: Turner syndrome: sonography showing fetal hydrops simulating hydramnios. AJR 135:846, 1980

60. Chervenak FA, Isaacson G, Blakemore KJ, et al: Fetal cystic hygroma: cause and natural history. N Engl J Med 309:822, 1983

61. Zarabi M, Mieckowski GC, Mazer J: Cystic hygroma associated with Noonan's syndrome. JCU 11:398, 1983

62. Bieber FR, Petres RE, McNamara Bieber J, et al: Prenatal detection of a familial nuchal bleb simulating encephalocele. Birth Defects 15(5A):51, 1979

63. Benacerraf BR, Frigoletto FD: Prenatal sonographic diagnosis of isolated congenital cystic hygroma, unassociated with lymphedema or other morphologic abnormality. J Ultrasound Med 6:63, 1987

64. Boue J, Boue A, Lazar P: Retrospective and prospective epidemiological studies of 1,500 karyotyped spontaneous abortions. Teratology 12:11, 1982

65. Doshi N, Surti U, Szulman AE: Morphologic anomalies in triploid liveborn fetuses. Hum Pathol 14:716, 1983

66. Wertelecki W, Graham JM, Sergovich FR: The clinical syndrome of triploidy. Obstet Gynecol 47:69, 1976

67. Edwards MT, Smith WL, Hanson J, et al: Prenatal sonographic diagnosis of triploidy. J Ultrasound Med 5:279, 1986

68. Porreco RP, Matson MR, Young PE, et al: Diagnosis of a triploid fetus at genetic amniocentesis. Obstet Gynecol 56:115, 1980

69. Broekhuizen FF, Elejalde R, Hamilton PR: Early-onset preeclampsia, triploidy and fetal hydrops. J Reprod Med 28:223, 1983

70. Crane JJP, Beaver HA, Cheung SW: Antenatal ultrasound findings in fetal triploidy syndrome. J Ultrasound Med 4:519, 1985

71. Benacerraf B: First trimester intrauterine growth retardation: associated with triploidy. J Ultrasound Med 7:153, 1988

72. Rubenstein JB, Swayne LC, Dise CA, et al: Placental changes in fetal triploidy syndrome. J Ultrasound Med 5:545, 1986

73. Benacerraf B, Barss, V, Saltzman D, et al: Percutaneous umbilical blood sampling under continuous ultrasound guidance. Radiology 166:105, 1988

74. Benacerraf BR, Barss VA, Saltzman DH, et al: Acute fetal distress associated with percutaneous umbilical blood sampling. Am J Obstet Gynecol 156:1218, 1987

75. Hobbins JC, Grannum PA, Romero R, et al: Percutaneous umbilical blood sampling. Am J Obstet Gynecol 152:1, 1985

76. Daffos F, Capella-Pavlovsky M, Forestier F: Fetal blood sampling during pregnancy with use of a needle guided by ultrasound: a study of 606 consecutive cases. Am J Obstet Gynecol 153:655, 1985

77. Benacerraf BR, Frigoletto FD: Amniocentesis under continuous ultrasound guidance: a series of 232 cases. Obstet Gynecol 62:760, 1983

3 Neural Tube Abnormalities

KYPROS NICOLAIDES
JAMES CAMPBELL

Spina bifida was among the first fetal abnormalities to be diagnosed by ultrasonography; during the past decade, several centers reported their experience with the diagnosis of this condition by examining the fetal spine.[1] More recent publications have focused on the identification of easily recognizable cranial and cerebellar signs that may improve the detection rate of spina bifida at the routine ultrasound scan.[2] The main emphasis of this chapter is on these recent studies.

BIOCHEMICAL SCREENING

The established screening test for fetal spina bifida is measurement of maternal serum α-fetoprotein (AFP) levels followed by amniocentesis in patients with elevated serum levels. A collaborative study in 1977 suggested that 79 percent of fetal spina bifidas would be detected at 16 to 18 weeks if the 95th centile were used as a cutoff point for serum screening.[3] Amniotic fluid AFP and acetylcholinesterase (AchE) testing increases the sensitivity to 99.5 percent.[4] However, in a population with a birth prevalence of 2 per 1,000 for open spina bifida, for every five fetuses with the anomaly that are correctly identified, one fetus will be lost as a result of spontaneous abortion after amniocentesis or elective abortion due to a false-positive diagnosis.[5]

ULTRASOUND SCREENING

During ultrasound examination, the fetal spine is visualized in its entire length both longitudinally and transversely. In the transverse view, the normal neural arch appears as a closed circle with an intact skin covering (Fig. 3.1), while in open spina bifida, the arch is U shaped, and there is a bulging

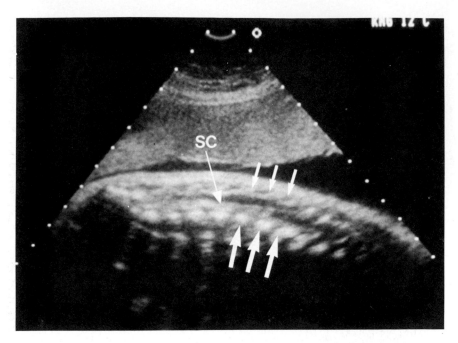

FIG. 3.1. Longitudinal section of the normal fetal spine demonstrating the complete skin covering of the spine (sc, spinal canal; large arrows, vertebral bodies; small arrows, neural arches). (Courtesy of Dr. Gianluigi Pilu, Bologna, Italy.)

myelocele or meningomyelocele (Fig. 3.2). The extent of the defect and of any associated kyphoscoliosis is best assessed in the longitudinal scan. The prognosis for the lesion is made by applying the same criteria as those suggested by Lorber[6] for postnatal assessment. However, limb movements and bladder function may appear normal, even with major lumbosacral lesions, and are therefore of no prognostic significance.

While the sensitivity and specificity of ultrasonographic assessment may be as high as 96 percent and 99.9 percent, respectively, few centers have personnel with the expertise necessary to achieve this degree of diagnostic accuracy.[7] Roberts examined the diagnostic accuracy of 2,509 scans performed between 1977 to 1982 in women considered at high risk of having a fetus with a neural tube defect.[8] During the first 3 years of the program, when the surgeons at University Hospital of Wales were relatively inexperienced and used less sophisticated equipment, the detection rate for spina bifida was 36 percent (5 of 14), the false-positive rate was 90 percent (45 of 50), and the false-negative rate was 1 percent (9 of 913). During the next 3 years of the study, as the same surgeons had become more experienced and the quality of their equipment had improved, the detection rate for spina bifida had risen to 80 percent (16 of 20) and the specificity to 99.7 percent (1,167 of 1,171).

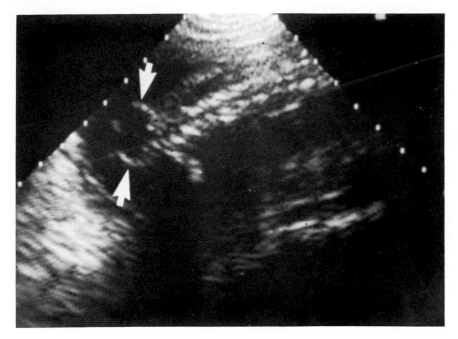

FIG. 3.2.   Longitudinal section of the spine in a fetus with lumbosacral myelomenin-gocele (arrows). From Jeanty P, Romero R: *Obstetrical Ultrasound*. McGraw-Hill, New York, with permission.)

Swedish Study

Routine ultrasound examination at 15 to 20 weeks gestation and measurement of maternal serum AFP were performed on 10,147 women with live singleton pregnancies.[9] The study was undertaken in Malmo during 1978 to 1981. There were nine fetuses with neural tube defects (five with open spina bifida, three with encephalocele, and one with anencephaly) and one with omphalocele. Screening by AFP alone detected 4 of 5 cases with open spina bifida, 2 of 3 with encephalocele, one anencephalic, and the one with omphalocele. Screening by routine ultrasound examination alone detected only 4 of 10 malformations. The investigators in this study did not specify which were the four defects detected by ultrasonography but stated that all were incompatible with extrauternie life. Therefore, assuming that the anencephalus and the three encephaloceles were detected, it is possible that all cases of open spina bifida were missed by routine ultrasound screening.

CRANIAL AND CEREBELLAR SIGNS

Cranial and cerebellar signs include cerebral ventriculomegaly, microcephaly, scalloping of the frontal bones of the fetal head (Fig. 3.3, the lemon sign), and absence or anterior curvature of the cerebellar hemispheres with simultaneous obliteration of the cisterna magna (Figs. 3.4 and 3.5, the banana sign).

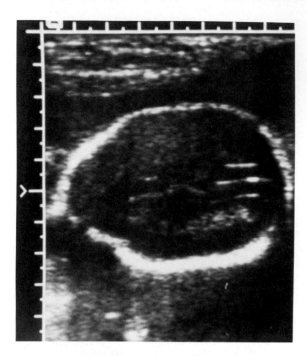

FIG. 3.3. Transverse section of the fetal head in a fetus with open spina bifida, demonstrating the "lemon" sign (scalloping of the frontal bones). (Courtesy of Dr. Roberto Romero, New Haven, CT.)

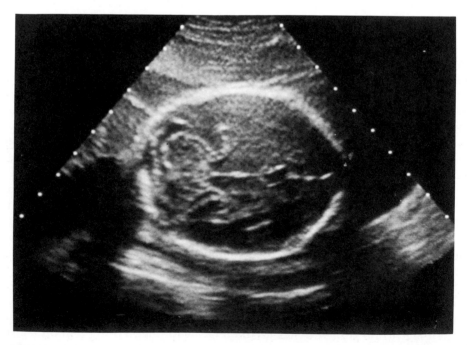

FIG. 3.4. Suboccipital bregmatic view of the fetal head at 18 weeks gestation, demonstrating the normal cerebellum. (Courtesy of Dr. Gianluigi Pilu, Bologna, Italy.)

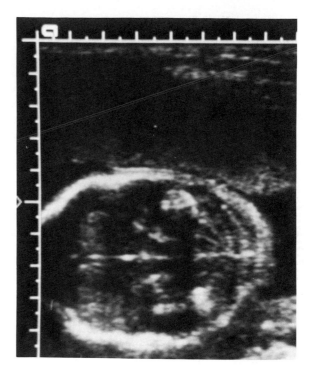

Fig. 3.5. Suboccipital bregmatic view of the fetus with open spina bifida, demonstrating the "banana" sign (anterior curvature of the cerebellar hemispheres and obliteration of the cisterna magna). (Courtesy of Dr. Roberto Romero, New Haven, CT.)

Cerebral Ventriculomegaly

In cranial sonograms obtained 2 to 4 days after birth in 29 neonates with meningomyeloceles, Babcock and Han[10] observed hydrocephalus in all but one case. Relative enlargement of the occipital or posterior horns of the lateral ventricles compared with the frontal or temporal horns was found in 19 cases. Zimmerman et al.[11] also described enlargement of the occipital horns on cranial CT scans in 89 percent (42 of 47) of children with a meningocele between the ages of 6 days and 15 years when studied.

Microcephaly

Wald et al.[12] originally reported that the biparietal diameter was 0.83 cm smaller when measured in the second trimester in 20 pregnancies complicated by spina bifida. These workers attributed this observation to fetal growth retardation. By contrast, Roberts and Campbell[13] demonstrated that the reduction in biparietal diameter was not due to growth retardation, as the abdominal circumference measurements in 15 fetuses with open spina bifida were within normal limits for the expected gestational age despite small biparietal diameters.

Arnold-Chiari Malformation

In 1891, Chiari described four malformations of the brain associated with congenital hydrocephalus.[14] Type 2, which is characteristic of open spina bifida, showed a variable displacement of the inferior vermis of the cerebellum into the upper cervical canal and was accompanied by a similar caudal displacement of the lower pons and medulla, together with an elongated fourth ventricle. In 1907, working in Arnold's laboratory, Schwalbe and Gredig[15] found these abnormalities to be regularly associated with spina bifida; they labeled them the Arnold-Chiari malformation, the name by which they are known today. More recently, Bell et al.[16] reported that seven of nine fetuses with open spina bifida, aborted at 14 to 23 weeks gestation, demonstrated the Arnold-Chiari malformation at postmortem examination. An equal number exhibited hydrocephaly. Arnold-Chiari complex may be attributed to tethering of the spinal cord at the site of the lesion with downward displacement of the brain as the fetus grows.[17] This process would reduce the contents of the cranium, leading to a decrease in biparietal diameter and head circumference. The scalloping of the frontal bones (the lemon sign) may be attributable to the same mechanism. The cerebellum, as it is displaced downward into the cervical canal, may become hypoplastic or may disappear from the cranium. In a study of 32 patients known to have Arnold-Chiari type 2 malformation, Naldick et al.[18] described an anteriorly pointed configuration of the cerebellar hemispheres on computed tomography. It is possible that downward traction on the spinal cord forces the cerebellum to wrap around the brain stem, creating the banana configuration.

Retrospective Study

The records of 70 fetuses with open spina bifida diagnosed in our unit by ultrasonography at 16 to 23 weeks gestation were examined.[2] Mothers were at increased risk of having a fetus with open spina bifida due to either a raised maternal serum AFP level (2.5 multiples of the median at 16 to 18 weeks gestation, $n = 49$) or suspicious ultrasound findings on routine screening at the referring hospital ($n = 21$). The diagnosis of open spina bifida was made on ultrasound evaluation and confirmed by postmortem examination after elective abortion in all 70 patients.

All patients underwent systematic real-time ultrasound study. The biparietal diameter was measured from the outer to outer edges of the fetal skull in a transverse section demonstrating a central midline echo broken in its anterior third by the septum cavum pellucidum. The anterior horn ventricular-hemisphere ratio (Va/H) was measured from the lateral border of the distal anterior horn of the lateral ventricle and compared with the hemisphere measurement from the midline to the inner table of the skull. The posterior horn ventricular-hemisphere ratio (Vp/H) was assessed by determining the distance from the medial to the lateral borders of the posterior horn and compared with the hemisphere measurement. The fetal head circumference and shape of the skull were also determined at the transverse section of the head used to measure the biparietal diameter. Fetal biparietal diameter, head circumference, Va/H, and Vp/H were compared with normograms established in our unit. The fetal cerebellum was examined by first obtaining the standard biparietal diameter image and then angling the transducer to achieve a suboccipital bregmatic view. The cerebellar hemispheres appear as symmetric spheres joined in the midline by the thin cerebellar vermis.[19]

The results of this study are shown in Table 3.1. The biparietal diameter and head circumference measurements fell below the 5th percentile for gestation in 61 percent (43/70) and 26 percent (17/66) of cases, respectively. The Va/H exceeded the 95th percentile in 77 percent (51 of 66) of these fetuses, and ventriculomegaly of the posterior horn of the lateral ventricle was observed in 86 percent (57 of 66) of cases. In eight (12 percent) fetuses, both ventricles were of normal size. In all 54 cases of open spina bifida in which pictures taken at the level of biparietal diameter were available for review, there was scalloping of the frontal bones. In 12 of 21 (57 percent) cases in which pictures of the suboccipital bregmatic view of the fetal cranium were obtained, the cerebellar hemispheres were banana shaped; in a further eight (38 percent) cases, the cerebellum was not visualized. The cerebellar hemispheres appeared normal in only one of the 21 (5 percent) fetuses with open spina bifida. Neither the lemon nor the banana nor absent cerebellum signs were observed in 100 consecutive patients presenting for routine ultrasound

TABLE 3.1. Cranial and cerebellar signs in spina bifida

Feature	Retrospective Study (N = 70)	Prospective Study (62 of 903)
Lemon sign (false positive)	70/70 (100%)	61/62 (98%)
	0/100 (0%)	10/841 (1.2%)
Cerebellum		
Banana shaped	12/21 (57%)	39/62 (63%)
Absent	8/21 (38%)	20/62 (32%)
Normal (false positive)	1/21 (5%)	5/62 (5%)
	0/100 (0%)	0/841 (0%)
Biparietal diameter <5th centile	43/70 (61%)	38/62 (61%)
Head circumference (<5th centile)	17/66 (26%)	24/62 (39%)
Ventricle/hemisphere >95th centile		
Anterior	51/66 (77%)	25/62 (40%)
Posterior	57/66 (86%)	38/62 (61%)

examinations in the second trimester. All the controls had biparietal diameter and head circumference measurements compatible with gestational age and normal values for Va/H and Vp/H. This retrospective study suggested that the lemon and banana or absent cerebellum signs could be useful in ultrasound screening for open spina bifida.

PROSPECTIVE STUDY OF HIGH-RISK PREGNANCIES

Ultrasound examinations were performed in 903 patients at 16 to 24 weeks gestation because the fetus was at increased risk of having open spina bifida (raised maternal serum AFP, suspicious findings on routine ultrasound examination of the fetus, and family or personal history of open spina bifida). Ultrasound was performed by obstetricians, research fellows, midwives, and radiographers. The ultrasonographers were instructed to comment on the shape of the fetal skull and cerebellum and to record the measurements biparietal diameter, head circumference, Va/H, and Vp/H before examining the fetal spine both longitudinally and transversely.

The results of this study are summarized in Table 3.1. The data for the first 436 patients were reported previously.[20] Open spina bifida was diagnosed in 62 cases and confirmed by postmortem examination after elective termination of pregnancy. In the cases of open spina bifida, the biparietal diameter was below the 5th percentile for gestation in 38 (61 percent) and the head circumference in 24 (39 percent). The Va/H and Vp/H were above the 95th percentile in 11 percent and 14 percent of cases, respectively. The lemon sign was present in 61 of 62 fetuses with spina bifida and in 10 of 841 fetuses with normal spines (false-positive rate 1.2 percent). In 9 fetuses, the cerebellum was absent and in 16 of the remaining 17 cases, the cerebellar hemispheres were banana shaped. The cerebellum was normal in only one fetus.

Although Bell et al.[16] report that isolated sacral defects are not associated with hydrocephalus or the Arnold-Chiari complex and that more brain abnormalities are found if the spinal defect is cephalad and extensive, we found that the lemon and banana or absent cerebellum signs were present in all 12 fetuses with sacral myelomeningoceles. These findings demonstrate that the cranial and cerebellar markers, in particular the lemon and banana signs, are consistant features of open spina bifida and are likely to help improve the diagnostic accuracy of ultrasonography in the evaluation of pregnancies at high risk for this fetal abnormality.

Multicenter Prospective Screening Study

We are currently investigating the value of the cranial and cerebellar signs in the detection of fetal spina bifida in a prospective multicenter study. At all 16 participating centers, ultrasound examination is offered routinely, at

TABLE 3.2. Multicenter ultrasound screening study of 5,541 women at 16 to 20 weeks gestation

| | Open Spina Bifida | |
| | Present | Absent |
Sign(s)	(6)	(5,536)
Lemon sign	6	13
Cerebellar signs	4	1

16 to 20 weeks gestation, to all patients booked for delivery. The ultrasonographers, including obstetricians, radiographers, and midwives, were instructed to record their assessment of the shape of the fetal skull and cerebellum before examining the fetal spine.

The preliminary results of this continuing study are summarized in Table 3.2. Ultrasound scans were performed in 11,136 pregnancies, and open spina bifida was diagnosed in 11 cases; in all cases, the diagnosis was confirmed by postmortem examination after elective termination of pregnancy. Of the 11,136 patients, 5,541 have now completed their pregnancies; there were no cases of undiagnosed spina bifida. In this group of completed pregnancies, the lemon sign was present in all six cases of open spina bifida, but also in 13 unaffected fetuses (false-positive rate 0.2 percent). The cerebellum was banana shaped or absent in 4 of 6 cases with open spina bifida, but also in one of the unaffected fetuses (false positive rate 0.02 percent).

Other Studies

Penso et al.[20] examined the shape of the fetal skull in 36 cases of hydrocephalus diagnosed by ultrasonography at 15 to 40 weeks gestation. In 24 fetuses, there was an associated open spina bifida; in all 13 cases diagnosed at 15 to 22 weeks and in 3 of 11 examined at 27 to 40 weeks, there was pointing of the frontal bones. In all 12 cases with isolated hydrocephalus, the shape of the fetal skull was normal.[20]

Pilu et al.[21] examined the posterior fossa of 19 fetuses with open spina bifida and noted that in all cases there was a downward displacement of the cerebellum and obliteration of the cisterna magna. In six cases, the cerebellum could not be visualized, and in 13 the transverse cerebellar diameter was below the 2.5th percentile of normal range. Furthermore, in all 19 cases, there was an elongation of the cerebral peduncles. None of these findings was observed in 17 fetuses with isolated hydrocephalus.

CONCLUSION

In the hands of experienced operators, prenatal diagnosis of spina bifida by ultrasonographic examination of the fetal spine is reliable. Nevertheless, ultrasonography has not had widespread success in the detection of this abnormality during routine screening. It appears that the lemon, banana, or absent cerebellum signs are easily recognizable markers of underlying open spina bifida. The demonstration of these signs does not require the same high level of ultrasound expertise necessary in the examination of the fetal spine. Indeed, all features, other than those relating to the cerebellum, are visible in the standard view obtained to measure biparietal diameter, which is a part of every routine ultrasound examination. The presence of abnormal cranial or cerebellar signs should therefore alert the ultrasonographer to the possibility of an underlying open spina bifida and thus stimulate detailed examination of the fetal spine. Such a policy should improve the diagnostic accuracy of ultrasonography in the detection of open spina bifida in both high- and low-risk pregnancies.

REFERENCES

1. Campbell S, Pryse-Davies J, Coltard TM, et al: Ultrasound in the diagnosis of spina bifida. Lancet 1:1065, 1975
2. Nicolaides KH, Gabbe SG, Guidetti R, Campbell S: Ultrasound screening for spina bifida: Cranial and cerebellar signs. Lancet 1:72, 1986
3. UK collaborative study on alpha-fetoprotein in relation to neural tube defects. Maternal serum-alpha-fetoprotein measurement in antenatal screening for anencephaly and spina bifida in early pregnancy. Lancet 1:1323, 1977
4. UK Collaborative Study on Alpha-Fetoprotein in Relation to Neural Tube Defects: Amniotic fluid alpha-fetoprotein measurements in antenatal diagnosis of anencephaly and open spina bifida in early pregnancy. Lancet 2:652, 1979
5. Wald NJ, Cuckle HS: Open neural-tube defects. p. 25. In Wald NJ (ed): Antenatal and Neonatal Screening. Oxford University Press, Oxford, 1984
6. Lorber J: Results of treatment of myelomeningoceles. An analysis of 524 unrelated cases, with special reference to possible selection for treatment. Dev Med Child Neurol 3:79, 1971
7. Nicolaides KH, Campbell S: Diagnosis of fetal abnormalities by ultrasound. p. 521. In Milunsky A (ed): Genetic Disorders and the Fetus: Diagnosis, Prevention and Treatment. 2nd Ed. Plenum Press, New York, 1987
8. Roberts CJ, Evans KT, Hibbard BM, et al: Diagnostic effectiveness of ultrasound in detection of neural tube defect: the South Wales experience of 2509 scans (1977–1982) in high-risk mothers. Lancet 2:1068, 1983
9. Persson PH, Kullander S, Gennser G, et al: Screening for fetal malformations using ultrasound and measurements of α-fetoprotein in maternal serum. Br Med J 286:747, 1983
10. Babcock DS, Han BK: Cranial sonographic findings in meningomyelocele. AJR 136:563, 1981
11. Zimmerman RD, Breckbill D, Dennis MW, Davis DO: Cranial CT findings in patients with meningomyelocele. AJR 132:623, 1979

12. Wald N, Cuckle H, Boreham J, Stirrat G: Small biparietal diameter of fetuses with spina bifida: Implications for antenatal screening. Br J Obstet Gynaecol 87:219, 1980

13. Roberts AB, Campbell S: Small biparietal diameter of fetuses with spina bifida: implications for antenatal screening. Br J Obstet Gynaecol 87:927, 1980

14. Chiari H: Uber veranderungen des kleinhirns infolge von hydrocephalus des grosshirns. Dtsch Med Wochenschr 17:1172, 1981

15. Schwalbe E, Gredig M: Uber entwicklungsstorungen de kleinhirns, hirnstamms and halsmarks bei spina bifida. Beitr Pathol Anat 40:132, 1906

16. Bell JE, Gordon A, Maloney FJ: The association of hydrocephalus and Arnold-Chiari malformation with spina bifida in the fetus. Neuropathol Appl Neurobiol 6:29, 1980

17. Ingraham FD, Scott HW: Spinda bifida and cranium bifidum. V. The Arnold-Chiari malformation: A review of twenty cases. N Engl J Med 229:108, 1943

18. Naldich TP, Pudlowski RM, Naldich JB: Computed tomographic signs of Chiari II malformation. II. Midbrain and cerebellum. Radiology 134:391, 1980

19. Smith PA, Johansson D, Tzannatos C, Campbell S: Prenatal measurement of the fetal cerebellum and cisterna cerebellomedullaris by ultrasound. Prenat Diagn 1987

20. Penso C, Redline RW, Benacerraf BR: A sonographic sign which predicts which fetuses with hydrocephalus have an associated neural tube defect. J Ultrasound Med 6:307, 1987

21. Pilu G, Romero R, Goldstein I, et al: Subnormal cerebellum size in fetuses with spina bifida. Am J Obstet Gynecol 1987

4 Fetal Echocardiography in the Diagnosis and Management of Fetal Heart Disease

Joshua A. Copel
Charles S. Kleinman

The field of fetal diagnosis has undergone revolutionary changes over the past 15 years, due in large part to improvements in ultrasound imaging techniques. Detailed evaluation of both normal and abnormal anatomy is now possible with high-resolution real-time imaging. A wide variety of diagnoses have been reliably established in virtually every system of the body. Furthermore, investigation of fetal behavior has led to the description of the biophysical profile, as well as speculation about fetal neurologic examination in the future.

Early fetal ultrasound systems relied on A-mode imaging, which provided limited information about the fetus, and could not be used to diagnose fetal structural anomalies. The next step was to convert the signals to composite images in the compound, or B-mode scan. This static scan provided only still pictures. While high-quality images of the fetus could be obtained, movement could not be assessed. Cardiologists used ultrasonography for dynamic cardiac imaging with M-mode echocardiography. In the fetus, until concurrent information about variations in position and orientation could be provided, the application of M-mode echocardiography to the fetus was necessarily limited. Nevertheless, the first description of fetal echocardiography was based entirely on M-mode ultrasonography.[1]

More recently, the availability of high-quality two-dimensional real-time ultrasound has provided a tool for the detailed examination of the fetal heart. Both normal and abnormal anatomic findings have been described by a number of fetal echocardiography laboratories.[2–9] The equipment used has in-

cluded two-dimensional real-time sector scanners with simultaneous or duplex M-mode capability; recently, pulsed Doppler ultrasound has been
applied to the evaluation of the human fetal heart.

PRINCIPLES OF FETAL ECHOCARDIOGRAPHY

Fetal cardiac structural diagnosis is based on interpretation of the same tomographic sections relied on in pediatric and adult echocardiography (Table
4.1). The sectional anatomy of the normal fetal heart has been clarified by a
number of workers.[3,4,8] It is important to bear in mind several important
facts about the fetal heart before undertaking fetal cardiac studies.

The cardiovascular system of the fetus is significantly different from the
postnatal system. Although our understanding of the fetal circulation is generally based on the fetal lamb model,[10] similar patterns can be expected in
humans. The major difference is likely to relate to the larger size of the
human brain relative to total body weight, which may increase the relative
contribution of the left ventricle to the combined ventricular output compared
with the lamb. Preliminary human studies using Doppler ultrasound appear
to confirm the principles initially derived from ovine models.

The ventricles of the fetal heart work in parallel, as opposed to working
in series postnatally. Blood returning to the fetus from the placenta crosses
the ductus venosus, is briefly carried through the inferior vena cava, and is
preferentially shunted across the foramen ovale into the left atrium. Thus,
the more oxygenated blood is distributed to the ascending aorta, to perfuse
the coronary and cerebral beds. The majority of right ventricular output
enters the ductus arteriosus and is thereby carried to the descending aorta.
This less oxygenated blood is then transported to the placenta. The right
ventricle can therefore be considered the ventricle responsible for perfusing
the organ of respiration prenatally as well as postnatally.

There are two communications between the right and left sides of the
normal fetal heart. These shunts, the foramen ovale and the ductus arteriosus,
are not normally visualized postnatally. Failure to demonstrate their presence
may indicate pathology in the fetus.

Another consequence of the parallel circulation of the fetus is that pressures
in the two ventricles are very similar. In addition, the fetal ventricles normally

TABLE 4.1.   Standard echocardiographic views
used in fetal echocardiography

Four-chamber
Long-axis left ventricle
Short-axis ventricles
Short-axis great vessels
Aortic arch
Pulmonary artery/ductus arteriosus

appear nearly equal to each other in size when examined by two-dimensional ultrasound.

Finally, it is essential to remember that the fetus is constantly moving and that orientation must be established at the outset of the study by locating the fetal head, spine, and stomach, to ensure normal situs and to permit the sonologist to identify chambers and great vessels.

TECHNIQUE

Fetal echocardiography requires demonstration of the same tomographic planes used in pediatric and adult echocardiography (Table 4.1). We rely primarily on two-dimensional imaging, reserving M-mode for analysis of arrhythmias, and measurement of septal thickness in diabetic pregnancies. Other investigators have suggested that M-mode-based measurement of cardiac chambers and structures take a greater role in the diagnosis of fetal structural cardiac anomalies.[11]

The examination can be conducted with either sector or linear array scanning equipment, although we find that sector transducers provide greater flexibility in approaching the fetal heart from the necessary angles. We currently use an electronic phased array scanner with a 5-MHz transducer for virtually all examinations (Hewlett-Packard 77020A Ultrasound Imaging System, Hewlett-Packard, Andover, MA). In selected patients, we use a variety of other techniques, including linear array (GE RT 3600, General Electric, Milwaukee WI), or mechanical sector scanners (ATL UltraMark 4, Advanced Technology Laboratories, Bellvue, WA; Interspec XL, Conshohocken, PA).

The simplest and easiest view to obtain is the four-chamber view, which includes both atria and ventricles, along with the atrioventricular valves. It can usually be found by starting from the image of the abdomen used for calculation of the abdominal circumference and angling the transducer cephalad (on the fetus). This view is especially useful for assessment of the relative sizes of the cardiac chambers, the anatomy of the atrioventricular valves, and the presence or absence of pericardial fluid (Fig. 4.1). To differentiate the chambers, the more posterior (left) atrial chamber should be seen to contain the flap of the foramen ovale, and the more anterior (right) ventricle should contain the moderator band. The apex of the heart should be on the same side of the body as the stomach. The atrioventricular valves should each have separate fibrous insertion rings, and the tricuspid valve insertion should appear to be slightly apical to that of the mitral valve.

The four-chamber view must be seen in relationship to the fetal stomach, spine, liver, and vena cavae in order to ascertain situs. We find that it is easiest to maintain our maternal anatomic orientation (i.e., looking from right to left, or feet toward head on the mother), regardless of the orientation of the heart on the screen, in order to adjust the transducer position on the mother's abdomen more easily when necessary.

Further experience will permit the examiner to adjust the transducer to obtain other necessary views. We include a long-axis view of the left ventricle,

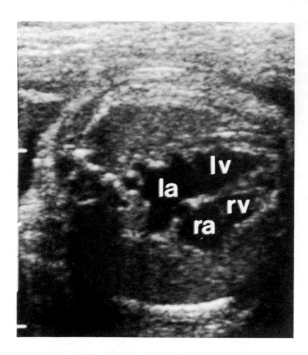

FIG. 4.1. Normal view of four-chamber anatomy. The fetal heart is oriented with the apex to the right. The two ventricular chambers (lv and rv) and the two atrial chambers (la and ra) are roughly equal in size. The foramen ovale is seen as a defect in the interatrial septum. The interventricular septum is intact, and the insertion points of the mitral and tricuspid valves into the central fibrous body of the heart are identified.

short-axis views of the ventricles and great vessels, and an aortic arch view in each examination. The maneuvers needed to produce each of these will vary with fetal position.

As in postnatal echocardiography, each tomographic section provides information about a specific portion of cardiac anatomy. The four-chamber view can demonstrate lesions of the atrioventricular valves and of the posterior atrioventricular septum and permits assessment of ventricular cavity enlargement or hypoplasia (Fig. 4.2). We have found the four-chamber view helpful as an initial screen for fetal heart disease. The long-axis view of the left ventricle is most important in the fetus for evaluation of septal-aortic continuity; failure to establish this relationship suggests override of the aorta. Should such a finding be suspected, serial evaluation of cardiac anatomy is essential, as the lesion may evolve in utero. We have seen several fetuses develop subpulmonic stenosis after aortic override was first appreciated, progressing to tetralogy of Fallot.

Evaluation of the great vessels, through the short axis, pulmonary artery/ductus, and aortic arch views, is important to ensure that the ventriculoarterial connections are correctly aligned. Determining which is the aorta and which the pulmonary artery can be difficult in utero, as the ductus arteriosus is quite large, and in continuity with the descending aorta. The complete scan must include demonstration of a bifurcating vessel leaving the anterior ventricle and entering the descending aorta (pulmonary artery), as well as the brachiocephalic, left carotid, and left subclavian arteries branching from the aortic arch.

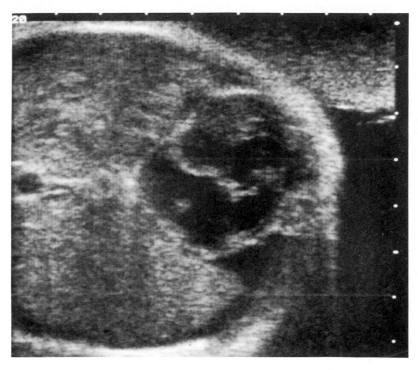

FIG. 4.2.   Abnormal four-chamber view of fetal heart with complete atrioventricular septal defect. The heart is oriented in the same fashion as the heart in Figure 4.1. Note the marked difference between the two cases. Here, a marked deficiency in interventricular septum, a large low-lying interatrial defect, and a single large atrioventricular valve (rather than two discrete valves) are seen.

In each view, it must be kept in mind that right and left ventricular outputs are not equal in utero (the right ventricular output appears to be slightly greater than the left).[12,13] As a result, the right ventricular dimension should be greater in size in utero than postnatally. A similar relationship holds for pulmonary versus aortic root size. Any major asymmetry suggests the presence of pathology.

CARDIAC RHYTHM

Throughout the anatomic examination, the sonologist should pay attention to the cardiac rate and rhythm. We have seen 554 fetuses for evaluation of the cardiac rhythm over 9 years. The distribution of diagnoses is shown in Table 4.2.

The normal fetal heart rate is 120 to 170, and regular. While sinus bradycardia may cause the fetal heart rate to be 100 to 120, if the rate is below 90, or above 180, careful evaluation of the rhythm is warranted. Often in fetuses with bradycardias, coexistent anatomic abnormalities are present.[14] If either

TABLE 4.2. Fetal arrhythmias (7/1/78–6/30/87)[a]

Abnormality	No. (percent)
Total fetuses referred	554
Dysryhythmia seen	446 (81)
Isolated extrasystoles	385 (69)
Supraventricular	336 (87)
Junctional/ventricular	37 (10)
Multiple sites	12 (3)
Developed SVT	4 (1)
Structural heart disease	7 (1.8)
Supraventricular tachycardia	32 (5.8)
Atrial flutter	6 (1)
Atrial fibrillation	2 (0.4)
Ventricular Tachycardia	3 (0.5)
Complete heart block	11 (2)
Structural abnormalities	5 (45)
Normal structure	6 (55)
Anti-Ro, + ANA	5[b]
Second-degree heart block	2 (0.4)
Sinus rhythm	114
Bradycardia	4
Tachycardia	2
Normal sinus rhythm	108 (19)

[a] One patient had atrial flutter and complete heart block and appears in both groups.
[b] ANA = antinuclear antibody. One patient diagnosed prior to anti-Ro assay availability at our institution.

second- or third-degree heart block is suspected based on M-mode or pulsed Doppler study, cardiac structures should be examined, and an assay for maternal connective-tissue autoantibodies, such as anti-Ro, is useful, as these markers for systemic lupus erythematosus are often present.[15–19] We have found structural heart disease in 5 of 11 fetuses with complete heart block (45 percent) and anti-Ro or antinuclear antibodies (ANA) in 5 of the remaining 6 seen in our institution over 9 years (in Table 4.2, the only patient with a normal heart and complete heart block was seen prior to the availability of anti-Ro testing at our institution).

The most common arrhythmia seen in our laboratory has been premature atrial extrasystoles,[20] found in 69 percent of fetuses referred for arrhythmias, and possibly having been present earlier in many of the patients referred for arrhythmias who were found to have normal sinus rhythm at evaluation (19 percent of total). These may be identified with either M-mode or pulsed

Doppler visualization of the premature atrial beat, which may or may not be conducted. While these are for the most part benign, they may precipitate supraventricular tachycardia in susceptible fetuses. While our experience has been that this occurred in 4 of 385 (1.04 percent), we are unable to determine a true denominator of fetuses at risk or to say that we know what rhythms were present in the fetuses presenting with supraventricular tachycardia prior to their referral.

When premature extrasystoles are found, we recommend weekly auscultation of the fetal heart to rule out runs of tachycardia, until they resolve. Isolated extrasystoles almost always resolve spontaneously before or just after birth (only 3 percent of fetuses had persistence to 5 days of age in our experience), so no treatment is recommended. Avoidance of possible cardiac stimulants, such as caffeine, sympathomimetics (including over-the-counter nasal decongestants as well as β-adrenergic tocolytics), and illicit drugs such as cocaine should be recommended, as these may worsen the dysrhythmia.

When supraventricular tachycardia is detected, appropriate management depends on the etiology and the gestational age. If fetal lung maturity is present as determined by well-established dates or amniocentesis, delivery may be prudent. For the preterm fetus, determination of the type of tachycardia is important in choosing the therapy. Fetal paroxysmal atrial tachycardia has responded well to digitalis as a first line of therapy in our experience. In those unresponsive to digitalis alone, we have added verapamil or propranolol. Digitalis and quinidine may be a good second line as well, since it would be appropriate treatment for atrial flutter, if that is the underlying disturbance in a resistant case. For this reason, we have recently favored digitalis and quinidine in this role. Fetal atrial flutter and fibrillation have been more difficult to control.[21] Treatment should be undertaken inhospital, at a center with experience in the management of these patients.

Pulsed Doppler ultrasound has proved helpful in evaluating fetal arrhythmias. The sample volume can be placed below the atrioventricular valves to examine diastolic flow into the ventricles. In contrast to the postnatal pattern of predominant passive flow, in the fetus most flow into the ventricles depends on atrial systole. This greater volume and greater velocity result in the a wave being higher than the e wave of atrial flow. In premature atrial extrasystoles, the early a wave can be identified.[22] Similar studies can be carried out in the fetus suspected of having supraventricular tachycardia.[23]

INDICATIONS FOR FETAL ECHOCARDIOGRAPHY

Fetal echocardiography is much more complex a procedure than is routine obstetric sonography. Although most congenital heart disease (CHD) occurs in children without identifiable risk factors, certain situations can be targeted as placing fetuses at particular risk of CHD. Our current list of indications for fetal echocardiography is shown in Table 4.3. We group these risk factors according to etiology: fetal, maternal, or familial.

TABLE 4.3. Proposed indications for fetal echocardiography

Fetal risk factors
  Extracardiac anomalies
    Chromosomal
    Anatomic
  Fetal cardiac arrhythmia
    Irregular rhythm
    Tachycardia (>200 BPM)
    Bradycardia (nonperiodic)
  Nonimmune hydrops fetalis
  Suspected cardiac anomaly on level I scan

Maternal risk factors
  Congenital heart disease
  Cardiac teratogen exposure
  Maternal metabolic disorders
    Diabetes mellitus
    Phenylketonuria
  Polyhydramnios
  Maternal infections
    Rubella
    Toxoplasmosis
    Coxsackie virus
    Cytomegalovirus
    Mumps

Familial risk factors
  Congenital heart disease
    Previous sibling
    Paternal
  Syndromes
    Noonan
    Tuberous sclerosis

The risk of CHD is increased significantly if a couple have had a previous child with CHD or if the mother herself has CHD. The general population risk for CHD is approximately 0.8 percent. If there has been a previous child with CHD, the risk rises to about 2 to 3 percent; if the mother herself has CHD, to about 5 to 10 percent.[24] If polygenic inheritance is assumed, the risk may be elevated slightly over that of the general population when the CHD has occurred in more distantly related individuals (e.g., the offspring of a patient's siblings), although the precise degree of incremental risk is unknown.

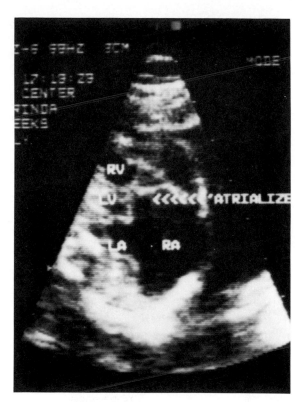

FIG. 4.3. Abnormal four-chamber anatomy in a fetus with the Ebstein malformation of the tricuspid valve. The tricuspid valve is displaced into the right ventricular cavity, resulting in a large area of "atrialized" right ventricle; the right heart chambers dwarf those of the left heart. The most striking abnormality is the remarkable dilation of the right atrium. Doppler color flow mapping and pulsed Doppler study demonstrated the presence of severe tricuspid regurgitation.

Maternal teratogen exposure constitutes an area of great concern to pregnant women.[25] Lithium carbonate has been associated with Ebstein anomaly of the tricuspid valve (Fig. 4.3). Synthetic progestins have also been implicated in some studies as potential teratogens, although this association is far from clear.[26] We recommend fetal echocardiography for any patient who has taken any of the drugs listed in Table 4.4, although to alleviate patient anxiety, women who have taken other medications are often scanned as well.

TABLE 4.4. Drugs suspected of cardiac teratogenicity

Lithium carbonate
Alcohol
Phenytoin
Valproic acid
Trimethadione
Isotretinoin
Amphetamines
Thalidomide
Sex steroids (synthetic progestins)

Insulin-dependent diabetic women (white class B and above) have a four-fold higher incidence of CHD in their offspring than that of nondiabetics.[27] There are two distinct fetal cardiac effects of maternal hyperglycemia: first-trimester exposure predisposing to structural CHD, and later exposure causing hypertrophic cardiomyopathy. All women with class B or greater diabetes are therefore offered fetal echocardiography at the same time as a general anatomic survey for other anomalies, approximately 20 to 22 weeks of gestation. Class A diabetics are not screened at the earlier time because they are not in danger of first-trimester hyperglycemia and should not be at higher risk of anomalies. Certainly, any patient diagnosed as having diabetes in the second trimester should be considered at risk of diabetic embryopathy, as she is likely to have had occult diabetes predating the pregnancy. We perform an additional scan between 30 and 32 weeks gestation to confirm the normal anatomy (Fig. 4.4), and detect hypertrophic cardiomyopathy.

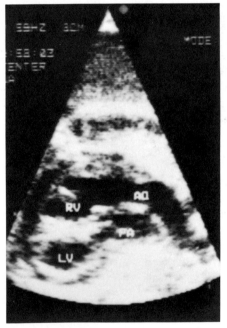 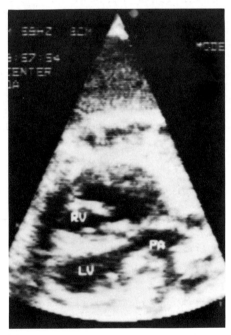

A B

FIG. 4.4. (A) Long-axis view of the right ventricular outflow tract of a 31-week fetus of a diabetic pregnancy. Despite the presence of normal four-chamber anatomy, this fetus was found to have a major anomaly that could only be detected by detailed evaluation of great artery anatomy. The anterior right ventricle gives rise to a transposed aorta (great arterial branches from the aortic arch are identified). (B) Long-axis view of the left ventricular outflow tract of the same fetus, demonstrating the origin of the bifurcating transposed pulmonary artery from the posterior left ventricular cavity. (AO, transposed aorta; PA, transposed pulmonary artery; LV, left ventricle; RV, right ventricle.)

Class A diabetics who have been difficult to control or who develop macrosomia early in the third trimester should be considered for fetal echocardiography to assess myocardial thickness.

Women with phenylketonuria who were successfully treated with dietary restrictions in childhood are now entering their own childbearing years. These women have often relaxed their diets, resulting in relatively high phenylalanine levels, which can cause cardiac and other anomalies.[28,29] As in the case of diabetics, these patients should receive preconception counseling regarding the need for strict dietary control during the first trimester, and should undergo careful scanning in the second trimester to seek any anomalies that may be present.[30]

Most of these "historical" risk factors result in slightly higher risks of CHD than found in the general population. By contrast, we find that fetuses with either an extracardiac anomaly detected on ultrasound examination, or with a suspected cardiac anomaly at the time of a general scan, are at much greater risk of CHD. Any fetus found to have an anomaly strongly associated with CHD should have a careful examination of the heart (unless the anomaly is itself invariably fatal), as the presence of CHD may influence the neonatal management and timing of any needed surgical procedures. These anomalies have been recently reviewed[30] (Table 4.5). We offer fetal echocardiography to all patients with an extracardiac anomaly, even if the particular anomaly is from a low-risk group. We scan these patients because the known risks are derived from pediatric data, and some severe anomaly combinations may not survive long enough to appear in pediatric series.

TABLE 4.5.   Extracardiac anomalies frequently associated with congenital heart disease

Abnormalities of cardiac position
Hydrocephalus[a]
Microcephaly[a]
Agenesis of corpus callosum
Encephalocele (Meckel-Gruber syndrome)
Ectopia cordis
Esophageal atresia/Tracheoesophageal fistula
Duodenal atresia
Situs abnormality (asplenia/polysplenia)
Omphalocele
Diaphragmatic hernia
Bilateral renal agenesis[b]
Conjoined twins

[a] Heterogeneous etiology, some causes associated with congenital heart disease, others not.
[b] Uniformly fatal, regardless of presence or absence of congenital heart disease.

Nonimmune hydrops has been described as fetal congestive heart failure.[31] It has further been found that the combination of structural heart disease, atrioventricular valve insufficiency and nonimmune hydrops carries an extremely poor prognosis.[32] The true frequency with which structural heart disease and arrhythmias cause nonimmune hydrops will vary somewhat with the population surveyed. We have found that about one-third of fetuses with nonimmune hydrops seen at Yale-New Haven Hospital have a cardiac etiology, although other centers have reported varying figures.[33–38] In many cases, this will be difficult to assess, as some fetal arrhythmias may cause hydrops and fetal death, leaving no signs at autopsy.

We have found CHD in a high percentage of fetuses referred because the heart "looked funny" during a routine scan.[20] In a study of 74 fetuses with heart disease, we found that 92 percent had abnormalities of the four-chamber view, suggesting that it may be useful as a screen for CHD.[39] It was clear that in many cases the full nature of the structural abnormality could not be determined from the four-chamber view alone, but downstream problems often caused sufficient deviations from the normal appearance to prompt more detailed evaluation (e.g., a fetus with pulmonic stenosis and secondary right atrial dilation). Preliminary results of a study testing the value of the four-chamber view as a screen for congenital heart disease have been encouraging.[40] Although a screening sonogram to detect fetal anomalies is not yet an accepted routine for all prenatal patients in the United States, a high enough percentage of patients are scanned at least once in the course of pregnancy that careful examination of the four-chamber view might be expected to increase the rate of detection of fetal heart disease.

Review of pediatric studies suggests that chromosomal abnormalities are found in 5 to 10 percent of cases of CHD.[30] We have found that a much higher number of cases of fetal heart disease have chromosomal abnormalities. In a series of 34 fetal diagnoses of heart disease, 11 (32 percent) had chromosomal abnormalities.[41] This incidence is similar to the findings of Wladimiroff and co-workers[42] in a smaller series. This finding has led us to pursue karyotype determination in all cases of fetal heart disease, regardless of the presence of extracardiac anomalies. After completion of our study of karyotype abnormalities in fetal heart disease, the message was emphasized even more by a patient who took lithium in the first trimester and who presented with a fetus showing the classic appearance of Ebstein anomaly of the tricuspid valve. The distortion of the cardiac anatomy obscured the atrioventricular canal defect; it was also present in this fetus, which had the typical dysmorphic features of trisomy 18 at birth.

There is an obvious need to perform fetal echocardiography in the fetus with an extracardiac anomaly or in the abnormal-appearing heart. We also believe that the reverse is true, as well: any fetus at risk of CHD also may be considered to be at risk of extracardiac structural anomalies. We therefore perform full anatomic screens and growth measurements in all fetuses referred for echocardiography.

IMPACT

Despite the potential future value of screening for fetal heart disease with the four-chamber view as alluded to above, there will still be a need for detailed fetal echocardiography in selected patients. Those with specific risk factors for fetal heart disease will continue to require such studies, which should be performed at centers with extensive experience, because of the time and expertise required. Since the greatest number of abnormalities occur in the absence of clear risk factors, many cardiac anomalies will continue to be identified during obstetric scanning for other purposes. The total impact of these diagnoses is complex to measure.

Some anomalies will be incompatible with postnatal survival, for example, the fetus with severe congenital heart disease and nonimmune hydrops fetalis. If found early in gestation, the parents may choose to terminate the pregnancy. If it is not identified until beyond the period in which termination is an option, or if the parents are opposed to such a course, there are still important benefits to be gained from the information obtained.

Many fetal cardiac diagnoses are made later in pregnancy. This reflects referrals because of suspicious-appearing hearts during obstetric sonograms and identification of extracardiac anomalies with concurrent heart disease. In such cases, accurate prenatal diagnosis permits honest counseling for the parents, as well as adequate medical planning for delivery and neonatal care (e.g., ensuring that prostaglandin E1 is mixed and ready in the nursery for the delivery of a fetus with a ductus-dependent lesion). Delivery of such fetuses in an institution equipped to provide comprehensive neonatal and cardiac care can be expected to improve the outcome for many infants. While our survival statistics for the first 150 fetuses with CHD diagnosed at Yale were not, by themselves, impressive (28 of 150 survivors, 19 percent), it is striking to note that 21 of the survivors had ductus-dependent lesions (75 percent). For this group, delivery at an institution with comprehensive neonatal cardiac care capabilities would be expected to improve outcome, as opposed to delivery at a community hospital with emergent transfer of the newborn.

Recently, the options for neonates with lesions previously considered inoperable have been widened. Both neonatal cardiac transplantation and the Norwood procedure have been offered for neonates with hypoplastic left heart syndrome. The complexities of supporting such critically ill newborns until transport is arranged to one of the few centers offering these procedures make transport difficult, so delivery would be best accomplished at an institution capable of providing comprehensive maternal and neonatal care. We also consider it important to allow the parents to consider their options. Informed consent for surgery is difficult in the best of circumstances, but with an unstable neonate at issue, it may be an impossibility. Education of the parents at one or more prenatal visits is essential for their active participation in deciding on expectant management versus transplant or the Norwood procedure for their infants.

We offer all parents of children with fetal heart disease information about the risks of chromosomal abnormalities and the option of karyotyping. If there is sufficient time prior to term, amniocentesis may be appropriate. In other situations, fetal blood sampling or placentocentesis (transabdominal chorionic villous biopsy) offers the possibility of karyotype results in just a few days. Waiting for delivery to assess facial morphology and other external factors or to obtain blood cells to karyotype may be fruitless, as many such infants will be stillborn, and important information regarding the likelihood of recurrence may be lost.

FUTURE DIRECTIONS

We can use fetal echocardiography to diagnose structural heart disease with a high degree of accuracy. We can also evaluate cardiac function, at least in terms of rhythm disturbances. Evaluation of cardiac pump performance remains as an important area of investigation. Preliminary studies have attempted to define such parameters as fractional shortening and ratios of ventricular dimensions.[11] Others have considered ventricular function through estimations of cardiac output based on planimetry measurements,[43,44] although such studies are confounded by two factors: (1) the parallel, rather than series, arrangement of ventricular function in utero; and (2) the difficulty in defining the geometric shape of the fetal ventricles needed for estimations of volume, based on two-dimensional images.

Another technique of great potential value is pulsed Doppler ultrasound, which permits sampling of a flow-velocity waveform from selected portions of the cardiovascular system. Mathematic manipulation of the waveform shape, including correction for factors such as the incident angle to the direction of blood flow and vessel diameter, permits estimation of blood velocity and volume flow. In order to reduce the random errors that may be introduced at each step in these calculations, various methods of relating velocities during different phases of the cardiac cycle have been proposed for study of flow in the umbilical cord and fetal descending aorta.[45] Similar angle-independent indices of flow during various parts of the cardiac cycle may prove useful in evaluating intracardiac blood flow (e.g., the relative peak velocities of passive and active ventricular filling, the e:a ratio).

Doppler echocardiography has already proved useful in the investigation of fetal arrhythmias and in detecting valvular regurgitation.[32,46] In the future, we may be able to measure the cardiac output of the fetus with Doppler,[13,47] although the technical difficulty of doing so and the large errors that may be randomly introduced continue to limit this technique to the research setting. It remains one of the most exciting areas of fetal research.

CONCLUSIONS

Prenatal diagnosis of structural heart disease is widely available. By identifying patients at risk, the frequency of unanticipated CHD can be diminished. Further improvement in the rate of identification may be possible through routine screening of the four-chamber view of the heart.[39,40] Any pregnancy with significant risk factors for fetal heart disease should be thoroughly evaluated with detailed fetal echocardiography rather than merely a screening four-chamber view, however (see Table 4.3). Particular attention should be paid to performing fetal echocardiography in pregnancies found to have other structural anomalies, as coexistent heart disease may suggest the presence of a syndrome with specific inheritance patterns and may alter neonatal management plans. Similarly, any fetus with structural heart disease should undergo a thorough examination of all systems. If fetal heart disease is found, parental counseling should include the strong possibility of chromosomal abnormalities and appropriate sampling for karyotype should be offered. Complete counseling, in our experience, is most easily accomplished with a team approach composed primarily of obstetricians and pediatric cardiologists. We further rely on frequent assistance from geneticists and on pediatric nursing specialists to provide information to the parents regarding realistic expectations about the care their infants will require.

ACKNOWLEDGMENTS

Dr. Copel is Kennedy-Dannreuther Fellow of the American Association of Obstetricians and Gynecologists Foundation. Dr. Kleinman is the recipient of Clinical Research Grant No. 6–225 from the March of Dimes Birth Defects Foundation, Mamaroneck, New York.

REFERENCES

1. Winsberg F: Echocardiography of the fetal and newborn heart. Invest Radiol 7:152, 1972
2. Kleinman CS, Hobbins JC, Jaffe CC, et al: Echocardiographic studies of the human fetus: Prenatal diagnosis of congenital heart disease and cardiac dysrhythmias. Pediatrics 65:1059, 1980
3. Allan LD, Tynan MJ, Campbell S, et al: Echocardiographic and anatomical correlates in the fetus. Br Heart J 44:444, 1980
4. Lange LW, Sahn DJ, Allen HD, et al: Qualitative real-time cross-sectional echocardiographic imaging of the human fetus in the second half of pregnancy. Circulation 62:799, 1980
5. Allan LD, Tynan M, Campbell S, Anderson RH: Identification of congenital cardiac malformations by echocardiography in the midtrimester fetus. Br Heart J 46:358, 1981
6. Wladimiroff JW, Stewart PA, Tonge HM: The role of diagnostic ultrasound in the study of fetal cardiac abnormalities. Ultrasound Med Biol 10:457, 1984
7. Allan LD, Crawford DC, Anderson RH, Tynan MJ: Echocardiographic and anatomical correlations in congenital heart disease. Br Heart J 52:542, 1984
8. Huhta JC, Hagler DJ, Hill LM: Two-dimensional echocardiographic assessment of normal fetal cardiac anatomy. J Reprod Med 29:162, 1984
9. Silverman NH, Golbus MS: Echocardiographic techniques for assessing normal and abnormal fetal cardiac anatomy. J Am Coll Cardiol 5:20S, 1985
10. Rudolph AM: Congenital Diseases of the Heart. Yearbook, Chicago, 1974
11. DeVore GR: The prenatal diagnosis of congenital heart disease: A practical approach for the fetal sonographer. J Clin Ultrasound 13:229, 1985

12. Rudolph AM, Heymann MA: Circulatory changes during growth in the fetal lamb. Circ Res 26:289, 1970

13. Reed KL, Meijboom EJ, Sahn DJ, et al.: Cardiac Doppler flow velocities in the human fetus. Circulation 73:41, 1986

14. Crawford D, Chapman M, Allan L: The assessment of persistent bradycardia in prenatal life. Br J Obstet Gynecol 92:941, 1985

15. Chameides L, Truex RC, Vetter V, et al: Association of maternal systemic lupus erythematosus with congenital complete heart block. N Engl J Med 297:1204, 1977

16. Esscher E, Scott JS: Congenital heart block and maternal systemic lupus erythematosus. Br Med J 1:1235, 1979

17. Scott JS, Maddison PJ, Taylor PV, et al: Connective-tissue disease, antibodies to ribonucleoprotein, and congenital heart block. N Engl J Med 309:209, 1983

18. Litsey SE, Noonan JA, O'Connor WN, et al: Maternal connective tissue disease and congenital heart block. N Engl J Med 312:98, 1985

19. Taylor PV, Scott JS, Gerlis LM, et al.: Maternal antibodies against fetal cardiac antigens in congenital complete heart block. N Engl J Med 315:667, 1986

20. Copel JA, Kleinman CS: The impact of fetal echocardiography on perinatal outcome. Ultrasound Med Biol 12:327, 1986

21. Kleinman CS, Copel JA, Weinstein EM, et al: In utero diagnosis and treatment of fetal supraventricular tachycardia. Semin Perinatol 9:113, 1985

22. Kleinman CS, Weinstein EM, Copel JA: Pulsed Doppler analysis of human fetal blood flow. Clin Diagn Ultrasound 17:173, 1986

23. Huhta JC, Strasburger JF, Carpenter RJ, et al: Pulsed Doppler fetal echocardiography. J Clin Ultrasound 13:247, 1985

24. Nora JJ, Nora AH: The genetic contribution to congenital heart diseases. In Nora JJ, Takao A (eds): Congenital Heart Diseases: Causes and Processes. Futura, Mount Kisco, NY, 1984

25. Zierler, S: Maternal drugs and congenital heart disease. Obstet Gynecol 65:155, 1985

26. Wilson JG, Brent RL: Are female sex hormones teratogenic? Am J Obstet Gynecol 141:567, 1981

27. Rowland TW, Hubbell JP, Nadas AS: Congenital heart disease in infants of diabetic mothers. J Pediatr 83:815, 1973

28. Levy HL, Waisbren SE: Effects of untreated maternal phenylketonuria and hyperphenylalaninemia on the fetus. N Engl J Med 309:1269, 1983

29. Lenke RL, Levy HL: Maternal phenylketonuria and hyperphenylalaninemia. N Engl J Med 303:1202, 1980

30. Copel JA, Pilu G, Kleinman CS: Congenital heart disease and extracardiac anomalies: Associations and indications for fetal echocardiography. Am J Obstet Gynecol 154:1121, 1985

31. Kleinman CS, Donnerstein RL, DeVore GR, et al: Fetal echocardiography for evaluation of in utero congestive heart failure: A technique for the study of non-immune hydrops fetalis. N Engl J Med 306:568, 1982

32. Silverman NH, Kleinman CS, Rudolph AM, et al: Fetal atrioventricular valve insufficiency associated with nonimmune hydrops: A two-dimensional echocardiographic and pulsed Doppler study. Circulation 72:825, 1985

33. Beischer NA, Fortune DW, Macafee J: Nonimmunologic hydrops fetalis and congenital abnormalities. Obstet Gynecol 38:86, 1971

34. Hutchison AA, Drew JH, Yu VYH, et al: Nonimmunologic hydrops fetalis: A review of 61 cases. Obstet Gynecol 59:347, 1982

35. Holzgreve W, Curry CJR, Golbus MS, et al: Investigation of nonimmune hydrops fetalis. Am J Obstet Gynecol 150:805, 1984

36. Romero R, Copel JA, Jeanty PJ, Hobbins JC: Causes, diagnosis and management of non-immune hydrops fetalis. Clin Perinatol 19:31, 1986

37. Allan LD, Chapman DC, Sheridan R, Chapman MG: Aetiology of non-immune hydrops: The value of echocardiography. Br J Obstet Gynecol 93:223, 1986

38. Gough JD, Keeling JW, Castle B, Iliff PJ: The obstetric management of non-immunological hydrops. Br J Obstet Gynecol 93:226, 1986

39. Copel JA, Pilu G, Green J, et al: Fetal echocardiographic screening for congenital heart disease: The importance of the four-chamber view. Am J Obstet Gynecol 157:648, 1987

40. Fermont L, deGeeter B, Aubry MC, et al: A close collaboration between obstetricians and pediatric cardiologists allows antenatal detection of severe cardiac malformations by two-dimensional echocardiography. p. 34. In Doyle EF, Engle MA, Gersony WM, et al (eds): Pediatric Cardiology: Proceedings of the Second World Congress. Springer-Verlag, New York, 1986

41. Copel JA, Cullen M, Green J, et al: The frequency of aneuploidy in prenatally diagnosed congenital heart disease: An indication for fetal karotyping. Am J Obstet Gynecol 158:409, 1988

42. Wladimiroff JW, Stewart PA, Sachs ES, Niermeijer MF: Prenatal diagnosis and management of congenital heart defect: Significance of associated fetal anomalies and prenatal chromosome studies. Am J Med Genet 21:285, 1985

43. Sahn DJ, Lange LW, Allen HD, et al: Quantitative real-time cross-sectional echocardiography in the developing normal human fetus and newborn. Circulation 62:588, 1980

44. Wladimiroff JW, Vosters R, McGhie JS: Normal cardiac ventricular geometry and function during the last timester of pregnancy and early neonatal period. Br J Obstet Gynecol 89:839, 1982

45. Griffin D, Cohen-Overbeek T, Campbell S: Fetal and utero-placental blood flow. Clin Obstet Gynecol 10:565, 1983

46. Maulik D, Nanda NC, Moodley S, et al: Application of Doppler echocardiography in the assessment of fetal cardiac disease. Am J Obstet Gynecol 151:951, 1985

47. Kenny JF, Plappert T, Doubilet P, et al: Changes in intracardiac blood flow velocities and right and left ventricular stroke volumes with gestational age in the normal human fetus: A prospective Doppler echocardiographic study. Circulation 74:1208, 1986

5 Fetal Anatomy in Ultrasonography

PHILIPPE JEANTY
TERRI L. DANIEL

To many, anatomy is a subject that brings back nightmares of medical school. Anatomy is one of the most difficult subjects to learn, since it does not lend itself to simplification by reasoning and can only be learned by memorization. This bias probably still affects a large number of those involved in performing obstetric ultrasound examinations, and it is likely that few readers will have rushed to this chapter after glancing at the table of contents in this volume.

Yet there are many reasons to master anatomy for fetal ultrasonography. To be able to identify the correct planes of scanning used to be one of the major reasons. However, with the improvement in the level of competence of those performing obstetric ultrasound examinations, this stage is probably acquired. Although not critical in most circumstances, better knowledge of anatomy avoids embarrassing mislabeling of structures (for example, the cavum of the septum pellucidum has been confused with the third ventricle, and the insula with the sylvian fissure).

Another reason that has progressively surfaced is to be able to distinguish normal from pathologic structures. Despite the fact that not everyone is willing to diagnose congenital malformations, one would prefer to avoid the embarrassment of referring a patient for a level II (or III?) examination to verify a finding that turns out to be a perfectly normal structure. It has been reported, for instance, that fetal ears had been confused with encephalocele. A case was referred to us in which a refraction artifact at the level of the rectus abdominis muscle of a young and fit woman produced a pseudo-encephalocele. In another case, prominent occipital horns particularly well seen through the posterior fontanel were thought to represent choroid plexus cysts. Finally, Dr. Callen demonstrated that what was previously thought to represent some artifactual ascites was the image of abdominal muscles of the fetus.

More recently, an unexpected reason for the interest in fetal anatomy has surfaced from an unanticipated front. A few years ago, a new company brought to the market a machine with what they considered vastly improved resolution compared to what other manufacturers were producing. To differentiate their equipment from the others, they qualified it as computed sonography, implying that their equipment used a computer and others did not. In fact, every ultrasound machine contains a fairly powerful computer. They also sold their equipment for a price considerably higher than the current price of other equipment, playing on the buyer's Bentley syndrome (i.e., if it is expensive and the "big guys" have one, I need one too). Ever since, ultrasonographers in major centers have been deluged with questions about the quality of this equipment and whether it is worth the difference in price. Differentiating between machines, to determine which is the most appropriate for one's needs, is a difficult and time-consuming task that exceeds the resources of most physicians in private practice. Therefore, they seek the advice of dedicated sonographers who use many kinds of machines and who might be better placed to judge the merit of various equipment.

Although machine performance can be to some extent judged from technical specifications, laboratory tests, phantom imaging, and so forth, the most useful test, in our opinion, is the resolution of the machine in real-life situations. Furthermore, one would like to be able to have some consistency in the results; not only should the machine perform well with thin patients, but its resolution should not drop dramatically with "normal-sized" patients.

Among all the subjects that can be imaged by ultrasonography, the fetus is by far the most challenging. Numerous tiny structures can serve to verify whether the equipment has the ability to image small structures or structures that differ only slightly in echogenicity. When dealing with such fine anatomic detail, a better understanding of the anatomy becomes necessary; hence the renewed interest in fetal anatomy.

Last but not least, there is an almost philosophic reason for a better understanding of fetal anatomy: the examinations are so much more interesting to perform when one knows what one is looking at. It can almost be compared with the fun of driving in good weather compared to driving in fog.

The following discussion includes a brief survey of interesting anatomic details. No efforts are made to be comprehensive: the literature contains numerous references that demonstrate the basic landmark of anatomy, and it is assumed that the reader is familiar with them.

Also, so that the reader can decide whether the resolution of "computed sonography" is necessary, we have elected to use images provided by low- or medium-cost machines and even some very old and discontinued machines (early 1980). We hope that it will be clear that some of these machines provide outstanding resolution and that as a general rule the limiting factor in the detection of anomalies does not lie in the equipment but in the user's knowledge of the anatomy and sensitivity to what is normal and what is not.

ANATOMY

Early Gestation

The most important advance in the high-resolution evaluation of the early fetuses is the more widespread use and improved resolution of transvaginal transducers. Fetal structures are easier to recognize, especially in obese patients (Fig. 5.1).

Face

Eyes

The different components of the eye that can be observed with ultrasonography are the globe (including the vitreous body), the lens, and the anterior chamber. In early gestation, a structure probably corresponding to the inter-

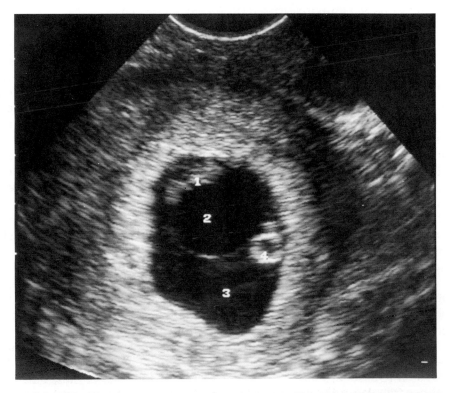

FIG. 5.1.   A 7-week-old fetus (1). The amniotic cavity (2) is separated from the extra-embryonic coelom (3) by the amnion. The localization of the secondary yolk sac (4) in the extraembryonic coelom is well demonstrated. The fetal heart is the hypoechoic structure on the left of the 1 marker.

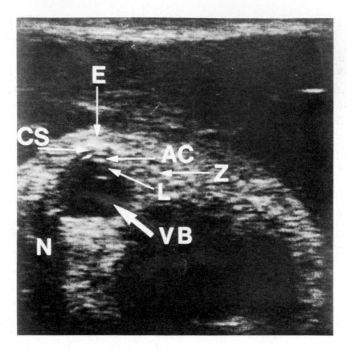

FIG. 5.2.   The different components of the eye that can be observed with ultrasound are the globe, including the vitreous body (VB), lens (L), anterior chamber (AC), cornea (tiny unlabeled arrow), eyelid (E), and, in early gestation, what probably corresponds to the interface of the conjunctival sac (CS). (Z, zygomatic bone; N, nasal cavity.) (From Jeanty P, Romero R, Hobbins JC: Fetal facial anatomy. J Ultrasound Med 5:607, 1986, with permission.)

face of the conjunctival sac can also be seen (Fig. 5.2). In the retro-orbital region, one can recognize the external (Fig. 5.3) and internal rectus muscles, as well as the superior oblique. The optic nerve (Fig. 5.3) and the ophthalmic artery (Fig. 5.4) are also discernible.

An equatorial section obtained in a fetus facing toward the transducer best demonstrates these structures. The vitreous body, lens, and anterior chamber can be seen in most circumstances. The conjunctival sac is formed by closure of the eyelids in front of the globe around the eighth week of menstrual age. It reopens around the seventh month. The lateral (or external) rectus muscle is seen as a thin hypoechogenic line, close to the orbital surface of the zygomatic bone (Fig. 5.3). The latter appears brightly echogenic (due to the acoustic enhancement behind the vitreous body), with distal shadowing. The internal (or medial) rectus muscle can be seen along the orbital plate of the ethmoid bone.

When the plane of section is slightly asynclinal, some of the other extraocular muscles can be imaged. The easiest to demonstrate is the superior oblique muscle, which is slightly more medial and superior to the medial rectus muscle. When the section is obtained high in the orbit, the complex of the superior rectus muscle and the levator palpebrae superioris are seen. Identifi-

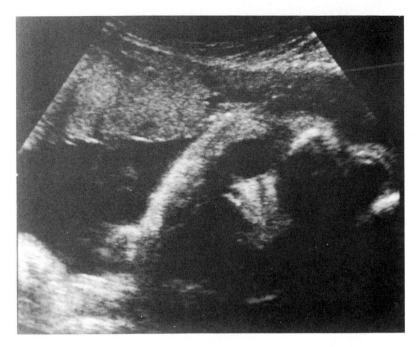

FIG. 5.3. The lateral (or external) rectus muscle is seen as a thin hypoechoic line close to the orbital surface of the zygomatic bone. The optic nerve has "fuzzy edges" and is perpendicular to the back of the orbit wall.

cation of the extraocular muscle is greatly facilitated by fetal eye movements. the pulling action of the muscles is then clearly differentiated from the passive tail-waving movement of the optic nerve.

The optic nerve is easily recognized in the equatorial section (Fig. 5.3) as a hypoechogenic structure exiting the globe opposite to the lens. Its contours are more fuzzy than those of the muscles, and its medial course in the conus region helps distinguish it from muscle. The pulsation of the ophthalmic artery can also be recognized (Fig. 5.4). The ophthalmic artery has a "train-track" appearance (two bright echoes surrounding a lucency), instead of the homogeneous gray of the optic nerve and rectus muscles.

Ear

The helix, scaphoid fossa, triangular fossa, concha, anthelix, tragus, antitragus, intertragic incisure, and lobule can be seen (Fig. 5.5). The internal auditory canal, as well as the middle and inner ear, are concealed in the petrous bone and its acoustic shadow.

Nose and Lips

The tip of the nose, the alae nasi, and the columna are seen above the upper lip (Fig. 5.6). The observation of the fetal nose would be of little clinical interest if it were not for the diagnosis of cleft lip. In cleft lip, the

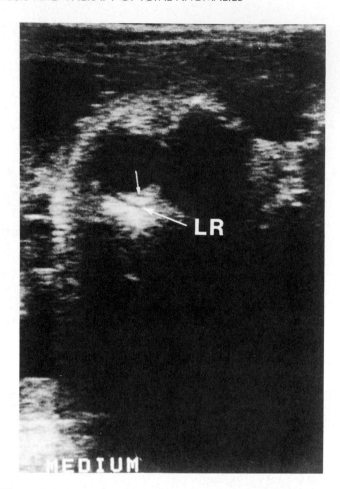

FIG. 5.4. The ophthalmic artery (small arrow) is recognized by its pulsations and its "train-track" appearance (two bright echos surrounding a lucency), which contrast to the homogeneous gray of the optic nerve and rectus muscles. (LR, = lateral rectus muscle.) (From Jeanty P, Romero R, Hobbins JC: Vascular anatomy of the fetus. J Ultrasound Med 3:113, 1984, with permission.)

nonunion of the maxillary process with the frontonasal process leaves a groove that extends from the nostril to the mouth (Fig. 5.7). Since cleft lip is a frequent malformation, and since the section demonstrating the nose and upper lip is easy to obtain, some degree of familiarity with the normal anatomy of the region is worthwhile.

Cheeks

In a transverse section of the cheek, one can recognize from medial to lateral, the tongue, buccinator muscle, and Bichat's fat pad (the corpus adiposum buccae) (Fig. 5.8). More posteriorly, the ascending branch of the mandible is seen medial and anterior to the masseter muscle.

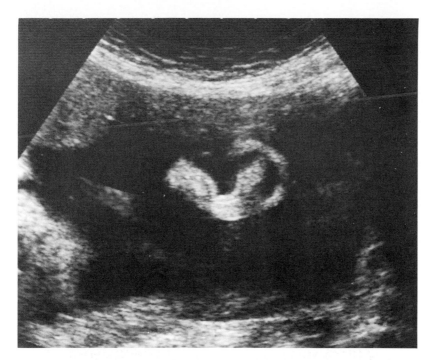

FIG. 5.5.   The pinna. The helix, scaphoid fossa, triangular fossa, anthelix, antitragus, Darwinian tubercle, and lobule can be seen.

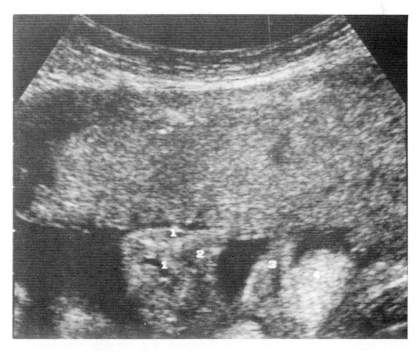

FIG. 5.6.   The tip of the nose, the alae nasi, the nostrils (1), and the columna are seen above the upper lip (2). 3, lower lip.

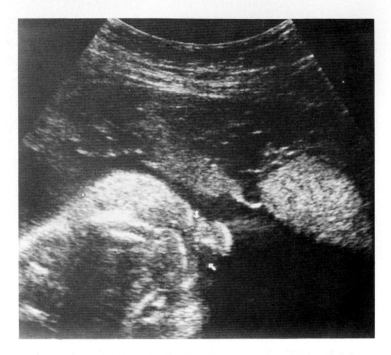

FIG. 5.7. In this case of bilateral cleft lip, the nonunion of the frontonasal process with the maxillary process is responsible for a groove on either side of the deformed columna (arrows).

Teeth

The tooth buds are enclosed in the dental sacs, which are rounded hypoechogenic areas (Fig. 5.9). The low echogenicity is probably due to the loose mesenchyme of the stellate reticulum surrounding the dental papilla. The bright echo that surrounds the tooth buds probably corresponds to the interface between the stellate reticulum and the gum, plus the adjacent interfaces produced by the gingival and glossal sulci. Tooth buds for the incisor, the canine, and the premolar are usually recognized. They begin calcifying between the fourth and fifth months. In a fetus with a cleft lip, failure to recognize the upper row of tooth buds is suggestive of a concomitant cleft palate. More posteriorly, the jugular vein and the carotid artery are seen anterior and lateral to the cartilaginous portion of the vertebral body.

Tongue, Epiglottis, and Larynx

The tongue can be seen both when moving and when at rest. The median sulcus is occasionally visible. At the root of the tongue, the epiglottis and the vestibulum of the larynx are seen (Fig. 5.8). The epiglottis is visible both in transverse scans of the base of the head and in coronal sections of the neck. The vestibulum of the larynx should not be confused with the

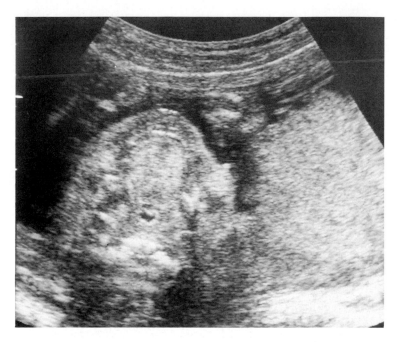

FIG. 5.8. In a transverse section of the cheek, one can recognize from medial to lateral, the tongue, buccinator muscle, and Bichat's fat pad (the corpus adiposum buccae). At the root of the tongue, the epiglottis and the vestibulum of the larynx are seen.

foramen magnum, which is more posterior. In a coronal section of the neck, the vocal cords are seen slightly below the larynx in the trachea.

Neck

The common carotids are roughly parallel and slightly posterior to the trachea in the neck. The jugular vein can be seen lateral to the carotid artery. The carotids have sharply defined walls, and their pulsation can be recorded. The jugular veins are closer to the skin than the carotid and are larger. The trachea is recognizable by its larger diameter. The vertebral arteries can be demonstrated along the cervical spine. They can be distinguished from the carotids by their more posterior course (Fig. 5.10). The course of the vertebral artery in the vertebral canal can be seen (Fig. 5.11), since the canal is only cartilaginous.

Chest

Heart

The cardiac anatomy has been exhaustively described (Fig. 5.12); the present discussion is limited to a few details pertinent to the demonstration of what high-quality equipment can demonstrate.

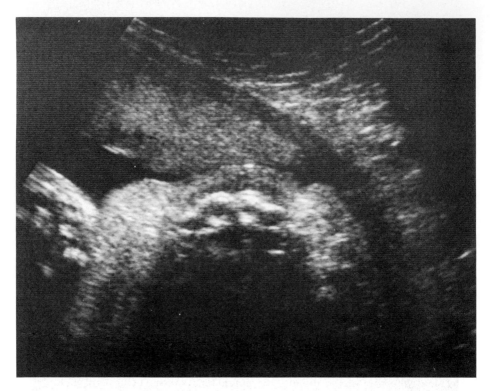

FIG. 5.9.   The tooth buds are enclosed in the dental sacs, seen as a rounded hypo-echogenic area. Tooth buds for the incisor, the canine, and the premolar are usually recognized.

The coronary arteries are sometimes visible by identifying the coronary ostium at the root of the aorta. In a basal section through the aortic cusps (Fig. 5.13), the two atria will appear posterior, and a small portion of the two ventricles will be seen anteriorly. The right coronary artery arises in front of the anterior semilunar valve (Fig. 5.13). The left coronary arises in front of the left posterior semilunar valve. The coronary arteries appear as well-delineated vessels. The ductus arteriosus (Fig. 5.14A) can be recognized from the aortic arch (Fig. 5.14B) by its much more abrupt bend and by the fact that the major cervical vessels do not originate from it. The superior vena cava is visible as it enters the right atrium (Fig. 5.15C).

Lungs

Bronchi and pulmonary vessels can be traced in the lung parenchyma. The pulmonary veins are easy to recognize since they terminate in the left atrium.

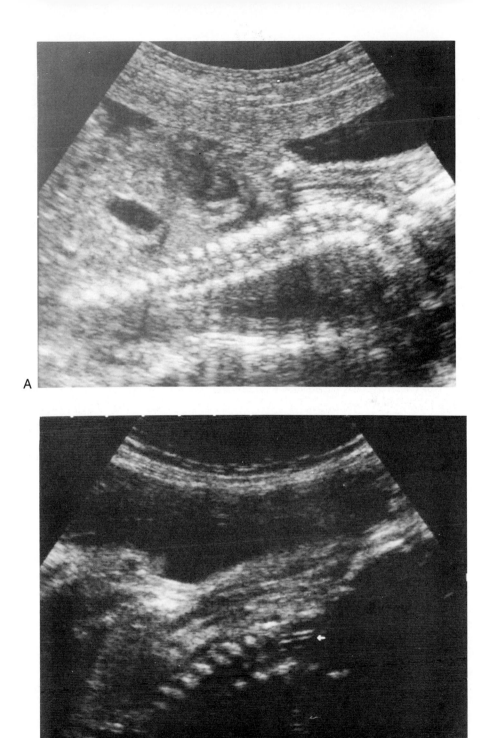

FIG. 5.10. Sagittal sections demonstrating the carotid artery (A), and the carotid artery with the vertebral artery dipping more posteriorly (B).

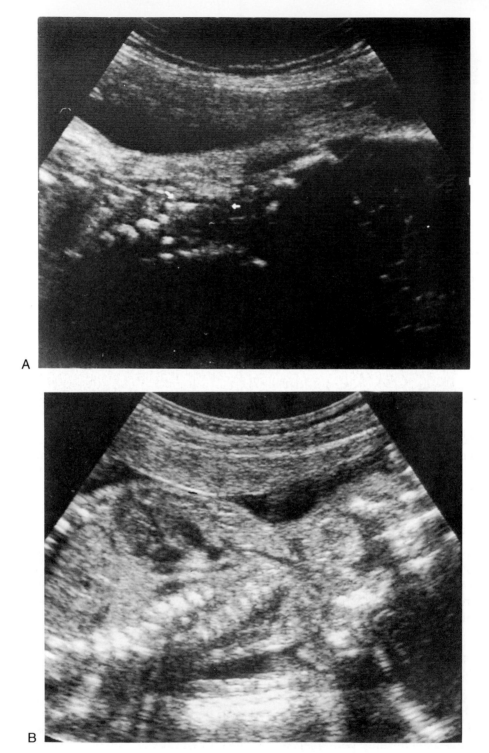

FIG. 5.11. The vertebral artery (arrows) is seen first outside of the vertebra canal (A), then inside (B).

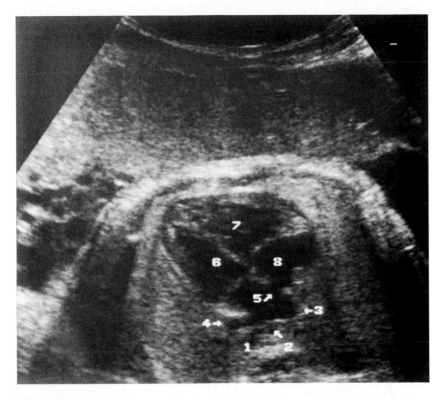

FIG. 5.12.   The fetal heart. Typical details identified in the four-chamber view include the right ventricle (7) with the moderator band, the left ventricle (6), both atria (8 and 5), the foramen ovale (arrow adjacent to the "5"), and the pulmonary veins (1, 3, 4). The descending aorta (2) can also be seen.

Thymus

The thymus is occasionally visible late in gestation, but it is often difficult to distinguish from lung parenchyma. It is conceivable that stressed fetuses react like newborns with a shrinking of the thymus. This could potentially provide an indicator of fetal stress, but more work needs to be done on this subject.

Vascular Anatomy

In the chest, one can also recognize the azygos vein (Fig. 5.15A) and azygos arch (Fig. 5.15B,C) joining the superior vena cava. The hemiazygos vein, which is smaller than the azygos vein, can be recognized on the other side of the aorta (Fig. 5.16). The subclavian artery can be recognized by its well-defined relationship with the clavicle. The humeral artery, which runs medial to the humerus, can be detected with oblique views. Segments of the distal humeral artery can also be seen.

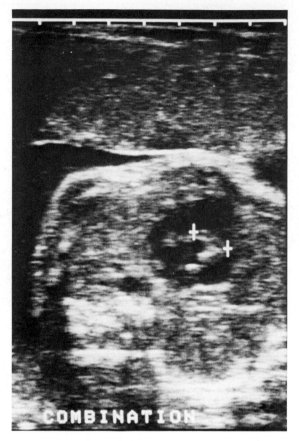

FIG. 5.13. The proximal segment of the right coronary artery (cursors) is visible in front of the anterior semilunar valve.

Abdomen

Vascular Anatomy

The celiac axis (Fig. 5.17) is apparent in a transverse section below the heart. The main landmarks are the stomach and the intra-abdominal part of umbilical vein. The celiac axis has the typical "seagull" shape seen in the adult, but the "legs of the seagull" (the celiac axis itself) are more visible because of the horizontality of the section. The hepatic artery makes a sharp bend to the right at the end of the celiac axis. The splenic artery is fairly straight in the fetus and courses behind the stomach to the splenic hilum.

The splenic artery can be differentiated from the splenic vein by its course and smaller size. The splenic vein is joined by the superior mesenteric vein to form the main portal vein. The splenoportal axis and its prolongation into the right and then right anterior branch of division can be imaged in a single plane. The pancreas is visible anterior to the splenic vessels and posterior to the posterior wall of the stomach. The more anterior position of the

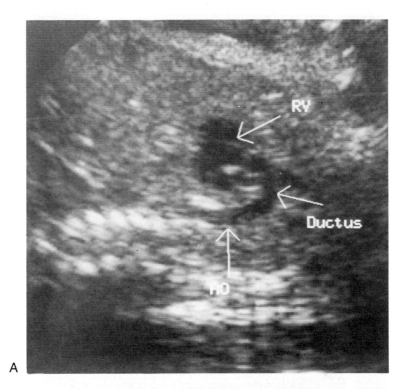

A

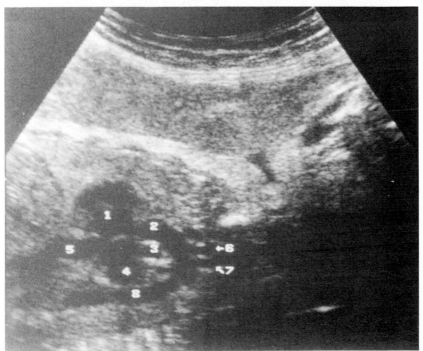

B

FIG. 5.14. The ductus arteriosus (A) has a more angular bend than the aortic arch (B), and the brachiocephalic vessels (6, 7) cannot be traced from it. (RV and 1, right ventricle; AO and 8, descending aorta; 2, ascending aorta; 3, ductus; 4, left atrium.)

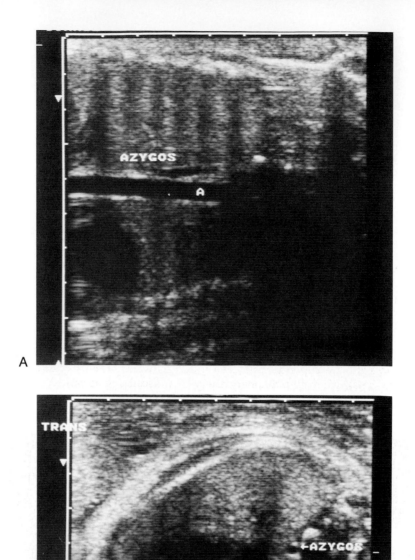

A

B

FIG. 5.15.   In a coronal section of the chest (A), the azygos vein can be seen roughly parallel to the descending aorta. There is no possible confusion with the inferior vena cava, which is larger and more anterior and has already joined the right atrium at this level. In a transverse scan (B), the proximity of the azygos vein and the aorta (A) is well seen. (*Figure continues.*)

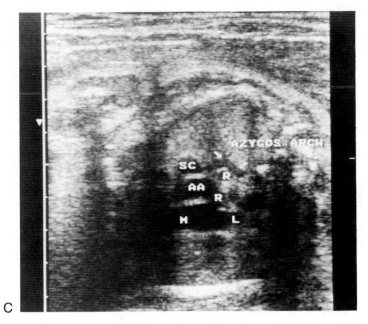

C

FIG. 5.15 (*Continued*).   At a higher level (C), the azygos arch (arrows) is visible at its junction with the superior vena cava (SC.) (R, right pulmonary artery; L, left pulmonary artery; M, main pulmonary artery; AA, ascending aorta.)

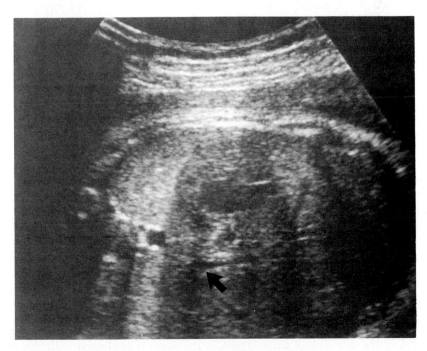

FIG. 5.16.   The hemiazygos vein (top) is thinner than the azygos vein, which is visible on the other side of the aorta. Note the confluence of the right and sagittal hepatic vein (arrow) which identifies the position of the vena cava.

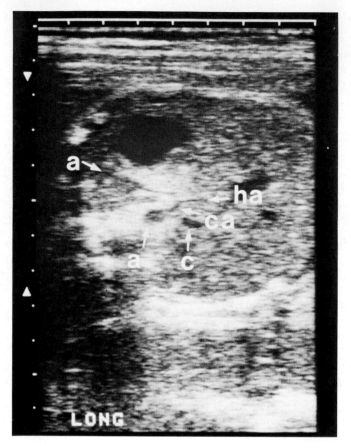

FIG. 5.17.   The celiac axis and its major branches. (a, aorta; ca, celiac axis; a, splenic artery; ha, hepatic artery; c, inferior vena cava.)

inferior vena cava (compared with the aorta), as it bends anteriorly to join the right atrium, can be appreciated at this level (Fig. 5.18).

Below the level of the celiac axis, one can observe the origin of the superior mesenteric artery (Fig. 5.19). The superior mesenteric artery has a straight departure from the anterior aortic wall. The superior mesenteric vein can be differentiated from the superior mesenteric artery by its larger caliber, its anterior position, and by the fact that it courses to the right of the superior mesenteric artery. The renal artery lies almost behind the vein on the left and runs behind the inferior vena cava on the right.

The bifurcation of the aorta and the common iliac arteries are easy to observe in a frontal plane of the retroperitoneal region. Their bifurcation into the internal and external branches can also be observed. They can then be traced into the femoral vessels (Fig. 5.20). Prolongation of the femoral artery into the popliteal, tibial, and finally into the plantar arteries is also visible. The

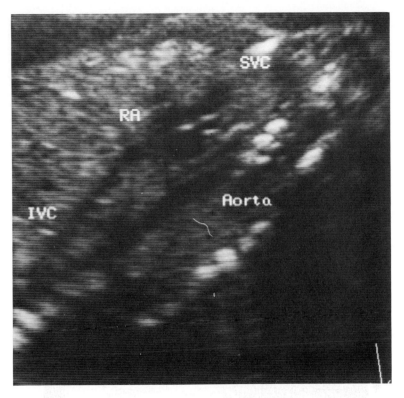

FIG. 5.18.   Oblique longitudinal view demonstrating how much anterior the inferior vena cava is compared with the aorta. (IVC, inferior vena cava; RA, right atrium; SVC, superior vena cava.)

intra-abdominal portion of the umbilical arteries is visible as they travel along both sides of the fetal bladder (Fig. 5.21).

On the venous side of the circulation, one can demonstrate the inferior vena cava entering the right atrium. The junction of the hepatic veins (the left, right, and sagittal vein) is visible close to the right atrium.

The anatomy of the intrahepatic circulation is best described by following the flow in the umbilical vein. The umbilical vein enters the abdominal wall and makes a sharp cephalic bend (Fig. 5.22) and travels along the free margin of the suspensory ligament of the liver to reach the transverse fissure. When the umbilical vein penetrates the liver, it becomes the umbilical portion of the left portal vein. Vena advehentes (Fig. 5.23) can be seen branching from the umbilical portion of the left portal vein. The blood then flows either to the ductus venosus (Fig. 5.24) or to the portal system. The ductus venosus, which is the persistent proximal part of one of the vitelline veins, anastomoses the portal circulation with the left hepatic vein or directly with the inferior vena cava. The main portal vein is composed by the confluence of the splenic and the superior mesenteric vein. It enters the liver and divides into the

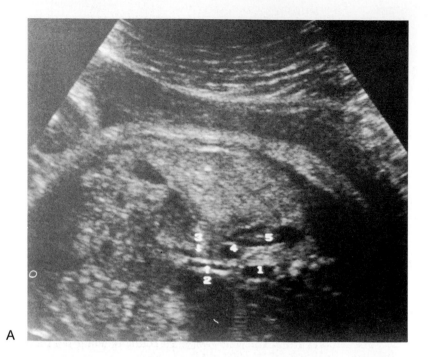

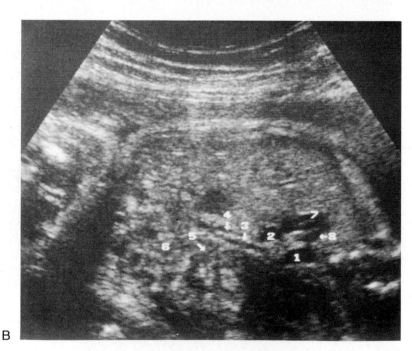

FIG. 5.19.   (A) The superior mesenteric artery (2) and vein (3) and their relationship to the aorta (1) and vena cava (4)(5, right adrenal). (B) Second-order branches (5) of the superior mesenteric artery can be seen on their way to small bowel (6).

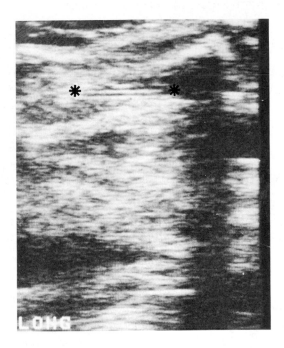

FIG. 5.20. The femoral artery and vein (asterisks coursing along the inner side of the left femur.

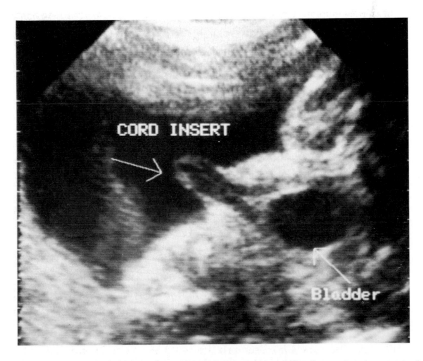

FIG. 5.21. The intra-abdominal portion of the two umbilical arteries (arrows) alongside the bladder.

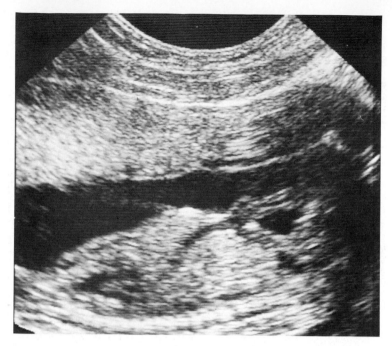

FIG. 5.22. Longitudinal section of the fetus. The vertical segment of the intra-abdominal portion of the umbilical vein is demonstrated.

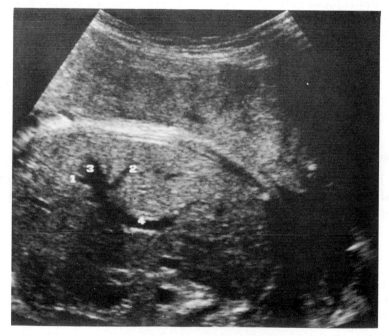

FIG. 5.23. Vena advehentes (1,2) at the umbilical portion of the left portal vein (3). 4, bifurcation of the main portal vein into the left and right branches.

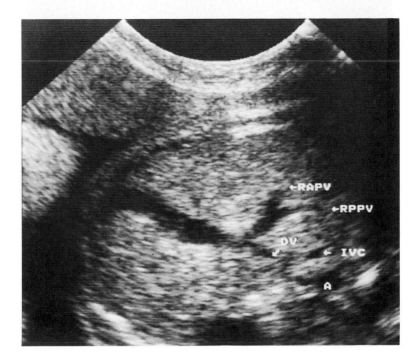

FIG. 5.24.   The ductus venosus (dv) and the left, right anterior (rapv), and right posterior (rppv) portal veins are demonstrated. Notice that the ductus venosus does not anastomose directly with the inferior vena cava (ivc) but with the left hepatic vein (not imaged in this plane). (a, aorta.)

right and the left portal vein (Fig. 5.23). This division of the main portal vein is the landmark used to measure the abdominal perimeter. The right portal vein divides into an anterior and a posterior branch. The left portal vein receives the umbilical portion of the umbilical vein.

Gastrointestinal and Genitourinary Anatomy

At the level of the stomach, the pylorus and bulb can be seen. The rest of the gastrointestinal and genitourinary anatomy has been described at length and need not be repeated here.

Limbs

Filly demonstrated that the cartilaginous portion of the long bones (Fig. 5.25), as well as the cartilaginous bone of the wrist, could be imaged (Fig. 5.26). He also demonstrated the tendons of the hands. Birnholz showed that the fingernails (Fig. 5.27) could be imaged. One can also image the palmar skin creases, a subject of potential interest in the noninvasive diagnosis of trisomy 21 (Fig. 5.28).

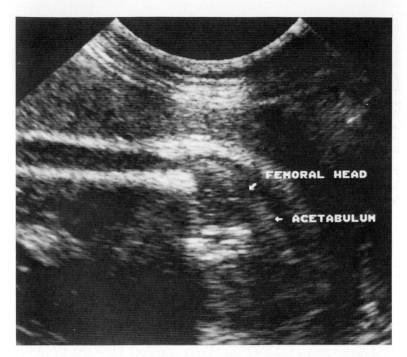

FIG. 5.25.   Cartilaginous portion of the femoral head. Note that the acetabulum is also visible. In fetuses with meningomyelocele, the dislocable hip can sometimes be imaged.

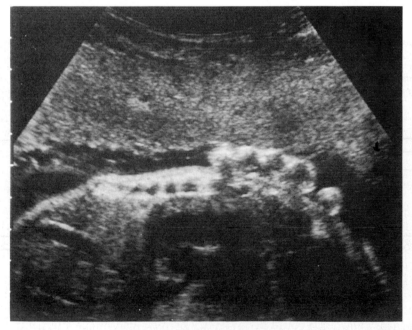

FIG. 5.26.   This section passes through the cartilaginous portion of the five fingers of the left hand and the chondrocostal junctions.

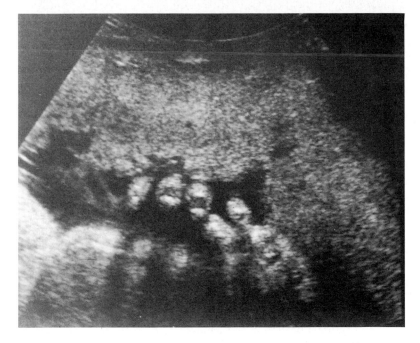

FIG. 5.27.   The fingernails of the fetus are visible.

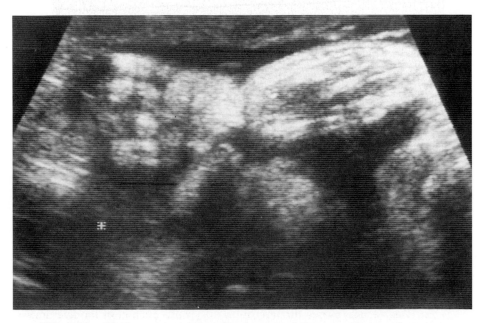

FIG. 5.28.   Simian crease. Note the absence of the normal second crease.

CONCLUSION

This brief survey of the fetal anatomy is not intended to demonstrate the entire extent of the current state of the art but to highlight the fact that a large number of very small structures can indeed be seen with current equipment. The sharpness of current images has improved since some of these images were obtained. Some images, such as images of the coronary artery and celiac axis, were obtained in 1983 with a transducer that had only 64 crystals (most current transducers have 128) and recorded on instant film. The machine used (a Toshiba SAL 50A) has long since been discontinued, yet these images demonstrated excellent detail. More recent images, such as that of the simian crease, were obtained with a very reasonably priced machine (Toshiba SAL 77).

In real life, the question is not whether one wants the best resolution to provide accurate diagnosis. The question is whether money is wisely spent on overpriced equipment, when for the same price one could get two or three machines with the degree of resolution demonstrated above. We hope to have provided the reader with some reference point to use in judging whether a conventional ultrasound scanner will fit his or her need or whether to pay the premium price to get "computed sonography."

SUGGESTED READINGS

Arey LB: Developmental Anatomy WB Saunders, Philadelphia 1974

Birnholz JC: The development of fetal eye movement patterns. Science 213:679, 1981

Chinn DH, Filly RA, Callen PW: Ultrasonic evaluation of fetal umbilical and hepatic vascular anatomy. Radiology 144:153, 1982

Fink IJ, Chinn DH, Callen PW: a potential pitfall in the ultrasonographic diagnosis of fetal encephalocele. J Ultrasound Med 2:313, 1983

Hamilton WJ, Mossman HW: Human Embryology. Williams & Wilkins, Baltimore, 1972

Jeffrey RB, Laing FC: High-resolution realtime sonography of fetal cardiovascular anatomy. J Ultrasound Med 1:249, 1982

6 Fetal Intrathoracic and Gastrointestinal Anomalies

REBECCA G. PENNELL
ALFRED B. KURTZ

Ultrasound is able to detect fetal intrathoracic and gastrointestinal (GI) anomalies with increasing accuracy due to technologic improvements in resolution and technique. This chapter reviews anomalies of these systems as detected by prenatal ultrasound examination.

NORMAL ANATOMY

The fetal thorax and abdomen are often evaluated using the same ultrasound scanning technique. Accurate detection of anomalies in the chest is based on their differentiation from normal fetal organs. The nonaerated fetal lung and mediastinal structures are homogeneously hyperechoic and fill the thorax. The heart normally lies in the midline with the apex toward the left. It is the only normal hypo- to anechoic structure within the chest and is easily identified by its configuration and motion (Fig. 6.1). The determination of cardiac situs is important for the evaluation not only of congenital cardiac disease but of noncardiac thoracic anomalies as well.

In the abdomen, the normal fetal GI anatomy has been well documented, and certain features should be appreciated on each ultrasound examination. The stomach appears as a spherical or semilunar anechoic structure in the left upper quadrant[1] (Fig. 6.2). It enlarges linearly with gestational age, from $4 \times 6 \times 9$ mm at 13 to 15 weeks to $16 \times 20 \times 32$ mm by 37 to 39 weeks.[2] The stomach fills and empties unpredictably and may rarely be empty during an ultrasound examination.[3,4] The pylorus of the stomach and duodenum may also be visualized and should not be construed as necessarily abnormal when the stomach bubble appears to cross the midline. Abdominal visceral situs may be established by determining the position of the stomach on the normal left side.

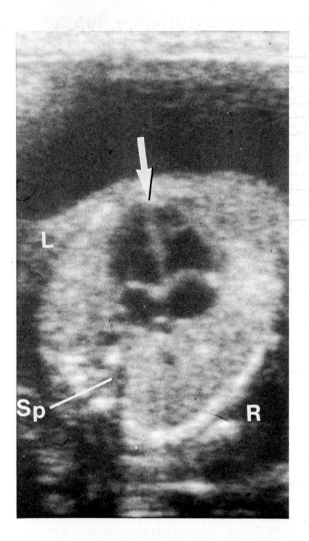

FIG. 6.1 Transaxial view of the fetal thorax shows four chambers of the heart in correct situs with the apex (arrow) pointing toward the left (L). Note the homogeneously hyperechoic fetal lung, which fills the remainder of the thorax. (R, right side of fetus; Sp, spine.)

The upper fetal abdomen is dominated by the liver, its largest organ. The liver is homogeneously hyperechoic, usually of similar or slightly less echogenicity than the fetal lung. Abdominal measurements are based on a transaxial diameter or circumference at the midpoint of the liver.[5] The intrahepatic vessels, particularly the umbilical portion of the left portal vein (portal sinus), are used as a landmark to identify the correct place to take these measurements.[6] From the beginning of the second until the middle of the third trimester (from 12 to 33 weeks), the biparietal diameter and average body diameter are within 5 mm of each other. Later in the third trimester, the body increases to as much as 15 mm larger than the head.[7] There are no well-established measurements for the thorax.

The gallbladder is frequently imaged on transaxial scans as an ovoid or

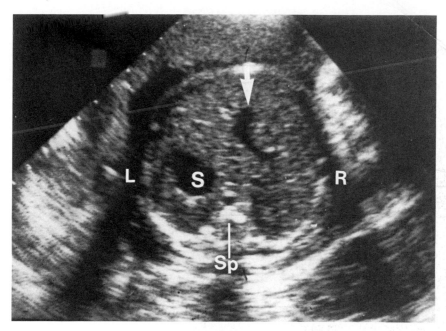

FIG. 6.2   Transaxial view of the fetal abdomen shows the normal fluid-filled stomach (S) in the left upper abdomen. The remainder of the abdomen is filled with the homogeneously hyperechoic fetal liver. Note midline umbilical portion of left portal vein or portal sinus (arrow). (Sp, spine; L, left side of fetus; R, right side of fetus.)

teardrop-shaped anechoic structure parallel and to the right of the portal sinus. The gallbladder and the portal sinus may be confused. Serial transverse scans tracing the midline umbilical vein inferiorly into the umbilical cord insertion at the anterior abdominal wall will help differentiate the two. The remainder of the biliary system is not routinely demonstrated.

The normal sonographic appearance of fetal small bowel and colon was reported in a prospective study of 130 fetuses and correlated with gestational age and fetal maturity.[8,9] The small bowel is usually identified as areas of increased echogenicity in the central mid- and lower portions of the abdomen below the fetal liver.[10] Fluid-filled small bowel loops may sometimes be seen in the central portion of the abdomen surrounded by hyperechoic mesentery. Normally, the segments should measure less than 7 mm in diameter and 15 mm in length, with peristalsis occasionally observed on real-time examination.[8]

The fetal colon is identified as a tubular structure located below the liver around the perimeter of the fetal abdomen. It is imaged as early as 22 menstrual weeks and routinely seen after 28 weeks[8,9] (Fig. 6.3). Sometimes the colon is only identified in short segments close to the kidneys or urinary bladder. The sigmoid colon may be visualized as a tubular structure deep in the pelvis. As the fetus matures, the echogenicity of the meconium content

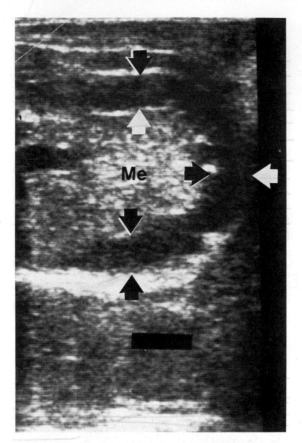

FIG. 6.3 The normal colon (arrows) is a homogeneously hypoechoic structure most often visualized along the perimeter of the lower fetal abdomen. Note that the meconium within the bowel is not completely anechoic. (Me, mesentery.)

of the bowel increases, and the haustra may become apparent late in pregnancy.[9] The colon diameter can be linearly related to menstrual age with a maximum of 18 mm at term.[8]

The diaphragm is situated between the fetal chest and abdomen. This thin muscle is convex toward the lungs, no more than 2 to 3 mm in thickness (Fig. 6.4). It is recognized both by its position between the adjacent and more hyperechoic liver and lung and by its motion on real-time examination, an important aspect of fetal well-being representing the respiratory part of the fetal biophysical profile.[11] With state-of-the-art sonographic equipment, the diaphragm is imaged as a curvilinear hypoechoic reflector, seen only segmentally where the transducer is perpendicular to the muscle. It resembles in echogenicity and thickness the anterior abdominal wall musculature.[12]

Swallowing, another normal in utero activity, may also be visualized during routine real-time sonography. It is normally seen intermittently and limited to one or two movements of the fetal pharynx or mandible per minute.[13] Increased swallowing activity has been seen in cases of polyhydramnios.[14] Cases of apparent vomiting have also been observed in fetuses with upper GI tract obstruction.[13]

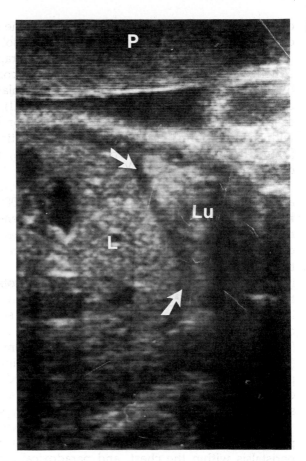

FIG. 6.4. The normal diaphragm (arrows) is identified in the long axis view of the fetus as a thin hypoechoic curvilinear structure between the more hyperechoic liver (L) and lung (Lu). (P, placenta.)

INTRATHORACIC ANOMALIES

Abnormalities of the fetal heart and great vessels are discussed in Chapter 4. Extracardiac thoracic anomalies can be detected by two changes: a mass effect altering the position of the cardiovascular structures, and different echogenicity from the hyperechoic lungs and mediastinum. If a hyperechoic solid thoracic mass is isoechoic with the lungs and mediastinum, detection is difficult, and a shift of the normal mediastinal structures (particularly the heart) may be the only clue to its presence. If the mass is large, regardless of its echogenicity, hydropic changes may occur as a secondary feature caused by compression of the cardiovascular structures.

Most fetal intrathoracic masses are benign. Their detection is not always associated with a poor prognosis. We have observed thoracic masses, detected in early prenatal life, that do not grow or that grow more slowly than the fetus and therefore shrink relative to the size of the thorax. The primary life-threatening neonatal complications of fetal chest masses are pulmonary hypoplasia secondary to compression and hydrops secondary to obstruction of venous return to the heart. If the mass is not too large, these complications may either not occur or may resolve as the fetus grows.

Fetal intrathoracic anomalies may be sonographically evaluated based on either of two appearances: (1) a complex mass containing cystic and/or mixed hypoechoic densities, which includes posterolateral diaphragmatic hernia, cystic adenomatoid malformation (types I and II), and bronchogenic or duplication cysts; or (2) a solid mass, isoechoic or hyperechoic in comparison with adjacent normal lung, which includes cystic adenomatoid malformation (type III), anteromedial diaphragmatic hernia, and bronchopulmonary sequestration.

Congenital diaphragmatic hernias are the most common intrathoracic anomaly, occurring once in every 2,100 to 5,000 live births.[15–18] There is a high association with other anomalies, between 16 and 56 percent.[18,19] The more common posterolateral diaphragmatic hernia is caused by herniation of abdominal viscera through the Bochdalek foramen, with the left side seven times more often involved than the right, and rarely bilateral. This foramen is formed by incomplete migration of the pleuroperitoneal membrane during the tenth week of embryonic life.[20] The most common organs to be found in this type of diaphragmatic hernia include the stomach, small bowel, spleen, colon, and left lobe of the liver.[17] Associated anomalies are cardiovascular (13 percent), neural tube defects (28 percent), omphalocele (20 percent), renal (15 percent), and chromosomal abnormalities, including the trisomies.[21] Diaphragmatic hernias have been reliably detected prenatally.[17,19,22] However, even with good perinatal management, there is at least an 80 percent mortality secondary to the high association with lung hypoplasia.[16,19,23]

The most specific prenatal ultrasound characteristics of posterolateral diaphragmatic hernias include heart displacement, real-time evidence of bowel peristalsis within the chest, and paradoxical diaphragmatic motion during fetal breathing.[15,17] Less specific ultrasound findings include cystic or solid masses in the chest, absent intra-abdominal stomach bubble, and a decreased abdominal diameter.[15,17] Polyhydramnios is a late finding, usually not observed before 25 weeks[15,22] (Fig. 6.5). Visualization of a normal diaphragm does not exclude a diaphragmatic hernia, since defects of the muscle have not been identified in utero.

Anteromedial diaphragmatic defects are difficult to detect. They are the rarer type of diaphragmatic hernias, located anteromedially in the region of the Morgagni foramen.[17] In neonates, this type of herniation rarely presents with fluid-filled bowel above the diaphragm, but instead contains part of the liver.[24] The embryology of mediastinal hernias involves maldevelopment of the septum transversum in the retrosternal area.[26] Fifty percent or more of infants with anteromedial hernias have associated congenital anomalies, including chromosomal abnormalities, mental retardation, and cardiovascular defects. Some of these hernias do not present until later in life.[24,25] Morgagni foramen hernias usually have an echogenicity equal to that of the adjacent lung and mediastinum,[15] since the most common organ within the hernia is the liver.[25] The mediastinal contents are only infrequently displaced, contributing to the difficulty in detection.

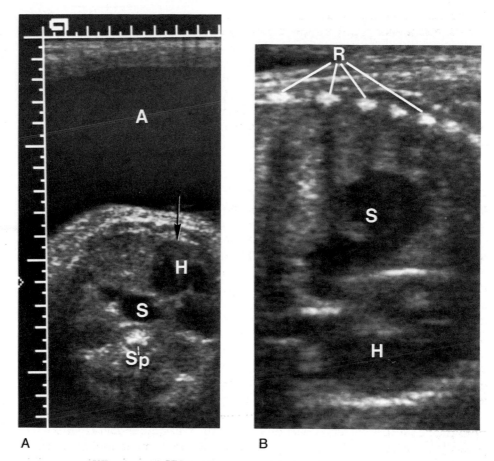

A B

FIG. 6.5.   Posterolateral diaphragmatic (Bochdalek) hernia. (A) Transaxial image through the region of the fetal thorax reveals an anechoic structure, the stomach (S), adjacent to and displacing the fetal heart (H) toward the right. Arrow marks cardiac apex (Sp, spine). Note the presence of increased amniotic fluid characteristic of polyhydramnios (A). (B) Parasagittal image through the fetal thorax shows the S configuration of the fetal stomach (S) within the thorax, adjacent to the cardiac border (H). (R, ribs.)

The pitfalls in diagnosing a diaphragmatic hernia are many. Even when the mass is cystic or complex, the ultrasound findings are nonspecific unless peristalsis is present. Amniography alone or incorporated with a subsequent computed tomogram (CT) may be helpful to demonstrate the presence of abdominal viscera within the chest.[17] Lack of a cystic mass in the chest does not exclude a posterolateral diaphragmatic hernia.[17] If there is an absence of swallowing activity secondary to a severe central nervous system (CNS) or very high GI obstructive lesion, with or without coexisting oligohydramnios, there will not be any fluid within the stomach. In these cases, the differentiation from esophageal atresia may only be made by the demonstration of a solid mass within the chest or atypical diaphragmatic motion.

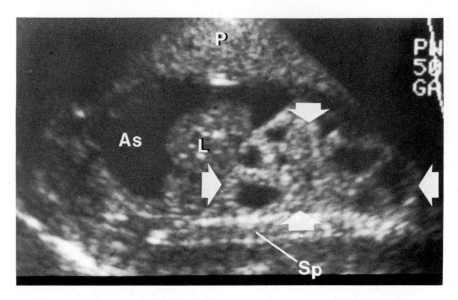

FIG. 6.6   Cystic adenomatoid malformation, type I (arrow). Note the anechoic cysts throughout the fetal thorax with interspersed lung parenchyma. Fetal ascites (As) is noted below the diaphragm. (L, liver; Sp, spine; P, placenta.)

In a prenatal ultrasound study of more than 94 cases,[19] two rare tumors in the thorax were confused with diaphragmatic hernias due to their complex solid and cystic appearance: a lung leiomyosarcoma and a mediastinal cystic teratoma. In addition, although also rare, a mesenchymal hamartoma or teratoma may arise in the region of the mediastium or thorax.[27] These tumors may appear solid or complex sonographically and must be considered in the differential diagnosis of fetal intrathoracic masses.[27,28]

Theoretically, although not reported in utero, diaphragmatic eventration should be differentiated from diaphragmatic hernia. There are two forms, congenital and acquired, both more common on the right.[29] The congenital type is a developmental abnormality characterized by muscular aplasia, causing a thin diaphragm with partial (65 percent) or complete prolapse into the thorax. The acquired cases are due to either birth trauma or postoperative injury to the phrenic nerve.[30] In both types, while diaphragmatic prolapse occurs, the abdominal contents do not transgress the diaphragm. Pulmonary hypoplasia has not been reported, and in general the prognosis is good. Nevertheless, eventration has been reported to be associated with chromosomal abnormalities, Beckwith syndrome, arthrogryposis, and congenital heart disease.[17,30]

Cystic adenomatoid malformation (CAM) is a rare dysplastic anomaly of the lung, classified pathologically into three types.[31] All types contain multiple communicating epithelium-lined cysts, usually involving one lobe. In one-third of cases, more than one lobe is involved,[32] the middle lobe rarely being affected. There is a low incidence of associated fetal anomalies.[33,34]

The usual neonatal presentation of CAM includes hydrops, polyhydramnios, prematurity, neonatal distress, and sometimes delayed symptoms of pulmonary infection.[35]

Type I CAM is characterized by multiple cysts, 3 to 7 cm in diameter.[36] It often (75 percent) causes mediastinal displacement and has the best survival rate of the three types[36] (Fig. 6.6). Type II CAM contains multiple cysts of less than 1.5 cm in size.[31] These have a lower incidence (12 percent) of mediastinal shift.[36] When the mass is cystic, the sonographic differential diagnosis includes a dilated, atretic, or obstructed esophagus or bronchus, bronchogenic cyst, duplication cyst, and diaphragmatic hernia.[32,37–42]

The rarest type, type III, typically presents as a solitary hyperechoic fetal lung mass that, on pathologic examination, contains multiple cysts, less than 5 mm in diameter[34,43,44] (Fig. 6.7). Type III abnormalities tend to be very large and cause mediastinal shift with compression of the heart. A wide

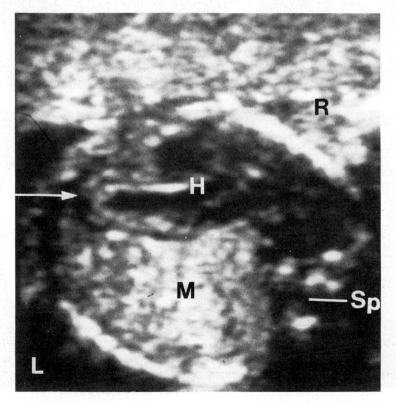

FIG. 6.7. Cystic adenomatoid malformation, type III. A hyperechoic mass (M) is noted within the fetal thorax on this transaxial image. Note that the cardiac silhouette (H) is displaced toward the right (R), although the apex (arrow) still points toward the left. The cysts (less than 5 mm diameter) were not resolvable by this ultrasound technique, hence the hyperechoic appearance of the mass. (Sp, spine; L, left side of fetus.)

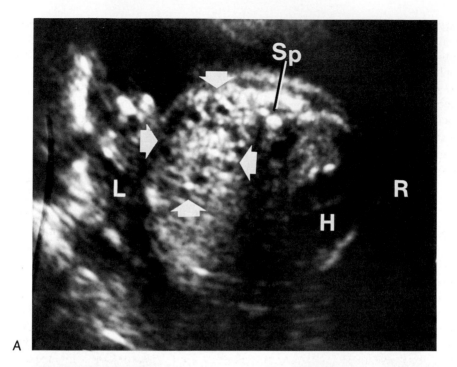

A

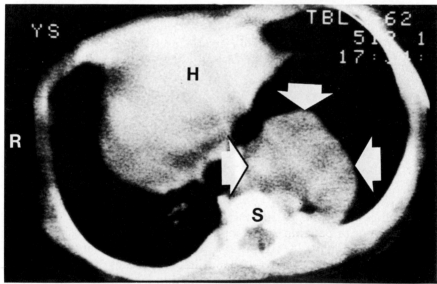

B

FIG. 6.8.   Bronchopulmonary extralobar sequestration. (A) Transaxial scan at the level of the fetal thorax reveals a predominantly solid mass with some cystic components within the left hemithorax posteriorly (arrows). Note that the heart (H) is displaced entirely into the right hemithorax (R). (L, left side of fetus; Sp, spine.) (B) Postnatal CT scan shows the collapsed mass (arrows) in the left lower lobe. Displacement of the heart (H) towards the right (R) is still evident. (S, spine.)

range, 25 to 90 percent, are associated with hydrops,[43] with high mortality rates of 80 to 100 percent.[36]

Extralobar pulmonary sequestration is a rare disorder, usually presenting as a hyperechoic mass in the left posterior costophrenic sulcus[39,40,45] (Fig. 6.8). Associated defects include diaphragmatic hernia and pericardial and vertebral defects. Two cases of an abnormally hyperechoic lung segment associated with bronchial atresia have presented as hyperechoic fetal chest masses.[37,38]

GASTROINTESTINAL ANOMALIES

Major fetal malformations occur in 1 percent of pregnancies,[46] with 9 percent being of GI origin. These include gastroschisis, esophageal atresia, duodenal obstruction, omphalocele, and small bowel obstruction. Clinically, many GI anomalies present as accelerated growth of the uterus (58 percent)[47] caused by polyhydramnios.[47] Polyhydramnios is most common in upper GI obstruction, omphalocele, and gastroschisis.

In terms of ultrasound detection, 15 to 20 percent of all fetal anomalies involve the GI system.[47] Ultrasound accuracy varies with the type of GI anomaly. The overall detection rate is 53 percent, the best accuracy for omphalocele and duodenal atresia.[47] The most difficult to detect is esophageal atresia with fistula and diaphragmatic hernia. In 66 percent of cases, associated multiple anomalies are present, especially in the cases of duodenal atresia and omphalocele.[47,48]

The following types of anomalies are discussed in greater detail: (1) obstructive lesions of the GI tract, (2) complications of meconium spillage into the peritoneal cavity, and (3) extrusive defects of the abdominal wall.

Obstruction

Obstructive GI lesions are commonly imaged as fluid-filled dilated bowel loops. In addition, polyhydramnios, which has a high incidence with upper GI tract obstructions,[47,49,50] frequently aids in the detection of these anomalies due to the large sonic amniotic fluid window.

The incidence of esophageal atresia is 3,000 to 4,500 live births.[51] Approximately 50 percent of patients with esophageal atresia have associated major anomalies, including the VACTERL complex of vertebral, anal (atresia), cardiac (30 percent), renal (12 percent), and limb anomalies.[52] It may also be associated with other GI anomalies, including duodenal atresia and esophageal duplication cysts.[41,53–55]

The most common ultrasound finding in esophageal atresia is the detection of polyhydramnios (62 to 91 percent). Esophageal atresia without tracheoesophageal fistula (10 percent of cases) can be diagnosed by demonstrating an absent or very small stomach in the presence of polyhydramnios.[56,57] In the other 90 percent associated with a fistula, ultrasound will detect only the one-third of cases in which the stomach is absent.[57] In both types, with or without a tracheoesophageal fistula, the stomach may appear very small, presumably containing only secretions.[51,56] In addition, it is possible that when the fistula is present, the amniotic fluid may enter the stomach by the trachea. Finally, in esophageal atresia some investigators have reported visualization of fetal vomiting by real-time examination.[13,42,50]

Obstruction of the bowel may be either complete (atresia) or partial (stenosis). Atresia is the most common cause of congenital intestinal obstruction.[48] Most intestinal obstructions (25 percent) occur at the duodenal level, 5 percent occurring in the colon and the remainder within the jejunum and ileum.[48]

The main findings in cases of proximal fetal bowel obstruction are

1. *Polyhydramnios:* Increased amniotic fluid may be present in 50 percent of duodenal or proximal jejunal atresias.[49,58,59]
2. *Dilated fluid-filled loops:* These preobstructed segments may not be detectable early in gestation, since significant fetal swallowing and GI peristalsis do not begin until after 25 weeks. Serial scans are therefore recommended to look for dilated loops when polyhydramnios is present without a cause.
3. *Progressive increase in bowel peristalsis:* This may be best visualized on real-time examination during the later stages of pregnancy.
4. *Associated anomalies:* In addition to looking for anomalies with ultrasound, an amniocentesis should be performed in all cases of fetal intestinal obstruction to rule out chromosomal abnormalities.

Duodenal obstruction may be due to partial or complete obliteration of the lumen either proximal or distal to the level of the ampulla. Twenty-one percent of duodenal atresias have an associated annular pancreas that is not the cause of the obstruction.[48] It is associated with the VACTERL syndrome, polyhydramnios, (45 percent) and premature birth (54 percent).[60] Twenty-two percent also have bowel malrotation. The cardiac abnormalities (20 percent) associated with duodenal atresia include ventricular septal defect, patent ductus arteriosus, and endocardial cushion defect. Since duodenal atresia has a high (30 percent) association with Down syndrome, the prenatal scans should therefore include a detailed examination of the fetal heart. In addition, it has been reported that the skin in the nuchal region of the neck may be thickened to 6 mm or greater.[61]

The prenatal ultrasound diagnosis of duodenal atresia is based on the detection of polyhydramnios and the visualization in the upper abdomen of two anechoic structures representing the dilated stomach and proximal duodenum (Fig. 6.9), the latter not often detected until the third trimester.[60,62–64] Although extremely rare, duplication of the stomach may mimic this appearance.[65] In postnatal life, infants with duodenal atresia present with vomiting of bilious material hours to days after delivery. With incomplete stenosis, the symptoms may be delayed. The infant may have a distended abdomen and present with poor feeding, failure to thrive, chronic vomiting, and aspiration. Prenatal diagnosis is important to ensure that the

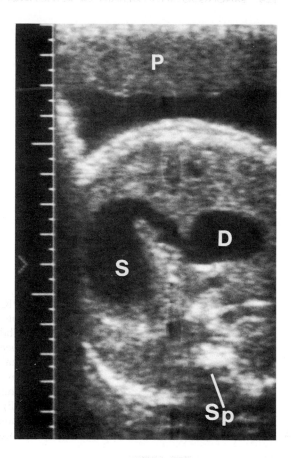

FIG. 6.9. Transaxial image of the fetal abdomen reveals dilation of the stomach (S) and proximal duodenum (D) in a case of duodenal atresia. Note the contracted portion of gastric antrum. (Sp, spine, P, placenta.)

fetus is born at a tertiary care center and is not fed until surgical repair has been performed.

Jejunoileal atresias are the second most common site of bowel obstruction in the neonate. The incidence of atretic segments is evenly distributed throughout the bowel. Four types have been described: a cordlike segment (35 percent), a diaphragm (20 percent), an atresia with a separation of blind ends and a large mesenteric defect (35 percent), and multiple atresias of the small bowel (6 percent).[48] Pathologically, the distal bowel is unused and is potentially normal, although it may appear small. There is always a marked disparity of luminal size between the pre- and postobstructed segments. Associated anomalies include volvulus, microcolon, omphalocele or gastro-schisis, and meconium ileus (20 percent), which frequently presents with signs of meconium peritonitis.[48]

On ultrasound examination, fetal jejunoileal atresia may exhibit cystic structures within the fetal abdomen surrounded by the hyperechoic mesentery (Fig. 6.10). One case of jejunal atresia presented at 32 weeks with dilated abdominal bowel loops without polyhydramnios.[66] Serial scanning revealed progressive dilation of these loops and real-time evidence of strong peristaltic

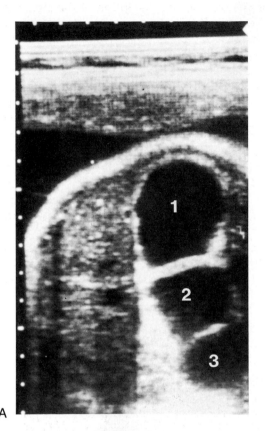

A

FIG. 6.10. Jejunal atresia. (A) Multiple cystic structures within the fetal abdomen (1,2,3) are the typical appearance for the dilated loops of jejunal atresia. The loops are surrounded by hyperechoic mesentery. Note that the amount of amniotic fluid is normal. (B) Neonatal abdominal radiograph demonstrates gas only within the dilated preobstructed loops.

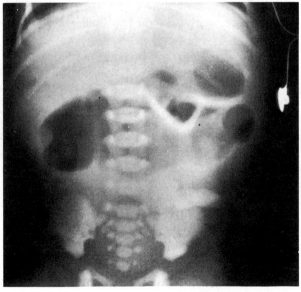

B

activity in the preobstructive loops. Uncommonly, distention of the stomach and polyhydramnios have been reported.[58] The diagnosis of lower small bowel atresias is difficult. In the absence of polyhydramnios and distended loops, lower GI obstruction cannot be reliably excluded.

Anal atresia may cause distal colonic obstructed loops in utero. The incidence is 1 in 5,000 live births.[67] There is a high association with other anomalies, particularly the VACTERL syndrome and the caudal regression syndrome.[67] The predominant ultrasound finding is dilated distal colon after 27 menstrual weeks.[67-69] In a study of 12 cases of anal atresia, 5 showed an abnormally dilated V- or U-shaped loop of colon with a diameter of 18 mm, greater than 2 SD above the mean[67] (Fig. 6.11). In another case, scanned after 34 weeks, a dilated fetal bowel loop appeared to be folded.[68] No dilated loops were imaged before 26 weeks gestational age. These loops may enlarge and show active peristalsis on serial scans. Polyhydramnios was present in only one of these cases.[67]

The differential diagnosis of ileal or colonic atresia/obstruction includes Hirschprung disease, meconium plug syndrome, meconium ileus, and megacystis microcolon intestinal hypoperistalsis syndrome. Hirschprung disease,

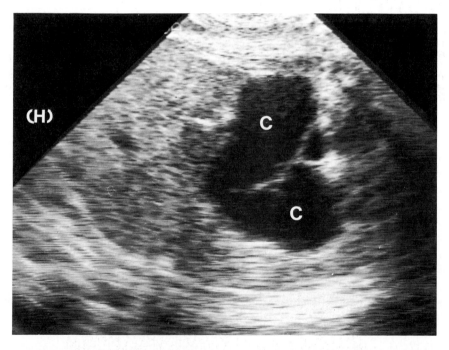

FIG. 6.11.   Coronal view of the fetal abdomen shows segmental dilation of the colon (C). The loops are greater than 2 SD above the mean, measuring 22 mm in diameter. The dilated loops are folded in a V configuration. This fetus was shown to have anorectal atresia with multiple other anomalies. (From Harris et al.,[67] with permission.)

or total aganglionosis, has been diagnosed prenatally by ultrasound examination.[70] This entity is a common cause of neonatal bowel obstruction. The ultrasound findings, not different from those of obstruction, include polyhydramnios, increased abdominal diameter, and diffusely dilated bowel loops with increased diameter on serial studies.[70,71]

MECONIUM PERITONITIS

Meconium peritonitis is a sterile inflammatory reaction of the peritoneum. Most frequently, it is caused by bowel obstruction with perforation. The etiologies include idiopathic intestinal atresia or stenosis, volvulus, Meckel's diverticulum, and incarcerated internal hernia.[72–75] An additional common cause of meconium peritonitis is meconium ileus.[76] This etiology is important, as it occurs in almost 40 percent of babies with cystic fibrosis.[76] Conversely, 10 to 15 percent of all babies born with cystic fibrosis present with meconium ileus and peritonitis.[77] In meconium ileus, the meconium is thicker and more viscous than is normal. Although this viscous meconium does not cause a true mechanical obstruction, its thickness predisposes to an ileus, perforation, and peritonitis. Occasionally, sonography may demonstrate dilated fetal bowel filled with thickened meconium as the primary sonographic finding of cystic fibrosis.[78]

Three types of meconium peritonitis have been described pathologically: fibroadhesive, generalized or diffuse, and cystic.[79] The pathogenesis of meconium peritonitis is initiated with obstruction of bowel. The subsequent ischemia with necrosis leads to perforation and spillage of sterile meconium into the peritoneum. A sterile peritonitis develops that, upon healing, ends in fibrosis, with or without calcification.

The generalized type is characterized by diffuse peritoneal fibrotic thickening with calcium deposits. It sometimes coexists with the other forms, particularly the cystic type. Peritoneal calcifications have been observed both radiographically and sonographically in pre- and postnatal life[72,78,80,81] and, although not consistently present, are a diagnostic sign of this entity. The characteristic in utero ultrasound findings of diffuse meconium peritonitis include polyhydramnios (50 percent), fetal ascites (70 percent), and hyperechoic calcific foci with acoustical shadowing.[76] Diffuse peritoneal and abdominal wall thickening may also be observed.[72,75,82]

The ultrasound differential diagnosis of fetal abdominal calcifications includes peritoneal calcification from ruptured hydrometroculpos or urine ascites.[83] Intrahepatic and hepatic venous calculi may show diffuse shadowing, mimicking peritoneal calcifications.[77,83,84] Most hepatic calcifications are found within the portal venous system or in hepatic parenchyma in cases of TORCH infections (Fig. 6.12). Rarely, intra-abdominal tumors can calcify, although these are usually focal masses.[85] Intraluminal colon calcification has been seen in cases of anal atresia,[67] and calcified meconium plaques have been observed within obstructive neonatal bowel lumens.[80]

The second type, fibroadhesive, is the result of an intensified fibrotic reac-

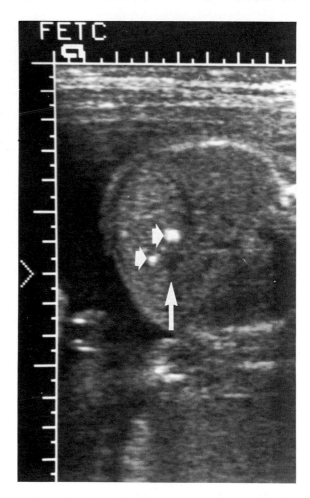

FIG. 6.12.   Hepatic calcification. Punctate calcifications (short arrows) within the hepatic parenchyma of the right lobe show some evidence of acoustic shadowing (long arrow). The etiology of the calcifications was unknown.

tion from the chemical peritonitis. This type is difficult to image with ultrasound, unless it produces obstruction of bowel loops by adhesive bands, usually at the site of perforation.[77] This may or may not develop into either the generalized or cystic form.

Meconium cyst, the third major type, is the best documented and has an incidence of 17 and 60 percent of all cases of meconium peritonitis.[72–74,83,85–87] The meconium cyst or pseudocyst is a collection of meconium and/or abnormal bowel loops surrounded by a wall of fibrogranulation tissue that may or may not be calcified.[74,79] In some cases, a giant meconium cyst may still communicate with the bowel lumen. This is often seen in cases of intestinal volvulus.[72] The walls are frequently calcified, contain hyperechoic debris, and are often associated with ascites or encapsulated ascites.[72] A high mortality is associated with meconium cysts.[72,74]

The most frequent ultrasound findings include a cystic or hypoechoic mass with good sound transmission and a hyperechoic and/or calcified rim. It is

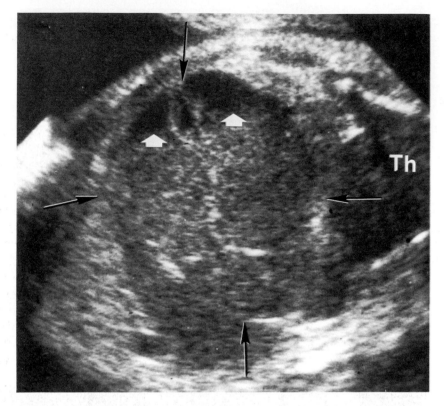

FIG. 6.13. Meconium pseudocyst. A large complex mass (long arrows) located in the mid-fetal abdomen has layering internal hyperechoic debris (short arrows). Also note septae within the mass. (Th, fetal thorax.)

usually well circumscribed and may contain debris[73,74,83,87,90] (Fig. 6.13). In most cases, there is accompanying ascites. This may cause massive abdominal distention so severe that a perinatal paracentesis is needed before delivery to prevent dystocia. These fetuses are not diffusely hydropic. The complicated ultrasound features help differentiate the meconium cyst from other uncomplicated cystic masses: ovarian cysts, cystic ovarian tumors, choledochal cysts, omental or mesenteric cysts, GI duplication cysts, urachal cysts, and hydrometroculpos.[65,74,87,89]

On occasion, a focal area of increased echogenicity can be imaged in the lower fetal abdomen, sometimes as early as the beginning of the second trimester.[10] Some observers believe that it represents normal collapsed bowel containing thick meconium[10]; other investigators have found that if calcification is related to the areas of increased echogenicity, it is most often abnormal.[84] One case was noted with very dense echoes, without shadowing, clustered in the anterior inferior abdomen in an infant found at birth to have cystic fibrosis with inspissated meconium in the terminal ileum.[76] This did not show calcification or shadowing on postnatal sonograms. From these cases, it can be stated that increased echogenicity in the lower fetal abdomen may represent normal bowel and mesentery; it may also be the first sign of uncomplicated meconium ileus in a fetus with cystic fibrosis.

EXOMPHALOS AND ANTERIOR WALL DEFECTS

The major fetal anomalies involving defects of the anterior abdominal wall include gastroschisis and omphalocele. Both involve herniation of various abdominal structures outside the fetal abdomen. These are rare anomalies with a frequency of approximately 1 in 5,000 live births.[91]

Omphalocele is more common and involves herniation of the abdominal viscera through an abdominal wall defect into the base of the umbilical cord[20] (Fig. 6.14). The herniated structures are covered by a membrane composed of amnion, peritoneum, and Wharton's jelly.[93] The umbilical cord inserts onto this membrane. Occasionally, the Wharton's jelly may form a cyst anterior to the defect. While this commonly ruptures at time of birth, its presence in utero is felt to be diagnostic of an omphalocele.[92] Rarely, the covering membrane may rupture, becoming sonographically inapparent. Embryologically the omphalocele results from failure of the lateral body folds to fuse in the midline in the region of the umbilical ring at approximately 10 men-

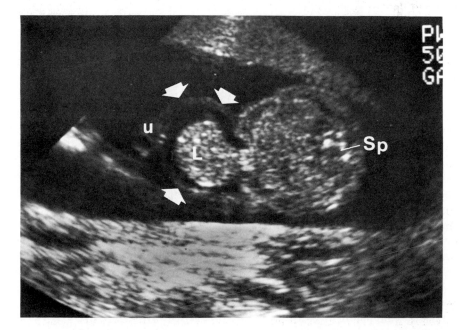

FIG. 6.14.   Omphalocele. This case illustrates the typical features, including mostly liver (L) within the defect, a well-defined membrane surrounding the extruded viscera (arrows) and umbilical vessels (U) inserting in the apex of the defect. (Sp, spine.)

strual weeks.[20] The organs most often contained within the hernia sac include the liver, gallbladder, small bowel, and rarely the stomach and colon. A high incidence (56 to 88 percent) of associated structural and chromosomal anomalies has been reported. These include malrotation, intestinal atresia, major chromosomal abnormalities (20 percent); complex abnormalities of the body fold (11 percent); Beckwith syndrome with omphalocele, organomegaly, macroglossia, and hypoglycemia (14 percent); and congenital heart disease (20 percent).[93,95] Other anomalies of the genitourinary, GI, musculoskeletal, and central nervous system have also been reported.[93–99]

Fetal omphalocele is also associated with ectopia cordis.[26,93] Ectopia cordis is a more extensive anomaly in the same spectrum of disease as the anterior abdominal wall defects, involving a defect of the lower sternum, diaphragm, and the anterior abdominal wall through which the heart protrudes outside the fetus, covered with skin or a thin membrane.[26,100] Its distinction from the less severe omphalocele is important since ectopia cordis is a lethal anomaly.

Gastroschisis is a paraumbilical defect, most commonly on the right side of the abdominal wall, that does not reveal a covering membrane over the herniated viscera. In gastroschisis the umbilical cord inserts into its normal location adjacent to the defect (Fig. 6.15). The embryologic etiology of gastroschisis is uncertain, but Hoyme et al.[97] believe that it may be due to early gestational interruption of the omphalomesenteric artery causing maldevelopment and interruption of the right portion of the abdominal wall. There is a much lower incidence of associated anomalies with gastroschisis, with most complications related to torsion of bowel malrotation and volvulus within the defect.[101] The size of the defect in gastroschisis tends to be smaller than that of omphalocele.[94] Gastroschisis is often seen in premature and low-birth-weight babies.[94,101]

In a study by Bair et al.,[93] the two types of defects were able to be differentiated on prenatal ultrasound in 75 percent of cases. However, there are many pitfalls that can occur. An inflammatory reaction around the loops of bowel in gastroschisis may mimic a covering membrane, and it is sometimes difficult to establish the relationship of the herniated mass to the insertion of the umbilical cord into the anterior abdominal wall[102] (Fig. 6.15). Early sonographic diagnosis is limited by the finding that there is normal exenterated bowel within the base of the cord before 13 weeks menstrual age.[103] Sometimes umbilical cord may be mistaken for extruded bowel.[91] In the presence of oligohydramnios, the thin overlying membrane of an omphalocele may be difficult to identify, making the differentiation from gastroschisis difficult[104–107] (Fig. 6.14 and 6.15).

The perinatal outcome of a fetus with an anterior wall defect is related to the other associated major anomalies and birth weight, rather than to the mode of delivery or type of anomaly.[94,101,108,109] The mortality rates are between 50 to 80 percent with all abdominal wall defects. Omphalocele death rates are higher because of the association with major anomalies.[93,98,101,108–111] The importance of diagnosing these anomalies in utero is to ensure delivery

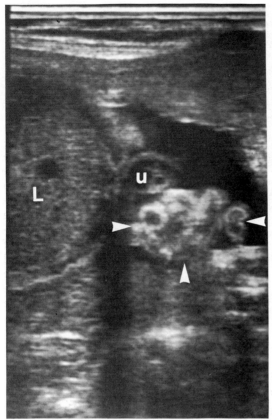

A

FIG. 6.15. Gastroschisis. (A) Transaxial view of the fetal abdomen reveals multiple thick-walled bowel loops (arrows) floating freely within the amniotic fluid. Note the normal umbilical cord (U) separate from the herniated viscera. (L, liver.) (B) This view details the appearance of the herniated bowel loops (arrows). Note the thickened bowel walls. (Ab, fetal abdomen.)

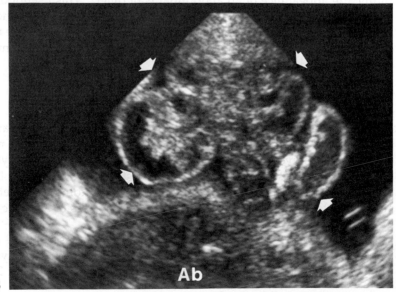

B

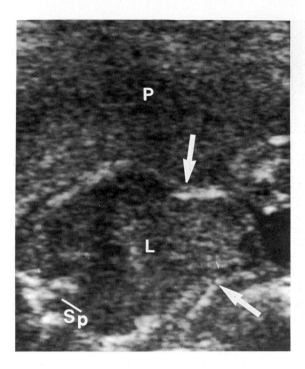

FIG. 6.16. Pseudo-ompha-locele. Transaxial image in the fetal abdomen shows a paucity of amniotic fluid due to the wedged position of the fetal body in the corner of the uterus adjacent to the placenta (P). A contour bulge of the anterior abdominal wall (arrows) is believed to be caused by compression by the uterus. Note its obtuse angle with the fetal abdomen. (Sp, spine, L, liver.)

at a tertiary hospital, as many of the fetuses may die postnatally of dehydration and heat loss.

Compression of the fetal abdomen between the walls of the uterus, in a corner of the uterus surrounded by little fluid, or in oligohydramnios may mimic the appearance of an abdominal wall defect. This pseudoomphalocele may be differentiated from a true omphalocele by changing the degree of compression, changing the scanning angle, and noting that there is an obtuse rather than acute angle of the defect in relation to the fetal abdominal wall[112] (Fig. 6.16).

HEPATOBILIARY SYSTEM

Although the literature details the examination of the fetal hepatic anatomy extensively, fetal hepatic mass lesions are extremely rare. The major cystic diseases of the liver in infancy and childhood include mesenchymal hemartoma and nonparasitic simple congenital cysts.[113] Tumors of the liver including hemangioma, hamartoma, hepatoblastoma, teratoma, and metastatic neuroblastoma can present as a complex mass with areas of acoustic shadowing suggesting calcification.[85,114]

Anomalies of the biliary system are also rarely observed in utero.[115,116] The antenatal observation of a choledochal cyst by sonography reports an enlarged cystic structure in continuity with the porta hepatis at 25 weeks of

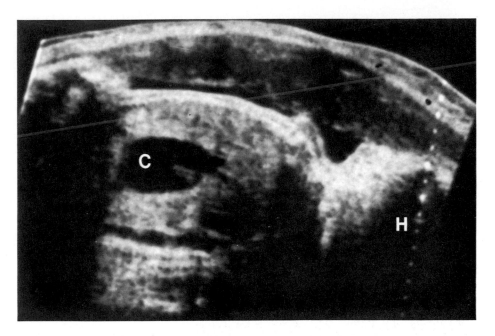

FIG. 6.17   Choledochal cyst. Coronal long-axis static sonogram shows a right mid-abdominal cystic structure (C). The superior elongation of the cyst is thought to represent the nubbin of the atretic bile duct. (H, fetal head.) (Courtesy of Dr. Harvey Nisenbaum, Philadelphia, PA.)

gestation.[115] Branching ducts may be observed entering the superior aspect of the cyst (Fig. 6.17).

In summary, complex anomalies of the fetal thorax and GI system are being detected with increasing accuracy by high-resolution prenatal sonography. Knowledge of their ultrasonographic appearances and differential diagnoses may further enhance antenatal and perinatal management of the affected fetus.

REFERENCES

1. Medearis AL, Shields JR: Normal fetal and pelvic anatomy. A cross-section review. Clin Obstet Gynecol 27:276, 1984

2. Goldstein I, Reece EA, Tarkoni S, et al: Growth of the fetal stomach in normal pregnancies. Obstet Gynecol 70:641, 1987

3. Bovicelli L, Rizzo N, Orsini LF, Pilu G: Prenatal diagnosis and management of fetal gastrointestinal abnormalities. Semin Perinatol 7:109, 1983

4. Farrant PT: The antenatal diagnosis of oesophageal atresia by ultrasound. Br J Radiol 53:1202, 1980

5. Campbell S, Wilkin D: Ultrasonic measurement of fetal abdomen circumference in the estimation of fetal weight. Br J Obstet Gynecol 82:689, 1975

6. Chinn DH, Filly RA, Callen PW: Ultrasonic evaluation of fetal umbilical and hepatic vascular anatomy. Radiology 144:153, 1982

7. Erikson PS, Secher NJ, Weis-Bentzon M: Normal growth of the fetal biparietal diameter and the abdominal diameter in a longitudinal study. Acta Obstet Gynecol Scand 64:65, 1985

8. Nyberg DA, Mack LA, Patten RM, Cyr DR: Fetal Bowel: Normal sonographic findings. J Ultrasound Med 6:3, 1987

9. Goldstein I, Lockwood C, Hobbins JC: Ultrasound assessment of fetal intestinal development in the evaluation of gestational age. Obstet Gynecol 70:682, 1987

10. Fakhry J, Reiser M, Shapiro LR, et al: Increased echogenicity in the lower fetal abdomen: A common normal variant in the second trimester. J Ultrasound Med 5:489, 1986

11. Manning FA, et al: Antepartum fetal evaluation: Development of fetal biophysical profile. Am J Obstet Gynecol 136:787, 1980

12. Hashimoto BE, Filly RA, Callen PW: Fetal pseudoascites: Further anatomic observations. J Ultrasound Med 5:151, 1986

13. Bowie JD, Clair MR: Fetal swallowing and regurgitation: Observation of normal and abnormal activity. Radiology 144:877, 1982

14. Abramovich DR, Gardena A, Janrial LB, Page KR: Fetal swallowing and voiding in relation to hydramnios. Obstet Gynecol 54:15, 1979

15. Chinn DH, Filly RA, Callen PW, et al: Congenital diaphragmatic hernia diagnosed prenatally by ultrasound. Radiology 148:119, 1983

16. Soper RT, Pringle KC, Scofield JC: Creation and repair of diaphragmatic hernia in the fetal lamb: Techniques and survival. J Pediatr Surg 19:33, 1984

17. Comstock CH: The antenatal diagnosis of diaphragmatic anomalies. J Ultrasound Med 5:391, 1986

18. Puri P, Gorman F: Lethal nonpulmonary anomalies associated with congenital diaphragmatic hernia: Implications for early morphologic spectrum. Hum Pathol 8:155, 1977

19. Adzick NS, Harrison MR, Glick PL, et al: Diaphragmatic hernia in the fetus: Prenatal diagnosis and outcome in 94 cases. J Pediatr Surg 20:357, 1985

20. Langman J: Medical Embryology. Williams & Wilkins, Baltimore, 1963

21. David T, Illingworth C: Diaphragmatic hernia in the southwest of England. J Med Genet 16:244, 1976

22. Benacerraf BR, Adzick NS: Fetal diaphragmatic hernia: Ultrasound diagnosis and clinical outcome in 19 cases. Am J Obstet Gynecol 156:573, 1987

23. Harrison MR, Bressack MA, Churg AM, Lorimier AA: Correction of congenital diaphragmatic hernia in utero. II. Simulated correction permits fetal lung growth with survival at birth. Surgery 88:260, 1980

24. Korobkin MT, Miller SW, deLorimier AA, et al: Hepatic herniation through the morgagni foramen. Am J Dis Child 126:217, 1973

25. Merten DF, Bowie JD, Kirks DR, Grossman H: Anteromedial diaphragmatic defects in infancy: Current approaches to diagnostic imaging. Radiology 142:361, 1982

26. Haynor DR, Shuman WP, Brewer DK, Mack LA: Imaging of fetal ectopia cordis: Roles of sonography and computed tomography. J Ultrasound Med 3:25, 1984

27. Mark EJ: Mesenchymal cystic harartoma of the lung. N Engl J Med 315:1255, 1986

28. Thurkow AL, Visser GHA, Oosterhuis JW, deVries JA; Ultrasound observations of a malignant cervical teratoma of the fetus in a case of polyhydramnios: Case history and review. Eur J Obstet Gynecol Reprod Biol 14:375, 1983

29. Symbas PN, Hatcher CR Jr, Waldo W: Diaphragmatic eventration in infancy and childhood. Ann Thorac Surg 24:113, 1977.

30. Wayne ER, Campbell JB, Burrington JD, Davis WS: Eventration of the diaphragm. J Pediatr Surg 9:643, 1974

31. Stocker JT, Madewell JE, Drake RM: Congenital cystic adenomatoid malformation of the lung, classification and morphologic spectrum. Hum Pathol 8:155, 1977

32. Panicek DM, Heitzman ER, Randall PA, et al: The continuum of pulmonary developmental anomalies. Radiographics 7:747, 1987

33. Gerald B, Merenstein MC: Congenital cystic adenomatoid malformation of the lung, report of a case and review of the literature. Am J Dis Child 118:772, 1969

34. Morcos SF, Lobb MO: The antenatal diagnosis by ultrasonography of type III congenital cystic adenomatoid malformation of the lung. Case report. Br J Obstet Gynecol 93:1002, 1986

35. Hartenberg MA, Brewer WH: Cystic adenomatoid malformation of the lung: Identification by sonography. AJR 140:693, 1983

36. Diwan RV, Brennan JN, Philipson EH, et al: Ultrasonic prenatal diagnosis of type III congenital cystic adenomatoid malformation of lung. J Clin Ultrasound 11:218, 1983

37. McAlister WH, Wright JR, Crane JP: Main-stem bronchial atresia: Intrauterine sonographic diagnosis. AJR 148:364, 1987.

38. Mayden KL, Tortora M, Chervenak FA, Hobbins JC: The antenatal sonographic detection of lung masses. Am J Obstet Gynecol 148:349, 1984

39. Knochel JQ, Lee TG, Melendez MG, et al: Fetal anomalies involving the thorax and abdomen. Radiol Clin North Am 20:297, 1982

40. Reece EA, Lockwood CJ, Rizzo N, et al: Intrinsic intrathoracic malformations of the fetus: Sonographic detection and clinical presentation. Obstet Gynecol 70:627, 1987

41. Claiborne AK, Blocker SH, Martin CM, McAlister WH: Prenatal and postnatal sonographic delineation of gastrointestinal abnormalities in a case of the VATER syndrome. J Ultrasound Med 5:45, 1986

42. Eyheremendy E, Pfister M: Antenatal real-time diagnosis of esophageal atresias. J Clin Ultrasound 11:395, 1983

43. Mendoza A, Wolf P, Edwards DK, et al: Prenatal ultrasonographic diagnosis of congenital adenomatoid malformation of the lung. Arch Pathol Lab Med 110:402, 1986

44. Johnson JA, Rumack CM, Johnson ML, et al: Cystic adenomatoid malformation: Antenatal demonstration. AJR 142:483, 1984

45. Romero R, Chervenak FA, Kotzen J, et al: Antenatal sonographic findings of extralobar pulmonary sequestration. J Ultrasound Med 1:131, 1982

46. Jassani MN, Gauderer MWL, Fanaroff AA, et al: A perinatal approach to the diagnosis and management of gastrointestinal malformations. Obstet Gynecol 59:33, 1982

47. Jouppila P, Kirkinen P: Ultrasonic and clinical aspects in the diagnosis and prognosis of congenital gastrointestinal anomalies. Ultrasound Med Biol 10:465: 1984

48. Touloukian RJ: Intestinal atresia. Clin Perinatol 5:3, 1978

49. Queenan JT, Gadow ED: Aminography for detection of congenital malformations. Obstet Gynecol 35:648, 1970

50. Pretorius DH, Meier PR, Johnson ML: Diagnosis of esophageal atresia in utero. J Ultrasound Med 2:475, 1983

51. Zimmerman HB: Prenatal demonstration of gastric and duodenal obstruction by ultrasound. J Can Assoc Radiol 29:138, 1978

52. Martin LW, Alexander F: Esophageal atresia. Surg Clin North Am 65:1099, 1985

53. Hayden CK, Schwartz MZ, Davis M, Swischuk LE: Combined esophageal and duodenal atresia: Sonographic findings. AJR 140:225, 1983

54. Jackson GH, Yiu-Chiu VS, Smith WL, Chiu LC: Sonography of combined esophageal and duodenal atresia. J Ultrasound Med 2:473, 1983

55. McCook TA, Felman AH: Esophageal atresia, duodenal atresia, and gastric distension: Report of two cases. AJR 131:167, 1978

56. Hobbins JC, Grannum PAT, Berkowitz RL, et al: Ultrasound in the diagnosis of congenital anomalies. Am J Obstet Gynecol 134:331, 1978

57. Pretorius DH, Drose JA, Dennis MA, Manchester DK, Manco-Johnson ML: J Ultrasound Med 6:509, 1987

58. Kjoller M, Holm-Nielsen G, Meiland H, et al: Prenatal obstruction of the ileum diagnosed by ultrasound. Prenat Diagn 5:427, 1985

59. Duenhoelter JH, Santos-Ramos R, Rosenfield CR, et al: Prenatal diagnosis of gastrointestinal tract obstruction. Obstet Gynecol 47:618, 1976

60. Nelson LW, Clark CE, Fishburne JI, et al: Value of serial sonography in the in utero detection of duodenal atresia. 59:657, 1982

61. Benacerraf BR, Frigoletto FD Jr, Laboda LA: Sonographic diagnosis of Down's syndrome in the second trimester. Am J Obstet Gynecol 153:49, 1985

62. Filkins K, Russo J, Flowers WK: Third trimester ultrasound diagnosis of intestinal atresia following clinical evidence of polyhydramnios. Prenat Diagn 5:215, 1985

63. Lees RF, Alford BA, Brenbridge AN, et al: Sonographic appearance of duodenal atresia in utero. AJR 131:701, 1978

64. Houlton MCC, Sutton M, Aitken J: Antenatal diagnosis of duodenal atresia. J Obstet Gynaecol Br Commonw 81:818, 1974

65. Bidwell JK, Nelson A: Prenatal ultrasonic diagnosis of congenital duplication of the stomach. J Ultrasound Med 5:589, 1986

66. Nikapota VLB, Loman C: Gray scale sonographic demonstration of fetal small-bowel atresia. J Clin Ultrasound 7:307, 1979

67. Harris RD, Nyberg DA, Mack LA, Weinberger E: Anorectal atresia: Prenatal sonographic diagnosis. AJR 149:395, 1987

68. Bean WJ, Calonje MA, Aprill CN, Geshner J: Anal atresia: A prenatal ultrasound diagnosis. J Clin Ultrasound 6:73, 1978

69. Barss VA, Benacerraf BR, Frigolotto FD: Antenatal sonographic diagnosis of fetal gastrointestinal malformation. Pediatrics 76:445, 1985

70. Vermesh M, Mayden KL, Confino E, et al: Prenatal sonographic diagnosis of Hirschsprung's disease. J Ultrasound Med 5:37, 1986

71. Wrobleski D, Wesselhoeft C: Ultrasonic diagnosis of prenatal intestinal obstruction. J Pediatr Surg 14:598, 1979

72. Clair MR, Rosenberg ER, Ram PC, Bowie JD: Prenatal sonographic diagnosis of meconium peritonitis. Prenatal diagnosis 3:65, 1983

73. Baxi LV, Yeh MN, Blanc WA, Schullinger JN: Antepartum diagnosis and management of in utero intestinal volvulus with perforation. N Engl J Med 308:1519, 1983

74. Bowen A, Mazer J, Zarabi M, Fujioka M: Cystic meconium peritonitis: Ultrasonographic features. Pediatr Radiol 14:18, 1984

75. Nancarrow PA, Mattrey RF, Edwards DK, Skram C: Fibroadhesive meconium peritonitis: In utero sonographic diagnosis. J Ultrasound Med 4:213, 1985

76. Dillard JP, Edwards DK, Leopold GR: Meconium peritonitis masquerading as fetal hydrops. J Ultrasound Med 6:49, 1987

77. Forouhar F: Meconium peritonitis. Am J Clin Pathol 78:208, 1982

78. Nyberg DA, Hastrup W, Watts H, Mack LA; Dilated fetal bowel: A sonographic sign of cystic fibrosis. J Ultrasound Med 6:257, 1987

79. Lorimer WS, Jr, Willis DG: Meconium peritonitis. Surgery 60:470, 1966

80. Ya-Xiong S, Lian-Chen S: Meconium peritonitis—Observations in 115 cases and antenatal diagnosis. Z Kinderchir 37:2, 1982

81. Glick PH, Harrison MR, Filly RA: Antepartum diagnosis of meconium peritonitis. (Letter to the editor.) N Engl J Med 3:1392, 1983

82. Dunne M, Haney P, Sun C-CJ: Sonographic features of bowel perforation and calcific meconium peritonitis in utero. Pediatr Radiol 13:231, 1983

83. Blumenthal DH, Rushovich AM, Williams RK, Rochester D: Prenatal sonographic findings of meconium peritonitis with pathologic correlation. J Clin Ultrasound 10:350, 1982

84. Lince DM, Pretorius DH, Manco-Johnson ML, et al: The clinical significance of increased echogenicity in the fetal abdomen. AJR 145:683, 1985

85. Nakamoto SK, Dreilinger A, Dattel B, et al: The sonographic appearance of hepatic hemangioma in utero. J Ultrasound Med 2:239, 1983

86. Hartung RW, Kilcheski TS, Greaney RB, et al: Antenatal diagnosis of cystic meconium peritonitis. J Ultrasound J Med 2:49, 1983

87. Carroll BA, Moskowitz PS: Sonographic diagnosis of neonatal meconium cyst. AJR 137:1262, 1981

88. Lauer JD, Cradock TV: Meconium pseudocyst: Prenatal sonographic and antenatal radiologic correlation. J Ultrasound Med 1:333, 1982

89. Schwimer SR, Vanley GT, Reinke RT: Prenatal diagnosis of cystic meconium peritonitis. J Clin Ultrasound 12:37, 1984

90. McGahan JP, Hanson F: Meconium peritonitis with accompanying pseudocyst: Prenatal sonographic diagnosis. Radiology 148:125, 1983

91. Lindfors KK, McGahan JP, Walter JP: Fetal omphalocele and gastroschisis: Pitfalls in sonographic diagnosis. AJR 147:797, 1986

92. Fink IJ, Filly RA: Omphalocele associated with umbilical cord allantoic cyst: Sonographic evaluation in utero. Radiology 149:473, 1983

93. Bair JH, Russ PD, Pretorius DH, et al: Fetal omphalocele and gastroschisis: A review of 24 cases. ARJ 147:1047, 1986

94. Seashore JH: Congenital abdominal wall defects. Clin Perinatol 5:61, 1978

95. Cohen MM Jr, Gorlin RJ, Feingold M, ten Bensel RW: The Beckwith-Wiedemann syndrome. Am J Dis Child 122:515, 1971

96. Grossfeld JL, Dawes L, Weber TR. Congenital abdominal wall defects: Current management and survival. Surg Clin North Am 61:1037, 1981

97. Hoyme HE, Jones MC, Jones KL: Gastroschisis: Abdominal wall disruption secondary to early gestational interruption of the omphalomesenteric artery. Semin Perinatol 7:294, 1983

98. Klein MD, Kosloske AM, Hertzler JH: Congenital defects of the abdominal wall. JAMA 245:1643, 1981

99. Nelson PA, Bowie JD, Filston HC, Crane LM: Sonographic diagnosis of omphalocele in utero. AJR 138:1178, 1982

100. Baker ME, Rosenberg ER, Trofatter KF, et al: The in utero findings in twin pentalogy of Cantrell. J Ultrasound Med 3:525, 1984

101. Carpenter MW, Curci MR, Dibbins AW, Haddow JE: Perinatal management of ventral wall defects. Obstet Gynecol 64:646, 1984.

102. Kluck P, Tibboel D, van der Kamp AWM, Molenaar JC: The effect of fetal urine on the development of the bowel in gastroschisis. J Pediatr Surg 18:47, 1983

103. Cyr DR, Mack LA, Schoenecker SA, et al: Bowel migration in the normal fetus: US detection. Radiology 161:119, 1986

104. Roberts C: Intrauterine diagnosis of omphalocele. Radiology 127:762, 1978

105. Yaghoobian J, Chaudary R, Pinck RL: Antenatal diagnosis of omphalocele by Ultrasound. J Reprod Med 26:274, 1981

106. Giulian BB, Alvear DT: Prenatal ultrasonographic diagnosis of fetal gastroschisis. Radiology 129:473, 1978
107. Cameron GM, McQuown DS, Modanlou HD, et al: Intrauterine diagnosis of an omphalocele by diagnostic ultrasonography. Am J Obstet Gynecol 131:821, 1978
108. Serman M, Benzie RJ, Pitson L, et al: Prenatal diagnosis and management of congenital defects of the anterior abdominal wall. Am J Obstet Gynecol 156:308, 1987
109. Hasan S, Hermansen MC: The prenatal diagnosis of ventral abdominal wall defects. Am J Obstet Gynecol 155:842, 1986
110. Kirk EP, Wah RM: Obstetric management of the fetus with omphalocele of gastroschisis: A review and report of one hundred twelve cases. Am J Obstet Gynecol 146:512, 1983
111. Smith LA, Telander RL, Cooney Dr, et al: Treatment of defects of the anterior abdominal wall in newborns. Mayo Clin Proc 58:797, 1983
112. Salzman L, Kuligowska E, Semine A: Pseudoomphalocele: Pitfall in fetal sonography. AJR 146:1283, 1986
113. Foucar E, Williamson RA, Yiu-Chiu V, et al: Mesenchymal hamartoma of the liver identified by fetal sonography. AJR 140:970, 1983
114. Nguyen DL, Leonard JC: Ischemic hepatic necrosis: A cause of fetal liver calcification. AJR 147:596, 1986
115. Frank JL, Hill MC, Chirathivat S, et al: Antenatal observation of a choledochal cyst by sonography. AJR 137:166, 1981
116. Greenholz SK, Lilly JR, Shikes RH, Hall RJ: Biliary atresia in the newborn. J Pediatr Surg 21:1147, 1986

7 Common Fetal Urinary Tract Anomalies

FRANK A. MANNING

Congenital anomalies affecting either a single or multiple organ system are a relatively common consequence of human fetal development occurring at a frequency of 1 to 2 percent of live births and up to 10 percent among stillborns.[1] Genitourinary tract anomalies are among the most common lesions reported, but the true incidence of these anomalies may not be determined with certainty. In prospective clinical studies, genitourinary tract anomalies account for about 18 percent of all lethal anomalies and occur at a frequency of about 1 per 1,000 live births.[2] Since most genitourinary anomalies (70 percent) do not result in perinatal death,[3] the true incidence of disease due to anomalies of this organ system is estimated to be not less than 3 per 1,000.

The advent of high-resolution dynamic ultrasound imaging methods and its now widespread application to perinatal medicine has had a profound impact on the relative clinical significance of congenital anomalies as a cause of death or damage of the perinate. Very specific recognition of the nonanomalous asphyxiated fetus, prompting timely intervention, has resulted in a significant fall in overall perinatal mortality while producing a relative increase in deaths attributed to lethal anomaly. Thus, for example, comparative studies in our population (N = 98,927 pregnancies) demonstrate a near 50 percent reduction in overall stillbirth rate (7.73 to 3.64 per 1,000), while stillbirths, due to anomaly, has increased nearly fivefold (10.2 to 56.6 percent).[1,2]

This increase in the relative importance of anomalies as a cause of perinatal morbidity and mortality has been paralleled by remarkable ultrasonographic-based advances in recognition of anomalies, monitoring of pathophysiology, accurate assignment of prognosis and in some instances implementation of effective therapy. Nowhere have these advances been more dramatic than in the assessment and management of anomalies of the fetal genitourinary tract. The object of this chapter is to review current status of ultrasound in the diagnosis, and more specifically the management, of the more common anomalies of this system.

PATHOPHYSIOLOGIC RELATIONSHIPS OF URINARY TRACT ANOMALIES

The unique structural-functional interrelationship of the fetal urinary tract renders this system especially amenable to in utero assessment by ultrasound methods. In its normal state, the fetal urinary tract is characterized by the near-continuous production of a product, fetal urine, and by the egress of this product through the collecting system to the amniotic fluid pool. Using contemporary ultrasound methods, the presence and the rate of production of fetal urine may be determined, the distribution within the collecting system determined, and the relative contribution to amniotic pool estimated. The ultimate clinical significance of any anomalous disruptions of this system is variable and complex; they may indirectly involve other vital organ systems, most notably the fetal lung. Abnormalities of fetal urine production are always a result of renal parenchymal disease, but such lesions may be either primary or secondary. Like most fetal anomalies, the etiology of anomalous renal parenchymal development is unknown. Renal parenchymal dysgenesis is characterized by gross histologic disruption of the glomerular unit with failure of communication with the collecting system. In a series of elegant experiments, using the chronic ovine fetal model, Harrison and co-workers showed that early (18-week human equivalent) complete obstruction of the ureter causes dysgenetic changes in the ipsilateral kidney and that release of the obstruction prevents the progression of these lesions.[4-7] In contrast to later obstruction (greater than 24 weeks human equivalent), the glomerular unit remains functionally intact showing only the effects of distention.[4,5] In pregnancies, sustained early (greater than 18 weeks gestation) obstruction to urine flow has been associated with renal dysgenesis,[8] but the effect is not uniform.[9] This relationship between functional and structural pathology is of some importance, since methods for in utero diversion of urine flow are now becoming available.[9,10] The cumulative data, while by no means conclusive, suggest that before some critical fetal age, obstruction causes renal dysgenesis, an irreversible and when bilateral a lethal process, whereas later obstruction may cause reversible and nonlethal compression effects only.

In most instances, the mechanism of death in fetuses with lethal renal anomalies is not renal but rather pulmonary[11] (Table 7.1). The relationship between conditions that cause absent urine production (eg. bilateral renal agenesis) or absent urine flow (bladder neck obstruction) and pulmonary hypoplasia is well known; virtually all liveborn infants with renal agenesis will die from pulmonary hypoplasia, and at least 80 percent of the neonatal deaths with obstructive uropathies are due to this complication.[11] The pathologic process connecting these two organ systems is unknown and may be variable. Both abnormalities in urine production and flow typically cause a reduction in amniotic fluid volume (oligohydramnios). Oligohydramnios due to nonrenal causes such as prolonged rupture of membranes[12] or to experimental manipulation in animal fetuses[13] is associated with increased incidence of pulmonary hypoplasia. The mechanism by which oligohydramnios alters

TABLE 7.1.   Fetal obstructive uropathy: classification of 43 deaths by primary etiology

| Etiology of Death | Time of Death | | | | | |
| | Prenatal | | Postnatal | | Total | |
	No.	%	No.	%	No.	%
Elective pregnancy termination	11	25.6	—	0	11	25.6
Associated anomalies	1	2.3	—	—	1	2.3
Procedure related	2	4.6	1	2.3	3	6.9
Pulmonary hypoplasia	—	0	27	62.8	27	62.8
Chronic renal failure	—	0	1	2.3	1	2.3
Total	14	32.5	29	67.5	43	100

(From Manning et al.,[11] with permission.)

lung growth is unknown but is suspected to be the result of direct thoracic compression by the uterus. Direct lung compression is known to inhibit normal lung growth.[14] There must also be other factors for this pathological association, however, as lethal pulmonary hypoplasia may be seen with incomplete obstruction to urine flow.[11]

In the normal fetus, the bladder is the only normal reservoir for fetal urine. Serial ultrasound observation of bladder volume demonstrates a pattern of filling and emptying and periodic active micturition[15,16] (Fig. 7.1). The observation of a fetal bladder strongly suggests that fetal urine production is present, but the observation of emptying and then refilling of the bladder virtually ensures that urine production is occurring. This observation is of some major clinical importance in differentiating oligohydramnios due to dysmature intrauterine growth retardation (IUGR) from that seen with renal agensis/dysgenesis syndrome. Obstruction of urine flow with the collecting system will cause progressive dilatation proximal to the obstruction; accordingly, the extent and site of obstruction can be deduced from the pattern of proximal dilatation.

SPECIFIC UROGENITAL TRACT ANOMALIES

Congenital Hydronephrosis

Hydronephrosis is a condition characterized by the abnormal accumulation of urine within the collecting system of the kidney and by definition always results from an obstructive process. In the fetus, isolated hydronephrosis is nearly always the result of a congenital functional stricture in the immediate proximal portion of the ureter. This disease process, termed ureteropelvic junction obstruction (UPJ syndrome) is the most common congenital urinary

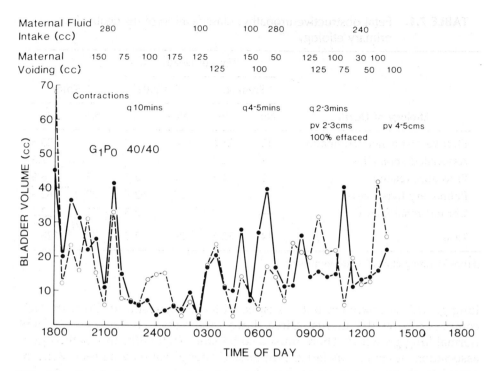

FIG. 7.1 Serial observation of fetal bladder volume made at 30-minute intervals over a 24-hour period in a low-risk primigravid patient at term. The matched paired observation reflects the results obtained by two independent observers. Both short-term and long-term (24-hour) periodic variation in bladder filling and emptying are seen. (From Chamberlain et al.,[15] with permission.)

tract lesion, accounting for up to 40 percent of recognized anomalies of this organ system.[3] The characteristic pathophysiology evolves as the result of a functional disturbance in either the initiation or the propagation of the normal peristatic activity within the ureter. In most cases, no anatomic stricture of the ureter may be identified. Histologic examination of the ureter reveals signs of chronic inflammation in the mucosa and submucosa and disruption and disorganization of collagen fibers and muscle in the wall of the ureter. The etiology for this functional derangement is unknown.

This disease process serves as a classic example of the interaction between function and structure in the kidney; the hallmark ultrasound signs are a result of this interaction. The obstruction produces proximal dilatation, the magnitude of which will vary with the degree of obstruction. In the normal state, the renal pelvis may be seen as a small echolucent area (less than 1 cm in diameter) and the proximal ureter is only occasionally seen, probably only during a peristaltic wave (Fig. 7.2). Mild functional obstruction causes renal pelvic dilatation only, usually best defined by a subjective impression, although a diameter of greater than 1 cm is used in some classifications.[3] Progressive degrees of obstruction cause further renal pelvis enlargement

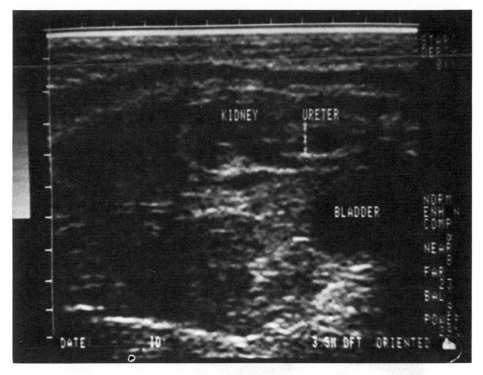

FIG 7.2.   Coronal scan of thorax and abdomen of a 32-week fetus. The fetal kidney is well visualized and renal parenchyma seen. The renal pelvis contains a small amount of urine, and the fetal ureter in its proximal portion is visualized. The fetal bladder is of normal size and contains fetal urine.

and dilation of major and minor calyces (Fig. 7.3). Thinning of the renal parenchyma and kidney enlargement are very unusual events with this disease and are signs of very severe obstruction. Marked reduction or absence of fetal urine production is not a feather of this disease process; accordingly, amniotic fluid volume reduction is not associated with the disease. This is of some clinical importance, since oligohydramnios with suspect UPJ disease implies either a second disease process (e.g., dysmature IUGR) or a misdiagnosis (e.g., bilateral multicystic dysplastic disease). Occasionally, increased amniotic fluid volume is reportedly assumed to be the result of extrinsic compression of the retroperitoneal portion of the duodenum by an enlarged renal pelvis.[17] Repetitive renocentesis has been used successfully to ameliorate this condition.[17,18]

The time of onset of ultrasound signs of the disease process is variable with most cases recognized in late mid-gestation (greater than 24 weeks). Similarly, the natural history of the disease process is variable. In our experience of the last 33 cases of UPJ disease diagnosed in utero, we noted that in 5 cases (15 percent) spontaneous resolution occurred, and in the remaining

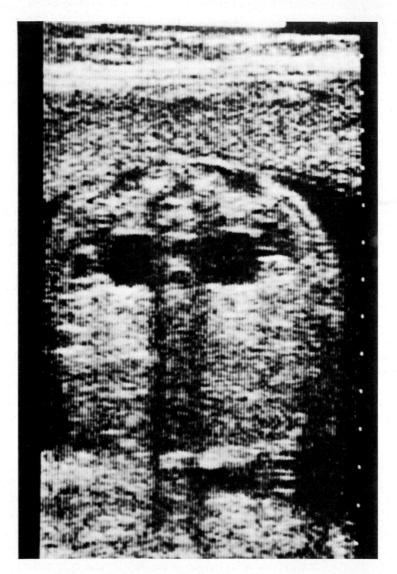

FIG. 7.3. Transverse scan of the fetal abdomen at the level of the kidneys. This fetus exhibits moderately severe bilateral ureteropelvic obstruction syndrome. Note that both renal pelvices are dilated (diameter 1.5 to 2.0 cm); dilation of the calyces is also evident. The kidney size is not increased and renal parenchymal architecture is normal. Amniotic fluid volume is normal, indicating adequate fetal urine production. The prognosis for such lesions is excellent, and intervention for fetal indications is only rarely indicated.

28 cases the disease either remained stable or progressed slowly. We did not have any cases in which rapid progression necessitated obstetrical intervention. The disease process was unilateral in most of these cases (82 percent). In the study group, we found no evidence of a hereditary basis for the disease although in other studies a multifactorial inheritance pattern has been suspected.[3]

Appropriate management of UPJ disease should include serial ultrasound monitoring at a frequency of 4 to 6 weeks and conservative management of nonprogressive or slowly progressive disease. Neonatal and infant follow-up is required for affected infants.

Primary Renal Anomalies: Ultrasound Characteristics

Congenital anomalies involving the kidney(s) may present as a broad spectrum of pathology ranging from isolated segmental lesions to diffuse bilateral lethal disease. Renal lesions present as among the most difficult diagnostic and management challenges. The functional unit, the glomerulus and the collecting system, develops concurrently from different primordia and eventually fuses to form the functioning urinary tract. Renal anomalies may involve the glomerular unit, the collecting system within the kidney, or both. Provided the glomerular unit is functioning, congenital anomalies of the kidney will always result in abnormal accumulation of urine within the kidney. However, if the glomerular unit is nonfunctioning, the characteristic features will be the absence of urine production, manifested in turn by the ultrasound signs of absence of fetal bladder filling and a reduction in amniotic fluid volume. These two types of pathology account for most of the pathologic ultrasound signs of renal parenchymal disease and form the basis for establishing the differential diagnosis.

Segmental anomalies of the glomerular units, which may be unilateral or bilateral and may be single or multiple, are characterized by the absence of communication of the glomerular unit and the collecting system. Localized disease will present as an isolated echolucent intrarenal cyst of variable size (Fig. 7.4). Multiple lesions will present as multiple cysts distributed throughout the renal parenchyma (Fig. 7.5). Differentiation of renal cyst(s) from UPJ disease is not difficult, achieved by noting the location of the cyst(s) and the absence of the typical pattern of renal pelvis and calyceal dilation. Simple renal cysts are not associated with increased echodensity of the noncystic parenchyma, nor are they associated with overall significant reduction in urine production and flow. Accordingly, single cystic disease is not characterized by either absence of bladder filling or oligohydramnios. Extensive simple cyst formation involving major portions of the renal prenchyma, can cause reduced amniotic fluid volume and may be associated with pulmonary hypoplasia.

Confirming these observations is of major importance in differentiating the condition from the much more serious and often lethal conditions of

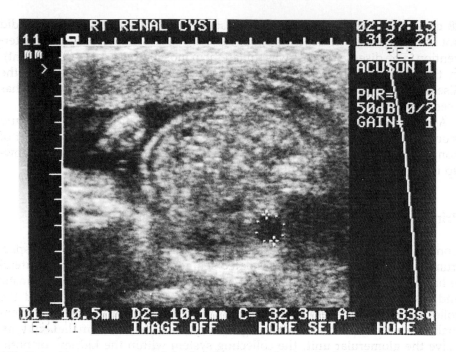

FIG. 7.4. Transverse scan of fetal abdomen at the level of the kidneys. The left kidney is normal, with normal parenchyma and the renal pelvis just visualized. In the right kidney, a single cyst of about 1 cm diameter is observed within the renal cortex. The remaining cortex and medulla are normal. Note the presence of a normal amount of amniotic fluid. Single renal cysts are not known to cause fetal compromise and are not an indication for intervention. The most likely etiology for these lesions is isolated obstruction of a minor calyx.

multicystic dysplastic disease. The appropriate fetal management of single renal cysts is observation only by serial ultrasound assessment. Obstetric intervention for fetal indication is not required.

Primary renal parenchymal anomalies are a result of abnormal glomerular unit development and presents as a wide clinical spectrum ranging from complete absence, renal agenesis, to varying degrees to glomerular unit disorganization, renal dysgenesis. Renal dysgenesis is characterized by the presence of heterotopic tissue and foci of reactive and metaplastic tubular and glomerular epithelium termed renal dysplasia. In its extreme form, renal dysplasia presents as nonfunctioning glomerular units; in less extreme forms, some function of the glomerular unit persists, creating multiple parenchymal cysts of varying size and distribution. Renal dysplasia may be focal, unilateral, or bilateral. Although unproved, it is most likely renal dysplasia as a pathologic consequence of obstruction to urine egress.[6,7] The ultrasound diagnosis of agenesis/dysgenesis syndromes is based on both assessment of renal parenchymal anatomy and/or the functional sequelae, absence of amniotic fluid volume.

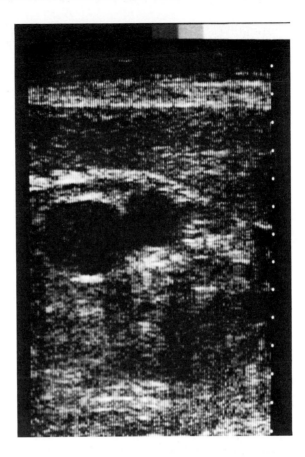

FIG. 7.5. Longitudinal view of a left fetal kidney demonstrating two large cysts within the renal parenchyma. On serial section, multiple simple cysts of varying size were distributed throughout the kidney. Note the absence of foci of increased echogenicity and the presence of oligohydramnios. These findings are typical of severe simple multicystic renal disease (polycystic kidney).

Renal agenesis, usually referred to clinically as Potter syndrome, manifests as a constellation of features invariably including IUGR; usually severe, pulmonary hypoplasia, and in later gestation (more then 16 weeks) by oligohydramnios that is often profound and associated with compression deformities of the fetal face and limbs. The pathognomonic feature of advanced disease and the usual ultrasound tipoff is the oligohydramnios reflecting the absence of the functional unit. The time of onset of oligohydramnios is variable, since up to about 14 to 16 weeks gestation, alternate sources of amniotic fluid including the fetal skin and umbilical cord surfaces are still active. Accordingly, a previous ultrasound report of normal amniotic fluid volume before 14 to 16 weeks does not exclude a subsequent diagnosis of renal agenesis. A filled fetal bladder may be seen from as early as 12 weeks gestation, and when observed at any stage of gestation, excludes the diagnosis of renal agenesis. Confirmation by ultrasonography of the presence of renal parenchyma can be difficult, since confusion with the adjacent fetal adrenal tissue can occur. Further definitive exclusion of renal tissue at the level of certainty needed to avoid any actions of fetal benefit is a very difficult and error-prone isolated ultrasound diagnosis. Finally, in later disease, the presence of oligohydramnios renders visualization of the renal fossae and their contents extremely difficult.

The more advanced the gestation, the more difficult the diagnosis of renal agenesis and the more critical the differential diagnosis. Before about 22 weeks gestation, the observation of sustained severe oligohydramnios due to causes other than rupture of membranes and amniotic fluid leakage carries an extremely poor perinatal prognosis. In our clinical experience, we have never seen fetal survival in such circumstances. This observation is of some practical clinical importance, as it implies that the degree of certainty by which the diagnosis of renal agenesis is made may be less critical in the younger fetus, with poor outcome almost certain. However, diagnosis of oligohydramnios beyond the fetal age of potential extrauterine survival (more than 24 weeks) requires thorough investigation to exclude the diagnosis of severe dysmature IUGR. This differentiation is crucial, since the prognosis, hence the management of the two conditions, is diametrically opposed. Aggressive intervention for fetal indications with severe dysmature IUGR may be life-saving, whereas any intervention for renal agenesis is without merit from the perinatal viewpoint. Both conditions are associated with abnormalities of the functional component, urine production, but for radically different reasons. Urine production with renal agensis is absent because the functional units are absent whereas with dysmature IUGR the units are present, but their function is severely depressed. With dysmature IUGR, the depression of functional activity is either a result of reduced perfusion (a consequence of hypoxemia induced aortic arch chemoreceptor-mediated redistribution of cardiac output) or a response to elevated vasopressin levels or both.[19,20] One major ultrasound-based key to this critical differentiation is observation of bladder filling and emptying.

Ultrasound detection of a fetal bladder, possible only when it contains fluid (urine), virtually excludes the diagnosis of renal agenesis. On a cautionary note, however, we have erroneously assumed a pelvic cystic mass to be fetal bladder and intervened; the neonate died of pulmonary hypoplasia and at autopsy demonstrate renal agenesis and a large solitary pedunculated hepatic cyst in the fetal pelvis (Manning FA, Harman CR: unpublished observation, 1986). Failure to observe a fetal bladder at initial examination does not exclude the diagnosis of severe dysmaturity, since with severe disease, fetal urine production may be extremely reduced. In such instances, serial observation at 30-minute intervals over a 4- to 6-hour period may be needed to exclude the presence of renal function confidently. In the normal fetus, the maximal interval for which the bladder did not contain urine and therefore was not visible by ultrasound was 30 minutes.[15] The administration of the potent diuretic, furosemide, to the mother in anticipation of transplacental passage and a direct stimulation of urine production by the fetal kidney has been reported as a diagnostic method to assess functional integrity of fetal renal parenchyma.[21,22] The clinical validity of this Lasix challenge test in differentiating congenital renal dysfunction from superimposed pathologic supression of function is subject to serious challenge. Wladimiroff[21] reported an 80 to 150 percent rise in fetal hourly urine production after the mother was given 60 mg of furosemide intravenously. Similar increase in bladder volume in the absence of maternal diuretics are reported by Chamberlain et al.[15] (Fig. 7.1). In the chronic fetal lamb model, maternal admistration of large doses of furosemide (up to 2 mg/kg) caused a significant increase in fetal urine osmolality and if anything a slight reduction in urine production.[23] Furthermore, furosemide could not be detected in the fetal sera. In the human, the placental pharmicokinetics of furosemide have not be studied systematically and, despite claims of some investigators,[22] the transplacental passage of this diuretic remains unproved. Finally, maternal furosemide may not provoke urine production in the compromised fetus or newborn.[24,25] Thus, the definitive test to exclude renal function and thereby confirm renal agenesis remains elusive. The advent of ultrasound-guided cordocentesis now renders direct fetal intravenous infusion of diuretics a diagnostic possibility. In the normoxic fetal lamb, furosemide given directly causes a prompt and significant diuresis.[23] The advantages, if any, of this method in the human fetus remain untested. The infusion of warmed normal saline into the amniotic cavity to improve visualization of the fetus and its renal fossae is an as yet unproved diagnostic method.

The multicystic dysplastic renal parenchymal anomaly falls within the spectrum of congenital renal dysgenesis and is characterized by the aberrant preservation of some glomerular functional units. The lesion, which may be focal, unilateral, or bilateral, is presumed to be the result of early and sustained obstruction to urine egress occurring within either the renal substance or the collecting system. Both the metaplastic and dysplastic histologic disruption of renal cortex creates the typical ultrasound features of the disease. The residual functional glomerular units continue to produce small quantities of fetal urine causing multiple cysts of varying size, shape, and location (Fig. 7.6). Renal parenchymal volume, hence kidney size, may be increased, and frequently the kidney appears to be lobulated with distorted surface architecture. Both the condensed metaplastic tissue and the foci of heterotopic tissue, often cartilaginous in structure, produce intense echodense areas within the kidney (Fig. 7.6). Occasionally, calcification of these sites occurs, creating very bright echodensities with acoustical shadowing.

The functional impact of multicystic dysplastic renal disease will vary directly with the extent of disease. Focal or unilateral disease will not alter amniotic fluid volume production significantly; accordingly, the lesion poses little direct threat to the fetus. In such cases, expectant fetal management is indicated. After delivery, detailed urologic investigation is needed, and excision is usually recommended. Bilateral disease presents in the same clinical manner as renal agenesis, that is, with oligohydramnios and an extreme risk of lethal pulmonary hypoplasia. Bilateral disease in the absence of overt extrarenal obstruction carries an extremely poor prognosis, active intervention for fetal indication is not recommended. Assessment and management of bilateral disease in the presence of overt extrarenal obstruction pose a more difficult clinical dilemma. In the ovine fetus, subsequent release of experimen-

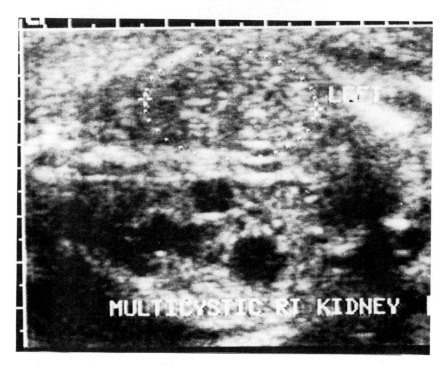

FIG. 7.6.   Tangential view of both kidneys in the coronal plane. Note that the left kidney exhibits normal size, surface architecture, and parenchymal structure. Multiple cysts of varying size, shape, and distribution are noted in the enlarged right kidney. The surface architecture of the right kidney is grossly abnormal, and the kidney is enlarged. The parenchymal architecture is distorted with areas of enchodensity. Amniotic fluid volume was normal. These findings are typical of unilateral multicystic dysplasia disease, a diagnosis confirmed after delivery of this fetus.

tal ureter obstruction can ameliorate the progression of multicystic dysplastic degeneration.[7] In the human fetus with bilateral disease and extrarenal obstruction, the major challenge is to determine whether sufficient normal renal function exists. Chemical constituent analysis of fetal urine obtained by ultrasound-guided vesicocentesis is advocated by some as a method of determining functional integrity of the kidney. Glick et al.[26] reported this experience with functional assessment in 20 human fetuses with congenital bilateral hydronephrosis, using serial aliquots of fetal urine obtained by placement of a temporary bladder catheter in utero. These workers noted uniform poor outcome when urine sodium was greater than 100 mEq/d1, urine chloride was greater than 90 mEq/dl and when urine osmolarity exceeds 210 mOsm. Fetal urine iodothalamate excretion and potassium and creatinine concentration were not found to be reliable markers. The predictive value of these fetal urine constituents in selecting those fetuses with good versus poor renal function is subject to serious challenge, as the studies are not controlled and intervention was based in part on these results.

Congenital infantile polycystic kidney is a familial condition of an autosomal-recessive inheritance pattern in which the collecting tubules within the medulla exhibit progressive obstruction. The characteristic ultrasound features are bilateral progressive symmetric renomegaly often of such massive proportion that the kidneys fill most of the abdomen and the preservation of normal, but generally echolucent, renal architecture. The obstructed tubules create microcysts that are not detectable by conventional ultrasound methods. Fetal urine production varies but is usually present, and amniotic fluid volume is normal or low normal. Maternal serum and amniotic α-fetoprotein (AFP) levels are usually markedly elevated. The perinatal prognosis is poor, and active intervention for fetal indication is not indicated.

Obstructive Uropathies

The ultrasound hallmarks of obstructive uropathy are fetal bladder enlargement, hydroureter, hydronephrosis either simple or with dysplastic degeneration, and frequently, but not invariably, a reduction in amniotic fluid volume. The diagnostic and management dilemmas are not in recognizing the presence of the disease process but are rather in determining the etiology and the pathophysiologic consequences. The significance of this assessment is now sharply focused, since active intervention in the form of chronic in utero urinary diversion therapy is now available. The true obstructive uropathies are almost always due to one of three conditions (Table 7.2). Posterior urethral valve syndrome (PUV disease) is a disease of male fetuses and results

TABLE 7.2.   Fetal obstructive uropathy: primary diagnosis and outcome in 73 treated cases[a]

Primary Diagnosis	No. of Cases	% of Total	No. of Survivors	% Survival by Diagnosis
Posterior urethral valve syndrome	21	28.8	16	76.2
Karyotype abnormality[a]	6	8.2	0	0
Renal dysplasia by ultrasound[a]	5	6.8	0	0
Urethral atresia	5	6.8	1	20
Prune belly syndrome	3	4.1	3	100
Unknown etiology	33	45.3	10	30.3
Total	73	100%	30	41%

[a] Elective pregnancy termination.
(From Manning et al.,[11] with permission.)

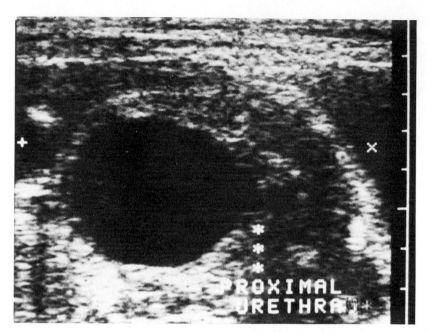

FIG. 7.7.   Expanded view of a distended fetal bladder and proximal urethra resulting from posterior urethral valve syndrome. Note the symmetry of the bladder distention, with an increase in bladder wall thickness. The dilated proximal urethra is well visualized.

from mucosal folds or values that occlude the proximal portion of the posterior urethra (Fig. 7.7). The obstruction may be complete or partial and may be sustained or transient. Characteristically, the proximal posterior urethra becomes dilated to the site of obstruction, and the fetal bladder wall becomes initially hypertrophied and ultimately distended and thin walled. The ureters become dilated and tortuous, and hydronephrosis is observed. With sustained obstruction, oligohydramnios is observed, and urachal cyst formation occasionally occurs. Urethral atresia is a result of failure of canalization of the urethra that affects both male and female fetuses. The obstruction is always complete, and therefore oligohydramnios is the rule. Massive bladder dilation and hydroureter occur and multicystic dysplastic renal parenchymal disease is common. *Persistent cloacal syndrome* is characterized by the development of a pelvic cystic mass, ambiguous genitalia, and progressive hydroureter/hydronephrosis. In our experience, urachal cyst formation is very common with this condition.

The natural history of these obstructive uropathies is not well studied to date. However, with at least two of these conditions, PUV syndrome and persistent cloacal syndrome, spontaneous resolution of the obstructive component may occur. We have observed complete resolution of posterior ureteral valve syndrome with intact perinatal survival and have also seen urachal cyst rupture with persistent cloacal syndrome with subsequent resolution of hydronephrosis and hydroureter and perinatal survival. Furthermore, the relationship among obstructive uropathies, amniotic fluid volume, and lethal pulmonary hypoplasia is unclear. Whereas most cases of pulmonary hypoplasia in these conditions are associated with oligohydramnios, lethal pulmonary hypoplasia is also reported when amniotic fluid volume is normal.[10] At least three nonobstructive anomalies of the genitourinary tract may present with similar ultrasound features of obstructive uropathy. Massive bilateral ureteral reflux may cause hydroureter and hydronephrosis. Fetal bladder size is usually normal in such cases, although bladder wall hypertrophy may be observed. Amniotic fluid volume is characteristically normal with ureteral reflux syndrome. The megalocystis-microcolon-intestinal hyperperistalsis syndrome (MMIH syndrome) is a rare uniformly lethal condition of unknown etiology affecting primarily female perinates and characterized by abnormalies of smooth muscle development. Ultrasound features include megacystis, hydroureter of usually massive proportions, and bilateral hydronephrosis. Amniotic fluid volume is characteristically normal. The lesion cannot be easily differentiated from partial obstructive uropathies. Finally prune belly syndrome, a condition characterized by megacystis, hydroureter, variable degrees of hydronephrosis, and absence of abdominal wall musculature, can masquerade as obstructive uropathy. The key in ultrasound recognition of this condition lies in assessing the abdominal wall. The presence of a thin, distended, and undulant abdominal wall is a key feature of this disease.

FETAL SURGERY FOR OBSTRUCTIVE UROPATHY: CASE-SELECTION CRITERIA AND METHODS

The selection of those very few fetuses who might benefit from in utero surgical urinary tract diversion procedures may be best achieved by the application of rigid exclusion criteria, few of which have been yet subjected to rigorous scientific scrutiny. Despite the optimistic enthusiasm of the fetal surgeon, there can be little doubt that neonatal repair of obstructive uropathies will almost always be a safer and more definitive procedure. Therefore, as the first principle, the fetus of sufficient age and maturity to sustain extrauterine survival should never be a candidate for in utero surgery. Whereas this point may now seem obvious, the reader is reminded that within the International Fetal Surgery Registry, in utero procedures for obstructive uropathy had been done at a gestational age as late as 36 weeks.[11] With hindsight, this would now seem quite inappropriate. A second principle should be that the therapy would only be considered in the fetus with bladder outlet obstruction and bilateral progressive renal disease. The primary aim of therapy is to prevent both the renal and the pulmonary sequelae. It can be said, albeit facetiously, that there is no fetal body cavity that cannot be reached, provided that the surgeon's needle and courage are long enough. However, striking the fetus with a needle, even when done by an experienced surgeon using the most sophisticated ultrasound guidance systems, is not without risk. Obstetricians have accumulated a large experience with needle penetration of the fetal peritoneal cavity and a lesser experience with bladder puncture; for either method, the fetal death rate directly attributable to the procedure is about 5 percent.[11,27] Therefore the issues must not be whether therapy is possible, for it nearly always is, but rather if such therapy will benefit the fetus and does this potential benefit outweigh any real fetal risk. Against this background the justification of prenatal therapy for unilateral disease, as has been reported[18] may be lacking, although in some cases an apparent amelioration of associated maternal disease has been described.[17,26]

The fetus with both obstructive uropathy and some other organ system structural anomaly or karyotypic anomaly should not be considered a candidate for prenatal therapy. This association is not uncommon; of 72 treated cases reported to the International Fetal Surgery Registry, five (7 percent) had multiple organ system anomalies, and six (8 percent) had karyotypic anomalies[11] (Table 7.2). Thus, 11 of 72 fetuses (15 percent) had lethal anomalies, a rate 15 to 30 times higher than that of the general population. Although maternal morbidity has not been described as a complication of in utero therapy for obstructive uropathy, severe maternal morbidity or death has been caused by other invasive intrauterine procedures such amniocentesis[29] and intrauterine transfusion.[30] Serious and potentially life-threatening maternal infection (chorioamnionitis) has been reported as a consequence of diagnostic or therapeutic maternal percutaneous placement of a fetal bladder catheter.[26] It follows that a very detailed and complete ultrasound fetal organ system review should be a prerequisite to any therapeutic efforts. In theory, such a review should detect all associated structural anomalies; in practice, the detection rate is about 90 percent.[2] Confirmation that the affected fetus considered for therapy had a normal karyotype has been a more difficult problem, since the traditional diagnostic method, amniocentesis for amniocyte culture, requires a waiting time of up to 4 weeks for results. Furthermore, in the presence of oligohydramnios, a frequent associated finding with obstructive uropathy, an amniotic fluid sample may not be obtainable. In such cases, fetal urine obtained by vesicocentesis may yield sufficient cells for culture,[9] but the reliability of this method is not uniform and, again, considerable delay is involved. The new technique of direct fetal umbilical vein blood sampling[31] yielding karyotype results as early as 2 days later will most certainly be the method to circumvent these problems. The clinical value, if any, of the measurement of fetal plasma creatinine or BUN, or of fetal glomerular filtration rate (GFR) measurement in selecting cases suitable for fetal surgery is unknown, but such determination is now technically feasible by this new method.

The relationship between amniotic fluid volume, as estimated by ultrasound, and outcome in fetuses with obstructive uropathy is unclear, therefore, the use of this variable for case selection remains controversial. Since fetal urine production is a major contributor to the dynamic amniotic fluid compartment in later pregnancy,[32] it would follow that significant fetal obstructive disease should be associated with a reduction or absence of amniotic fluid (oligohydramnios). The data contained in the International Fetal Surgery

TABLE 7.3. Relationship of amniotic fluid volume to perinatal survival in treated cases of fetal obstructive uropathy

Amniotic Fluid Volume	No. of Cases	% of Total Cases	No. of Survivors	% Survival
Normal	15	21	6	40
Oligohydramnios	57	78	23	41
No recorded	1	1	1	100

(From Manning et al.,[11] with permission.)

Registry do not support this supposition; whereas most fetuses with obstructive uropathy do have oligohydramnios (78 percent), survival rates are similar among treated fetuses with or without oligohydramnios (41 percent and 40 percent, respectively)[11] (Table 7.3). Furthermore, perinatal death due to pulmonary hypoplasia is observed among fetuses with obstructive uropathy and apparent normal amniotic fluid volume. The discrepancy between the predicted and observed relationships of amniotic fluid volume to perinatal outcome in fetuses with obstructive uropathy may be due to a variety of factors. Amniotic fluid volume determination by ultrasonography is often done by subjective assessment, and the use of objective criteria such as the largest fluid pocket measurement has not been uniform.[33] Under such subjective conditions, the true relationship remains uncertain. Alternately, in fetuses with partial or incomplete obstruction, there may be sufficient outflow impedance to cause proximal dilation and damage, while urine efflux may be enough to maintain some amniotic fluid. Pulmonary hypoplasia is by far the most common cause of perinatal death in obstructive uropathies, accounting for 81 percent of deaths among treated pregnancies.[11] Chronic oligohydramnios, both in the experimental animal model and in the human, is associated with an increased incidence of lethal pulmonary hypoplasia.[12,13] It is tempting to suggest that the high incidence of pulmonary hypoplasia seen in fetuses with obstructive uropathy is therefore caused by this oligohydramnios. In the experimental animal model, reversal of experimental oligohydramnios restores lung growth and prevents pulmonary hypoplasia,[13] and a similar recovery of lung growth is seen with corrected experimental obstructive uropathy.[5] The clinical human experience also clearly indicates that in utero diversion therapy resulting in the restoration of normal amniotic fluid volume may be associated with intact survival, even in the presence of pretreatment extreme oligohydramnios.[9,34] Thus, despite reported opinions to the contrary,[35] there is simply no evidence that oligohydramnios is a contraindication to therapy. However, the observation of lethal pulmonary hypoplasia with obstructive uropathy, even in the presence of normal amniotic fluid volume, indicates there must be more than one etiologic factor for pulmonary hypoplasia. Intrinsic pulmonary compression due to bladder and urinary

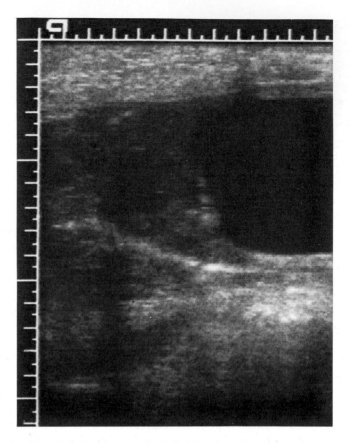

FIG. 7.8.   Coronal view of fetal chest and abdomen in a fetus with extreme bladder distention secondary to urethral atresia. The fetal kidneys are not well visualized, suggesting major renal dysgenesis/agensis. The fetal thorax is compressed by the abdominal mass. The fetal heart occupies most of the chest (approx. 70 percent) and minimal pulmonary tissue is seen. These findings are suggestive, but not diagnostic, of associated pulmonary hypoplasia.

tract dilation may be another cause; diaphragmatic hernia, either experimental or clinical, is known to cause pulmonary hypoplasia by this method[14] (Fig. 7.8). Again, in such circumstances, urinary tract decompression by in utero diversion therapy may be expected to enhance lung growth and therefore improve survival. An alternate explanation for the association of lung and urinary tract anomalies is that the primary insult, the nature of which remains entirely unknown, affects the endodermal lung primordia and the mesodermal genitourinary primordia simultaneously. Such a mechanism, while possible, is viewed as highly unlikely, since most teratogens affect either all germ cell layers or a single layer, but rarely if ever affect only two of the three layers. Nonetheless, if such a mechanism is indeed operant then the theoretical argument for urinary tract diversion to prevent pulmonary hypoplasia are without foundation.

We have now begun to learn, at a very rapid rate, how to evaluate fetal renal function; these data are becoming an integral part of individual case-selection criteria. Initial attempts to assess renal function were based on noninvasive measurement of fetal urine production rates.[16] These methods are not easily applied to the fetus with obstruction to the urinary tract and have not been of much benefit in case selection. Invasive evaluation of the fetal urinary tract, by ultrasound-guided percutaneous fetal bladder aspiration, is now the key step in individual case selection. Temporary external drainage of the fetal bladder permits accurate measurement of fetal urine production rates, estimation of fetal GFR by a creatinine or iothalamate excretion, and urine electrolyte composition.[26] These methods are being abandoned, however, since the risk of perinatal infection is high (6 percent)[26] and have been replaced by a single procedure of needle aspiration and urine electrolyte composition determination.[36] Fetal urine is produced from as early as 13 weeks gestation and is an ultrafiltrate of fetal serum made hypotonic by selective tubular absorption of sodium and chloride. In the fetus with intact renal function, the urinary sodium is always less than 100 mEq/dl the chloride less than 90 mEq/dl, and the osmolality less then 200 mOsm/L. Fetal urine values above these levels are associated with poor renal function and perinatal loss.[36] Methods for prenatal detection of lethal pulmonary hypoplasia remain to be elucidated, although preliminary results by determination of lung density by ultrasound appear promising (Harman CR: personal communication, 1986).

The question remains: Does the karyotypic and otherwise structurally normal immature fetus with sustained outflow tract obstruction and bilateral urinary tract dilation with known intact renal function and assumed pulmonary tissue benefit from in utero urinary tract diversion—so-called fetal surgery? The rationale for fetal surgery would be to prevent progression of associated renal and/or pulmonary damage, thereby reducing the risk of stillbirth or immediate neonatal death (pulmonary hypoplasia). The development of the field of perinatal medicine is now advanced to the point where such highly selected fetuses can be identified with some certainty. The empirical answer to the critical question, based on experimental ovine fetal models and anecdotal clinical reports, would be affirmative. The specific human data base to support this contention beyond refute does not exist. The 73 treated cases of fetal obstructive uropathy recently reported offer incomplete evidence to support this premise, since this group of fetuses have disease of diverse etiology and documentation.[11] Furthermore, the potential for bias in any voluntary registry must be taken into account. Within this larger group of fetuses, however, may be the subset that carries the critical information. Twenty-one (28.8 percent) of the 73 treated cases reported to the Registry had an unequivocal diagnosis of posterior urethral valve syndrome (Table 7.2). These cases may be the best model in which to evaluate the benefit if any of fetal therapy, since the etiologic lesion was isolated and well described, was not associated with other karyotypic or structural anomalies, produced bilateral renal disease, and was usually associated with oligohydramnios.

The survival rate for this subset of treated fetuses was 76.2 percent (16 of 21 cases). The survival rate of comparable but nontreated fetuses is unknown but cannot be 0 percent, since comparable patients are well known to the pediatrician. However, the survival rate in neonates born with posterior urethral valve syndrome is sharply different. Nakayama et al.[37] identified 11 neonates in whom the diagnosis of posterior urethral valves was made at birth. Since these neonates were subjected to aggressive resuscitative measures, it may be assumed that this population represents only a portion of those perinates born with the condition. Others may have been denied the resuscitative measures because of the observed anomalies at birth. Five of these anomalous fetuses died (45 percent) either within hours (three cases) or within days (two cases) from respiratory insufficiency due to proven (four cases) or assumed (one case) pulmonary hypoplasia. All those children who perished exhibited extreme oligohydramnios in utero. These data, when compared with the outcome data of similar fetuses treated in utero, demonstrated a nearly twofold difference in mortality (45 percent to 22.8 percent mortality, respectively). Survival rates for posturethral valve syndrome in both treated fetuses and neonates are much lower than those reported among older children with this condition.[38,39] The powerful influence of natural selection in the prenatal period no doubt accounts for these differences. The long-term morbidity of survivors in the two groups also varies sharply. All untreated survivors with this condition exhibited serious morbidity: four of six survivors had prolonged respiratory insufficiency suggestive of sublethal pulmonary hypoplasia, and five of six survivors had signs of chronic renal impairment as evidenced by azotemia, defects in fixed acid excretion, and growth failure. By contrast, none of the 16 survivors of in utero therapy exhibited clinical signs of respiratory insufficiency, and only one developed chronic renal failure. The long-term outcome of these cases is unknown and must be determined, since late-onset renal disease is described with this condition.[40] Comparison of the outcome data between these somewhat similar groups presents a powerful argument for the benefit of in utero surgery for the posterior urethral valve syndrome in this limited and carefully defined group of patients. It may be argued that, in view of the serious nature of the condition of the newborn, that the disease in utero is unlikely to be less severe. Whether such comparisons established the benefit of in utero therapy beyond a reasonable doubt remains a moot point. The definitive scientific evidence can only be garnered by a prospective trial in which diagnosed in utero cases are randomly assigned to a treated or nontreated category. However, in view of the rather clear animal experimental evidence delineating the pathophysiology of the condition, the observed differences in perinatal outcome between treated fetuses and neonates born with the condition, and anecdotal reports of successful outcome in treated fetuses, the ethics of such a trial for this specific condition may be seriously challenged. The issue is now before the medical community, to be resolved by collaborative communication among prenatal diagnosticians, therapists, and pediatric urologists.

The optimal method of in utero therapy, when elected, is not well defined. Percutaneous placement of a chronic vesico amniotic shunt would seem at first glance to be the method of choice. The procedure carries minimal maternal risks and does not require a reproductive debilitating uterine scar. The method is not without serious fetal risk, however, carrying a risk of fetal death of up to about 5 percent per procedure. In experienced hands, shunt placement is usually not difficult, but prolonged shunt patency remains a problem. These shunts are susceptible to occlusion, due to kinking, plugging with cellular debris, or tissue overgrowth. The shunts are also susceptible to migration with fetal growth and may even be removed by the fetus. Under dynamic ultrasound imaging, we have watched a fetus reach down, grasp, and pull out a vesicoamniotic shunt. Improving the shunt design by altering shape, size, and perforations and adding retaining flanges may overcome these technical problems.

Direct fetal repair or diversion is the alternate method of therapy. Methods that have been described include percutaneous ureterostomies[10] and vesicostomy.[36] Urethral valvectomy is theoretically possible but is yet to be reported. Direct fetal procedures require maternal general anesthesia, laparotomy, and hysterotomy, which no doubt carry real maternal risks. Furthermore, the hysterotomy scar will require operative delivery for all subsequent pregnancies, a serious concern in view of the low repetitive frequency of these fetal disorders. The fetal risks of an open procedure are not well defined but are likely to be considerable. Foremost among these risks is that of premature delivery due to the uterine incision. Although controversial, it would appear that the percutaneous method is the prudent route to consider.

SUMMARY

The role of ultrasound in detecting fetal anomalies in general and genitourinary tract anomalies in particular has undergone, and continues to undergo, remarkable changes. The diagnostic process began with a focus on the structural nature of anomalies and now has moved forward to include a detailed assessment of the functional nature and sequelae of these lesions. Concurrent with this shift in diagnostic emphasis has been the development of the role of ultrasonography in guiding invasive diagnostic procedures, such as percutaneous fetal blood sampling and fetal urine aspiration, and in guiding therapeutic procedures, such as chronic in utero vesicoamniotic shunt placement. These changes are occurring against a background of the role of ultrasound in assessing pathophysiology of the anomaly and assignment of prognosis, two decisions that profoundly influence pregnancy management. The challenge for the perinatal ultasonographer is now not only to recognize the lesion, but also to institute the further investigative steps upon which a rational management plan may be based. As illustrated in this brief review of the more common genitourinary tract anomalies, the range of outcome and the pathophysiologic progression of the disease are both wide and complex. Continued improvements in ultrasound technologies and application hold the key to the ultimate reduction in the clinical significance of these common fetal diseases.

REFERENCES

1. Morrison I, Olsen J: Weight-specific stillbirths and associated causes of death: An analysis of 765 stillbirths. Am J Obstet Gynecol 152:975, 1985

2. Manning FA, Morrison I, Lange IR, et al: Fetal assessment based on fetal biophysical profile scoring: Experience in 12,620 referred high risk pregnancies. I. Perinatal mortality by frequency and etiology. Am J Obstet Gynecol 151:343, 1985

3. Duval JM, Milon J, Coadou Y, et al: Ultrasonographic anatomy and diagnosis of fetal uropathies affecting the upper urinary tract. I. Obstructive uropathies. Anat Clin 7:301, 1985

4. Harrison MR, Ross N, Noall R, et al: Correction of congenital hydronephrosis in utero. I. The model: Fetal urethral obstruction produces hydronephrosis and pulmonary hyoplasia in fetal lambs. J Pediatr Surg 18:247, 1983

5. Harrison MR, Nakayama DK, Noall R, et al: Correction of congenital hydronephrosis in utero. II. Decompression measures the effects of obstruction on the fetal lung and urinary tract. J Pediatr Surg 17:965, 1982

6. Glick PL, Harrison MR, Noall R, et al: Correction of congenital hydronephrosis in utero. III. Early mid-trimester ureteral obstruction produces renal dysplasia. J Pediatr Surg 18:681, 1983

7. Glick PL, Harrison MR, Adzick NS, et al: Correction of congential hydronephrosis in utero. IV. In utero decompression prevents renal dysplasia. J Pediatr Surg 19:649, 1984

8. Avni EF, Rodesch F, Schulman CC: Fetal uropathies: Diagnostic pitfalls and management. J Urol 134:921, 1985

9. Manning FA, Harman CR, Lange IR, et al: Antepartum chronic fetal vesicoamniotic shunts for obstructive uropathy: A report of two cases. Am J Obstet Gynecol 145:819, 1983

10. Harrison MR, Golbus MS, Filly RA, et al: Fetal surgery for congenital hydronephrosis. N Engl J Med 306:591, 1982

11. Manning FA, Harrison MR, Rodeck C, et al: Catheter shunts for fetal hydronephrosis and hydrocephalus: Report of the International Fetal Surgery Registry. N Engl J Med 315:336, 1986

12. Nimrod CA, Varela-Gittings F, Machin G, et al: The effect of very prolonged membrane rupture on fetal development. Am J Obstet Gynecol 148:540, 1984

13. Nakayama DK, Glick PL, Harrison MR, et al: Experimental pulmonary hypoplasia due to oligohydramnios and its reversal by relieving thoracic compression. J Pediatr Surg 18:347, 1983

14. Harrison MR, Adzick NS, Nakayama DK: Fetal diaphragmatic hernia: Pathophysiology, natural history and outcome. Clin Obstet Gynecol 29:490, 1986

15. Chamberlain PF, Manning FA, Morrison I, et al: Circadian rhythm in bladder volumes in the term human fetus. Obstet Gynecol 64:657, 1984

16. Wladimiroff JW, Campbell S: Fetal urine production rates in normal and complicated pregnancies. Lancet 1:151, 1974

17. Seeds JW, Mandell J: Congenital obstructive uropathies: Pre and postnatal treatment. Urol Clin North Am 13:155, 1986

18. Kirkinen P, Joupila P, Tuononen S, et al: Repeated transabdominal renocentesis in a case of fetal hydronephrotic kidney. Am J Obstet Gynecol 142:1049, 1982

19. Cohn HE, Sacks EJ, Heyman MA, et al: Cardiovascular responses to hypoxemia and acidemia in fetal lambs. Am J Obstet Gynecol 120:817, 1974

20. Gomez AR, Meernick JG, Juehl WD, et al: Developmental aspects of the renal response to hemorrhage during fetal life. Pediatr Res 18:40, 1984

21. Wladimiroff JW: Effect of furosemide on fetal urine production. Br J Obstet Gynaecol 82:221, 1975

22. Barrett RJ, Rayburn WF, Barr M: Furosemide (Lasix) challenge test in assessing bilateral fetal nephrosis. Am J Obstet Gynecol 147:846, 1983

23. Chamberlain PF, Cumming M, Torschia M, et al: Ovine fetal urine production following maternal intravenous furosemide administration. Am J Obstet Gynecol 151:815, 1985

24. Harman CR: Maternal furosemide may not provoke urine production in the compromised fetus. Am J Obstet Gynecol 150:322, 1984

25. Yeh TF, Raval A, Shibili RS, et al: Poor diuretic response to furosemide in small premature infants (<2000 gms) with birth asphyxia. Proceedings of the Society of Pediatric Research, 1984 (abst)

26. Glick PL, Harrison MR, Golbus MS, et al: Management of the fetus with congenital hydronephrosis. II. Prognostic criteria and selection for treatment. J Pediatr Surg 20:376, 1985

27. Bowman JM, Manning FA: Intrauterine transfusion: Winnipeg 1982. Obstet Gynecol 61:203, 1983

28. Vintzileos AM, Nochimson DJ, Walzak MP, et al: Unilateral fetal hydronephrosis: Successful in utero surgical management. Am J Obstet Gynecol 145:885, 1983

29. Hasaart TA, Essed GG: Amniotic fluid embolism after transabdominal amniocentesis. Eur J Obstet Gynecol Reprod Biol 16:25, 1983

30. Bowman JM: Rh erythroblastosis foetalis 1975. Semin Hematol 12:189, 1975

31. Daffos F, Capella-Pavlovsky M, Forestier F: Fetal blood sampling during pregnancy with use of a needle guided by ultrasound. A study of 606 consecutive cases. Am J Obstet Gynecol 153:655, 1985

32. Seeds AE: Current concepts of amniotic fluid dynamics. Am J Obstet Gynecol 138:575, 1980

33. Chamberlain PF, Manning FA, Morrison I, et al: Ultrasound evaluation of amniotic fluid volume. I. The relationship of marginal and decreased amniotic fluid volume to perinatal outcome. Am J Obstet Gynecol 150:245, 1984

34. Shalev E, Weiner E, Feldman E, et al: External bladder-amniotic fluid shunt for fetal urinary test obstruction. Obstet Gynecol 63 (suppl):31, 1984

35. Thomas DF, Irving HC, Arthur RJ: Prenatal diagnosis: How useful is it. Br J Urol 57:784, 1985

36. Appelman Z, Golbus MS: The management of fetal urinary tract obstruction. Clin Obstet Gynecol 29:483, 1986

37. Nakayama DK, Harrison MR, de Lorimier AA: Prognosis of posterior urethral valve syndrome presenting at birth. J Pediatr Surg 21:43, 1986

38. Evins SC, Lorenzo RL: Posterior urethral valves: Current concepts in diagnosis and treatment. J Urol 121:76, 1979

39. Williams DI: Urethral valves: A hundred cases with hydronephrosis. Birth Defects 13:55, 1977

40. Warshaw BL, Edelbrook HH, Ehenger RB, et al: Progression to end stage renal disease in children with obstructive uropathy. J Pediatr 100:183, 1982

8 The Prenatal Diagnosis of Skeletal Dysplasias

ROBERTO ROMERO
MARINA SIRTORI

Skeletal dysplasias are a heterogeneous group of disorders of bone growth resulting in abnormal shape and size of the skeleton. The prenatal diagnosis of these disorders is a particularly challenging task. This chapter reviews the birth prevalence and classification of skeletal dysplasias and provides an approach to the diagnosis of conditions identifiable at birth.

BIRTH PREVALENCE AND CONTRIBUTION TO PERINATAL MORTALITY

The birth prevalence of skeletal dysplasias that are recognizable during the neonatal period has been estimated to be 2.4 per 10,000 births (95 percent confidence limits: 1.8 and 3.2 per 10,000 births).[1] These data come from an Italian multicentric monitoring system for birth defects in which newborns (stillbirths and live births) with limb shortness or limb trunk disproportion, delivered in 90 hospitals, were radiographed and photographed. The figures are based on 217,061 deliveries (215,392 live births and 1669 stillbirths). Among the 53 cases of skeletal dysplasias, 23 percent were stillbirths and 32 percent died during the first week of life. The overall frequency of skeletal dysplasias among perinatal deaths was 9.1 per 1,000 or 1 in 110.

The birth prevalence of the different skeletal dysplasias and their relative frequency among perinatal deaths is shown in Table 8.1.[1] The four most common skeletal dysplasias were thanatophoric dysplasia, achondroplasia, osteogenesis imperfecta, and achondrogenesis. Thanatophoric dysplasia and achondrogenesis accounted for 62 percent of all lethal skeletal dysplasias. The most common nonlethal skeletal dysplasia was achondroplasia.

TABLE 8.1. Birth prevalence (per 10,000 total births) of skeletal dysplasias

Skeletal Dysplasias	Birth Prevalence (per 10,000)	Frequency Among Perinatal Deaths
Thanatophoric dysplasia	0.69	1:246
Achondroplasia	0.37	—
Achondrogenesis	0.23	1:639
Osteogenesis imperfecta, type II	0.18	1:799
Osteogenesis imperfecta, other types	0.18	—
Asphyxiating thoracic dysplasia	0.14	1:3196
Chondrodysplasia punctata	0.09	—
Campomelic dysplasia	0.05	1:3196
Chondroectodermal dysplasia	0.05	1:3196
Larsen syndrome	0.05	—
Mesomelic dysplasia (Langer's type)	0.05	—
Others	0.46	1:800
Total skeletal dysplasias	2.44	1:110

(From Camera and Mastroiacovo,[1] with permission.)

CLASSIFICATION OF SKELETAL DYSPLASIAS

The existing nomenclature for skeletal dysplasias is complicated. There is a lack of uniformity about definition criteria. For example, some are referred to by eponyms (Ellis-van Creveld syndrome, Larsen dysplasia), by Greek terms describing a salient feature of the disease (*diastrophic* means twisted, *metatropic* means changeable), or by a term related to the presumed pathogenesis of the disease (osteogenesis imperfecta, achondrogenesis). The fundamental problem with any classification of skeletal dysplasias is that the pathogenesis of these diseases is largely unknown. Therefore, the current system relies on purely descriptive findings of either clinical or radiologic nature.

In an attempt to develop a uniform terminology, a group of experts met in Paris in 1977 and in 1982 and proposed an International Nomenclature for Skeletal Dysplasias. The system subdivides the diseases into five different groups: (1) osteochondrodysplasias (abnormalities of cartilage and/or bone growth and development), (2) dysostoses (malformations of individual bones, singly or in combination), (3) idiopathic osteolyses (disorders associated with multifocal resorption of bone), (4) skeletal disorders associated with chromosomal aberrations, and (5) primary metabolic disorders. Table 8.2 displays the International Classification of Constitutional Diseases of Bone.

TABLE 8.2. International classification for dysplasias[a]

	Inheritance	Frequency
Osteochondrodysplasias		
Abnormalities of cartilage and/or bone growth and development		
A. *Defects of growth of tubular bones and/or spine*		
a. *Identifiable at birth*		
α. Usually lethal before or shortly after birth		
1. Achondrogenesis type I (Parenti-Fraccaro)	AR	**
2. Achondrogenesis type II (Langer-Saldino)		**
3. Hypochondrogenesis		*
4. Fibrochondrogenesis	AR	*
5. Thanatophoric dysplasia		***
6. Thanatophoric dysplasia with cloverleaf skull		**
7. Atelosteogenesis		*
8. Short rib syndrome (with or without polydactyly)		
a. Type I (Saldino-Noonan)	AR	**
b. Type II (Majewski)	AR	*
c. Type III (lethal thoracic dysplasia)	AR	*
β. Usually nonlethal dysplasia		
9. Chondrodysplasia punctata		
a. Rhizomelic form autosomal recessive	AR	**
b. Dominant X-linked form; lethal in male	XLD	**
c. Common mild form (Sheffield)		***
Exclude: symptomatic stippling (warfarin, chromosomal aberration)		
10. Campomelic dysplasia	AR	**
11. Kyphomelic dysplasia	AR	*
12. Achondroplasia	AD	****
13. Diastrophic dysplasia	AR	***
14. Metatropic dysplasia (several forms)	AR, AD	**
15. Chondroectodermal dysplasia (Ellis-Van Creveld)	AR	***
16. Asphyxiating thoracic dysplasia (Jeune)	AR	**
17. Spondyloepiphyseal dysplasia congenita		
a. Autosomal-dominant form	AD	**
b. Autosomal-recessive form	AR	**
18. Kniest dysplasia	AD	**
19. Dyssegmental dysplasia	AR	*
20. Mesomelic dysplasia		
a. Type Nievergelt	AD	*
b. Type Langer (probable homozygous dyschondrosteosis)	AR	*
c. Type Robinow		*
d. Type Rheinhardt	AD	*
e. Others		***

(Table continues).

TABLE 8.2 (Continued).

21. Acromesomelic dysplasia	AR	**
22. Cleidocranial dysplasia	AD	****
23. Otopalatodigital syndrome		
a. Type I (Langer)	XLSD	**
b. Type II (André)	XLR	**
24. Larsen syndrome	AR, AD	**
25. Other multiple dislocation syndromes (Desbuquois)	AR	
b. Identifiable in later life		
1. Hypochondroplasia	AD	***
2. Dyschondrosteosis	AD	***
3. Metaphyseal chondrodysplasia type Jansen	AD	*
4. Metaphyseal chondrodysplasia type Schmid	AD	**
5. Metaphyseal chondrodysplasia type McKusick	AR	**
6. Metaphyseal chondrodysplasia with exocrine pancreatic insufficiency and cyclic neutropenia	AR	**
7. Spondylometaphyseal dysplasia		
a. Type Kozlowski	AD	**
b. Other forms		***
8. Multiple epiphyseal dysplasia		
a. Type Fairbank	AD	****
b. Other forms		***
9. Multiple epiphyseal dysplasia with early diabetes (Wolcott-Rallisson)	AR	**
10. Arthro-ophthalmopathy (Stickler)	AR	***
11. Pseudoachondroplasia		
a. Dominant	AD	***
b. Recessive	AR	**
12. Spondyloepiphyseal dysplasia tarda (X-linked recessive)	XLR	**
13. Progressive pseudorheumatoid chondrodysplasia	AR	**
14. Spondyloepiphyseal dysplasia, other forms		***
15. Brachyolmia		
a. Autosomal recessive	AR	*
b. Autosomal dominant	AD	*
16. Dyggve-Melchior-Clausen dysplasia	AR	**
17. Spondyloepimetaphyseal dysplasia (several forms)	AR	***
18. Spondyloepimetaphyseal dysplasia with joint laxity	AR	**
19. Otospondylomegaepiphyseal dysplasia (OSMED)	AR	*
20. Myotonic chondrodysplasia (Catel-Schwartz-Jampel)	AR	**
21. Parastremmatic dysplasia	AD	*
22. Trichorhinophalangeal dysplasia	AD	**

	Inheritance	Frequency
23. Acrodysplasia with retinitis pigmentosa and nephropathy (Saldino-Mainzer)	AR	**
B. Disorganized development of cartilage and fibrous components of skeleton		
1. Dysplasia epiphyseal hemimelica		**
2. Multiple cartilaginous exostoses	AD	****
3. Acrodysplasia with exostoses (Giedion-Langer)		**
4. Enchondromatosis (Ollier)		***
5. Enchondromatosis with hemangioma (Maffucci)		**
6. Metachondromatosis	AD	**
7. Spondyloenchondroplasia	AR	*
8. Osteoglophonic dysplasia		*
9. Fibrous dysplasia (Jaffe-Lichtenstein)		***
10. Fibrous dysplasia with skin pigmentation and precocious puberty (McCune-Albright)		***
11. Cherubism (familial fibrous dysplasia of the jaws)	AD	**
C. Abnormalities of density of cortical diaphyseal structure and/or metaphyseal modeling		
1. Osteogenesis imperfecta (several forms)	AR, AD	****
2. Juvenile idiopathic osteoporosis		**
3. Osteoporosis with pseudoglioma	AR	*
4. Osteopetrosis		
a. Autosomal-recessive lethal	AR	**
b. Intermediate recessive	AR	**
c. Autosomal dominant	AD	***
d. Recessive with tubular acidosis	AR	**
5. Pyknodysostosis	AR	***
6. Dominant osteosclerosis type Stanescu	AD	**
7. Osteomesopycnosis	AD	**
8. Osteopoikilosis	AD	***
9. Osteopathia striata	AD	***
10. Osteopathia striata with cranial sclerosis	AD	**
11. Melorheostosis		***
12. Diaphyseal dysplasia (Camurati-Engelmann)	AD	***
13. Craniodiaphyseal dysplasia	AR	**
14. Endosteal hyperostosis		
a. Autosomal dominant (Worth)	AD	**
b. Autosomal recessive (Van Buchem)	AR	**
c. Autosomal recessive (sclerosteosis)	AR	**
15. Tubular stenosis (Kenny-Caffey)	AD	*
16. Pachydermoperiostosis	AD	**
17. Osteodysplasty (Melnick-Needles)	AD	**
18. Frontometaphyseal dysplasia	XLR	**

(Table continues).

167

TABLE 8.2 (Continued).

19. Craniometaphyseal dysplasia (several forms)	AD	***
20. Metaphyseal dysplasia (Pyle)	AR or AD	**
21. Dysosteosclerosis	AR or XLR	**
22. Osteoectasia with hyperphosphatasia	AR	**
23. Oculodentoosseous dysplasia		
a. Mild type	AD	***
b. Severe type	AR	*
24. Infantile cortical hyperostosis (Caffey disease, familial type)	AD	**

Dysostoses

Malformation of individual bones, singly or in combination

A. Dysostoses with cranial and facial involvement

1. Craniosynostosis (several forms)		***
2. Craniofacial dysostosis (Crouzon)		***
3. Acrocephalosyndactyly		
a. Type Apert	AD	***
b. Type Chotzen	AD	**
c. Type Pfeiffer	AD	**
d. Other types		***
4. Acrocephalopolysyndactyly (Carpenter and others)	AR	**
5. Cephalopolysyndactyly (Greig)	AD	*
6. First and second branchial arch syndromes		
a. Mandibulofacial dysostosis (Treacher-Collins, Franceschetti)	AD	***
b. Acrofacial dysostosis (Nager)		**
c. Oculoauriculovertebral dysostosis (Goldenhar)	AR	***
d. Hemifacial microsomia		***
e. Others (Probably parts of a large spectrum)		***
7. Oculomandibulofacial syndrome (Hallermann-Streiff-François)		**

B. Dysostoses with predominant axial involvement

1. Vertebral segmentation defects (including Klippel-Feil)		**
2. Cervico-oculoacoustic syndrome (Wildervanck)		***
3. Sprengel anomaly		***
4. Spondylocostal dysostosis		
a. Dominant form	AD	**
b. Recessive forms	AR	**
5. Oculovertebral syndrome (Weyers)		*
6. Osteo-onychodysostosis	AD	***
7. Cerebrocostomandibular syndrome	AR	**

C. Dysostoses with predominant involvement of extremities

Entry	Inheritance	Rating
1. Acheiria	AR	**
2. Apodia		**
3. Tetraphocomelia syndrome (Roberts) (SC pseudothalidomide syndrome)	AR	**
4. Ectrodactyly		
a. Isolated		***
b. Ectrodactyly–ectodermal dysplasia, cleft palate syndrome	AD	**
c. Ectrodactyly with scalp defects	AD	**
5. Oroacral syndrome (aglossia syndrome, Hanhart syndrome)	AD	*
6. Familial radioulnar synostosis		**
7. Brachydactyly, types A, B, C, D, E (Bell's classification)	AD	****
8. Symphalangism	AD	***
9. Polydactyly (several forms)		****
10. Syndactyly (several forms)		****
11. Polysyndactyly (several forms)		***
12. Camptodactyly		****
13. Manzke syndrome		*
14. Poland syndrome		***
15. Rubinstein-Taybi syndrome		**
16. Coffin-Siris syndrome		**
17. Pancytopenia-dysmelia syndrome (Fanconi)	AR	***
18. Blackfan-Diamond anemia with thumb anomalies (Aase syndrome)	AR	**
19. Thrombocytopenia-radial-aplasia syndrome	AR	**
20. Orodigitofacial syndrome		
a. Type Papillon-Leage; lethal in males	XLD	**
b. Type Mohr	AR	**
21. Cardiomelic syndromes (Holt-Oram and others)	AD	***
22. Femoral focal deficiency (with or without facial anomalies)	AD	**
23. Multiple synostoses (includes some forms of symphalangism)	AD	***
24. Scapulo-iliac dysostosis (Kosenow-Sinios)	AD	**
25. Hand–foot–genital syndrome	AD	**
26. Focal dermal hypoplasia (Goltz); lethal in males	XLD	**

Idiopathic Osteolyses

Entry	Inheritance	Rating
1. Phalangeal (several forms)		**
2. Tarsocarpal		
a. Including François form and others	AR	**
b. With nephropathy	AD	**

(Table continues).

169

TABLE 8.2 (*Continued*).

3. Multicentric		
a. Hajdu-Cheney form	AD	**
b. Winchester form	AR	*
c. Torg form	AR	*
d. Other forms		**

Miscellaneous Disorders with Osseous Involvement

1. Early acceleration of skeletal maturation		
a. Marshall-Smith syndrome		*
b. Weaver syndrome		*
c. Other types		*
2. Marfan syndrome	AD	****
3. Congenital contractural arachnodactyly	AD	**
4. Cerebrohepatorenal syndrome (Zellweger)		**
5. Coffin-Lowry syndrome	SLR	**
6. Cockayne syndrome	AR	**
7. Fibrodysplasia ossificans congenita	AD	***
8. Epidermal nervus syndrome (Solomon)		**
9. Nevoid basal cell carcinoma syndrome		**
10. Multiple hereditary fibromatosis		**
11. Neurofibromatosis	AD	****

Chromosomal Aberrations

Primary Metabolic Abnormalities

A. Calcium and/or phosphorus

1. Hypophosphatemic rickets	XLD	****
2. Vitamin D dependency or pseudodeficiency rickets		
a. Type I with probable deficiency in 25-hydroxy vitamin D 1-α-hydroxylase	AR	**
b. Type II with target-organ resistancy	AR	**
3. Late rickets (McCance)		**
4. Idiopathic hypercalciuria		***
5. Hypophosphatasia (several forms)	AR	***
6. Pseudohypoparathyroidism (normo- and hypocalcemic forms, including acrodysostosis)	AD	***

B. Complex carbohydrates

1. Mucopolysaccharidosis type I (α-L-iduronidase deficiency)		
a. Hurler form	AR	***
b. Scheie form	AR	**
c. Other forms	AR	**
2. Mucopolysaccharidosis type II—Hunter (sulfoiduronate sulfatase deficiency)	XLR	***

Disorder	Inheritance	
3. Mucopolysaccharidosis type III—Sanfilippo		***
a. Type III B (*N*-acetyl-α-glucosaminidase deficiency)	AR	
b. Type III B (*N*-acetyl-α-glucosaminidase deficiency)	AR	
c. Type III C (α-glucosaminide-*N*-acetyl transferase deficiency)	AR	
d. Type III D (*N*-acetyl-glucosamine 6-sulfate sulfatase deficiency)	AR	
4. Mucopolysaccharidosis type IV		**
a. Type IV A—Morquio (*N*-acetylgalactosamine-6 sulfate sulfatase deficiency)	AR	
b. Type IV B (β-galactosidase deficiency)	AR	
5. Mucopolysaccharidosis type VI—Maroteaux-Lamy (arylsulfatase B deficiency)	AR	**
6. Mucopolysaccharidosis type VII (β-glucuronidase deficiency)	AR	**
7. Aspartyl glucosaminuria (aspartylglucosaminidase deficiency)	AR	**
8. Mannosidosis (α-mannosidase deficiency)	AR	**
9. Fucosidosis (α-fucosidase deficiency)	AR	**
10. GMI-Gangliosidosis (β-galactosidase deficiency) (several forms)	AR	**
11. Multiple sulfatases deficiency (Austin-Thieffry)	AR	**
12. Isolated neuraminidase deficiency, several forms including	AR	**
a. Mucolipidosis I		
b. Nephrosialidosis		
c. Cherry red spot myoclonia syndrome		
13. Phosphotransferase deficiency; several forms including		**
a. Mucolipidosis II (I cell disease)	AR	
b. Mucolipidosis III (pseudopolydystrophy)	AR	
14. Combined neuraminidase β-galactosidase deficiency	AR	*
15. Salla disease	AR	*
C. *Lipids*		
1. Niemann-Pick disease (sphingomyelinase deficiency) (several forms)	AR	***
2. Gaucher disease (β-glucosidase deficiency) (several types)	AR	****
3. Farber disease lipogranulomatosis (ceraminidase deficiency)	AR	**

(Table continues).

TABLE 8.2 (*Continued*).

D. Nucleic acids		
1. Adenosine-deaminase deficiency and others	AR	**
E. Amino acids		
1. Homocystinuria and others	AR	***
F. Metals		
1. Menkes syndrome (e.g., kinky hair syndrome)	AR	**

[a] Estimates of the relative frequency of these conditions are based on the compilers' experience and a review of the literature.
[b] Mode of transmission.
[c] Frequency.
AR, autosomal recessive; XLD, X-linked dominant; AD, autosomal dominant; XLR, X-linked recessive; SLR, sex-linked recessive; **** 1000 + cases; *** 100–1000 cases; ** 20–100 cases; * fewer than 20 cases.
(From Kozlowski et al.,[6] with permission.)

A comprehensive description of these diseases is beyond the scope of this chapter, and the interested reader is referred to genetic textbooks for a full discussion on the subject. This chapter focuses primarily on those osteo-chondrodysplasias that are recognizable at birth. Although more than 200 skeletal dysplasias have been described, and more will probably be described, the number that can be recognized with the use of sonography during the antepartum period is much less. Most of these disorders result in short stature, and the term *dwarfism* has been used to refer to this clinical condition. Unfortunately, this term carries a negative connotation, and for this reason the term *dysplasia* has been substituted.

EMBRYOLOGY OF THE SKELETON

The skeletal system develops from mesoderm. In most bones (e.g., the long bones), ossification is preceded by cartilage (endochondral ossification). However, cartilage does not become bone; rather, it is destroyed, and bone is formed in its place. In other cases, such as flat bones, ossification develops directly in the mesenchyme without cartilage formation (intramembranous ossification).

In long bones, ossification proceeds in an orderly fashion. It first begins in the shaft, or diaphysis, and extends from the middle toward both ends (epiphyses) where two areas of cartilage are left. During the last weeks of gestation and the first weeks of neonatal life, ossification centers appear in the epiphyses and lead to bone formation. However, between the diaphysis and the epiphyses persists an area of cartilage, metaphysis, which represents the growing portion of the bone. Once adult size is achieved, this area ossifies and the diaphysis joins permanently to the epiphyses. The terms *diaphysis*, *epiphysis*, and *metaphysis* are frequently employed in the description of the pathology of bone diseases.

BIOMETRY OF THE FETAL SKELETON IN THE DIAGNOSIS OF BONE DYSPLASIAS

Long bone biometry has been used extensively in the prediction of gestational age. Nomograms available for this purpose use the long bone as the independent variable and the estimated fetal age as the dependent variable. However, the type of nomogram required to assess the normality of bone dimensions uses gestational age as the independent variable and the long bone as the dependent variable. For the proper use of these nomograms, the clinician must have accurate knowledge of the gestational age of the fetus. Therefore, patients at risk of skeletal dysplasias should be advised to seek prenatal care at an early stage to assess all clinical estimators of gestational age. Tables 8.3 and 8.4 present nomograms for the assessment of limb biometry for the upper and lower extremities, respectively. For those patients presenting with uncertain gestational age, comparisons between limb dimensions and the

TABLE 8.3. Normal values for the arm

Week	Length of Humerus (mm)			Length of Ulna (mm)			Length of Radius (mm)		
	Percentile			Percentile			Percentile		
	5th	50th	95th	5th	50th	95th	5th	50th	95th
12	—	9	—	—	7	—	—	7	—
13	6	11	16	5	10	15	6	10	14
14	9	14	19	8	13	18	8	13	17
15	12	17	22	11	16	21	11	15	20
16	15	20	25	13	18	23	13	18	22
17	18	22	27	16	21	26	14	20	26
18	20	25	30	19	24	29	15	22	29
19	23	28	33	21	26	31	20	24	29
20	25	30	35	24	29	34	22	27	32
21	28	33	38	26	31	36	24	29	33
22	30	35	40	28	33	38	27	31	34
23	33	38	42	31	36	41	26	32	39
24	35	40	45	33	38	43	26	34	42
25	37	42	47	35	40	45	31	36	41
26	39	44	49	37	42	47	32	37	43
27	41	46	51	39	44	49	33	39	45
28	43	48	53	41	46	51	33	40	48
29	45	50	55	43	48	53	36	42	47
30	47	51	56	44	49	54	36	43	49
31	48	53	58	46	51	56	38	44	50
32	50	55	60	48	53	58	37	45	53
33	51	56	61	49	54	59	41	46	51
34	53	58	63	51	56	61	40	47	53
35	54	59	64	52	57	62	41	48	54
36	56	61	65	53	58	63	39	48	57
37	57	62	67	55	60	65	45	49	53
38	59	63	68	56	61	66	45	49	54
39	60	65	70	57	62	67	45	50	54
40	61	66	71	58	63	68	46	50	55

TABLE 8.4. Normal values for the leg

Week	Length of Tibia (mm)			Length of Fibula (mm)			Length of Femur (mm)		
	Percentile			Percentile			Percentile		
	5th	50th	95th	5th	50th	95th	5th	50th	95th
12	—	7	—	—	6	—	4	8	13
13	—	10	—	—	9	—	6	11	16
14	7	12	17	6	12	19	9	14	18
15	9	15	20	9	15	21	12	17	21
16	12	17	22	13	18	23	15	20	24
17	15	20	25	13	21	28	18	23	27
18	17	22	27	15	23	31	21	25	30
19	20	25	30	19	26	33	24	28	33
20	22	27	33	21	28	36	26	31	36
21	25	30	35	24	31	37	29	34	38
22	27	32	38	27	33	39	32	36	41
23	30	35	40	28	35	42	35	39	44
24	32	37	42	29	37	45	37	42	46
25	34	40	45	34	40	45	40	44	49
26	37	42	47	36	42	47	42	47	51
27	39	44	49	37	44	50	45	49	54
28	41	46	51	38	45	53	47	52	56
29	43	48	53	41	47	54	50	54	59
30	45	50	55	43	49	56	52	56	61
31	47	52	57	42	51	59	54	59	63
32	48	54	59	42	52	63	56	61	65
33	50	55	60	46	54	62	58	63	67
34	52	57	62	46	55	65	60	65	69
35	53	58	64	51	57	62	62	67	71
36	55	60	65	54	58	63	64	68	73
37	56	61	67	54	59	65	65	70	74
38	58	63	68	56	61	65	67	71	76
39	59	64	69	56	62	67	68	73	77
40	61	66	71	59	63	67	70	74	79

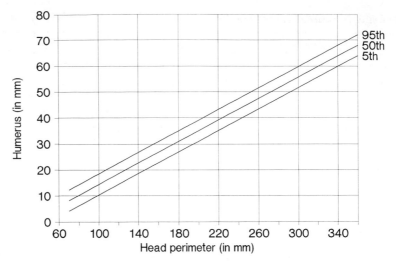

FIG. 8.1.   Relationship between head perimeter and humerus length.

head perimeter can be used (Figs. 8.1 and 8.2). Other investigators have employed the biparietal diameter for this purpose. The head perimeter has the advantage of being shaped independently. A limitation of this approach is that it assumes that the cranium is not involved in the dysplastic process, and this may not be the case in some skeletal dysplasias.

The nomograms and figures in this chapter provide the mean, 5th, and 95th percentiles of limb biometric parameters. The reader should be aware that 5 percent of the general population will fall below the boundary. Ideally,

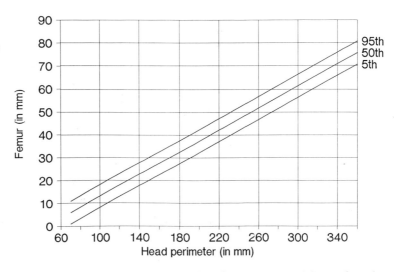

FIG. 8.2.   Relationship between head perimeter and femur length.

a more stringent criterion such as the 1st percentile limb growth for gestational age should be used for the diagnosis. Unfortunately, none of the currently available nomograms have been based on enough patients to provide an accurate discrimination between the 5th and the 1st percentile. However, most skeletal dysplasias diagnosed in utero or at birth are associated with dramatic long bone shortening and, under these circumstances, the precise boundary used (1st or 5th percentile) will not be critical. An exception to this is achondroplasia, in which limb biometry is mildly affected until the third trimester when abnormal growth can be detected by examining the slope of growth of femur length.[2]

TERMINOLOGY FREQUENTLY USED IN THE DESCRIPTION OF BONE DYSPLASIAS

Shortening of the extremities can involve the entire limb (micromelia), the proximal segment (rhizomelia), the intermediate segment (mesomelia), or the distal segment (acromelia). The diagnosis of rhizomelia and mesomelia requires comparison of the dimensions of the bones of the leg and forearm with those of the thigh and arm. Figures 8.3 and 8.4 display the relationship between the humerus and ulna, and the femur and tibia and can be used

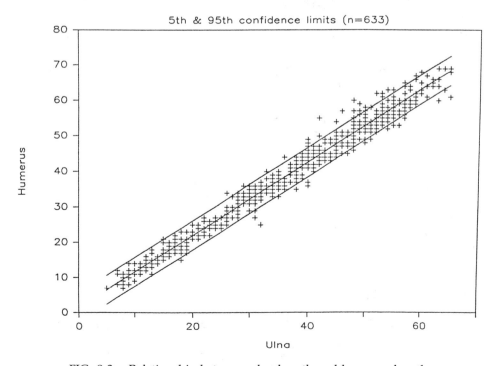

FIG. 8.3.   Relationship between ulna length and humerus length.

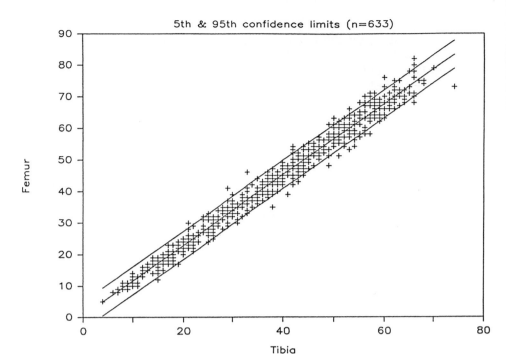

FIG. 8.4.   Relationship between tibia length and femur length.

in the assessment of rhizomelia and acromesomelia. Table 8.5 presents skeletal dysplasias characterized by rhizomelia, mesomelia, acromelia, and micromelia.

Several skeletal dysplasias feature alteration of the hands and feet. Polydactyly refers to the presence of more than five digits. It is classified as postaxial if the extra digits are on the ulnar or fibular side and as preaxial if they are located on the radial or tibial side. Syndactyly refers to soft tissue or bony fusion of adjacent digits. Clinodactyly consists of deviation of a finger(s). The most common spinal abnormality seen in skeletal dysplasias is platyspondyly, which consists of flattening of the vertebrae (Fig. 8.5). The antenatal detection of this abnormality has not been reported. Kyphosis and scoliosis can be identified in utero (Fig. 8.6). Prenatal diagnosis of congenital hemivertebra (Fig. 8.7) has also recently been reported.[3]

CLINICAL PRESENTATION

The challenge of the antenatal diagnosis of skeletal dysplasias generally presents itself in one of two ways: (1) patient who has delivered an infant with a skeletal dysplasia and who wants antenatal assessment of a subsequent

TABLE 8.5. Classification of skeletal dysplasias by rhizomelia, mesomelia, acromelia, and micromelia

Rhizomelia
> Thanatophoric dysplasia
> Atelosteogenesis
> Chondrodysplasia punctata (rhizomelic type)
> Diastrophic dysplasia
> Congenital short femur
> Achondroplasia

Mesomelia
> Mesomelic dysplasia (Langer, Rheinhardt, and Robinow types)
> COVESDEM association

Acromelia
> Ellis-van Creveld syndrome (chondroectodermal dysplasia)

Micromelia
> Achondrogenesis
> Atelosteogenesis
> Short rib-polydactyly syndrome (types I and II)
> Diastrophic dysplasia
> Fibrochondrogenesis
> Osteogenesis imperfecta (type III)
> Kniest dysplasia
> Dyssegmental dysplasia
> Roberts syndrome

pregnancy, or (2) the incidental finding of a shortened, bowed, or anomalous extremity during a routine sonographic examination. The task is easier when a particular phenotype is looked for in a patient at risk. The inability to obtain reliable information about skeletal mineralization and the involvement of other systems (e.g., skin) with sonography is a limiting factor in the establishment of an accurate diagnosis after the identification of an incidental finding. Another limitation is the paucity of information about the in utero natural history of these disorders.

Despite these difficulties and limitations, there are good medical reasons for attempting an accurate prenatal diagnosis of skeletal dysplasias. A number of these disorders are uniformly lethal, and a confident antenatal diagnosis would present options for the termination of the pregnancy. Table 8.6 lists such disorders. Other skeletal dysplasias are associated with mental retardation, and this information is important in prenatal counseling.

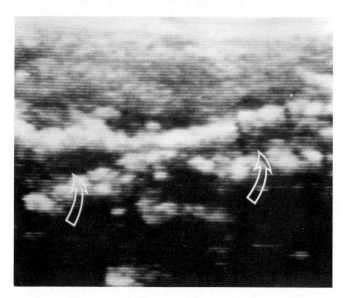

FIG. 8.5. Coronal section of the spine of a fetus with Jarcho-Levin syndrome at 23 weeks. Note the shortening of the spine and flaring of the vertebral canal (arrows).

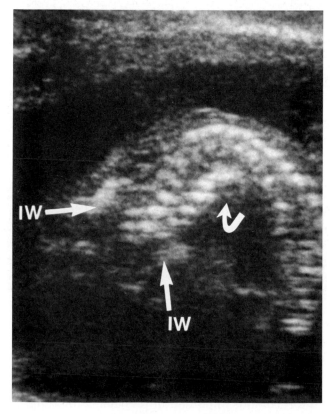

FIG. 8.6. Coronal scan demonstrating severe scoliosis (curved arrow). (IW, iliac wings.)

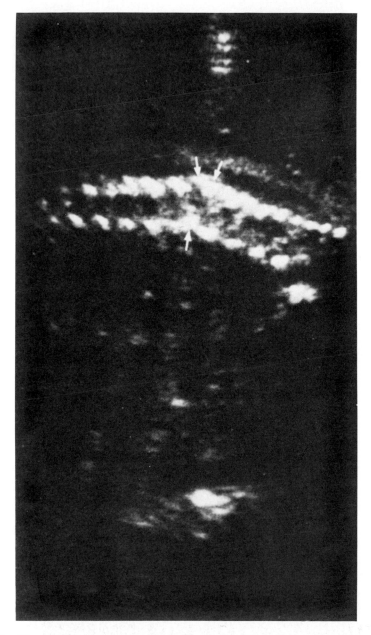

FIG. 8.7. Hemivertebra. Longitudinal view of the lower thoracic spine showing the two abnormal ossification centers of the posterior elements, opposite a single ossification center. (From Benacerraf et al.,[3] with permission.)

TABLE 8.6. Lethal skeletal dysplasias

Achondrogenesis
Thanatophoric dysplasia
Short rib-polydactyly syndromes (types I, II, and III)
Fibrochondrogenesis
Atelosteogenesis
Homozygous achondroplasia
Osteogenesis imperfecta, perinatal type
Hypophosphatasia

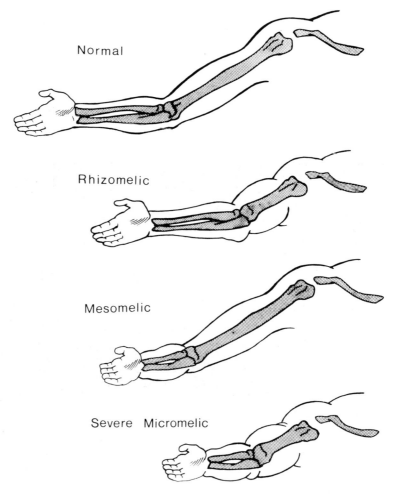

FIG. 8.8. Varieties of short limb dysplasia according to the segment involved.

APPROACH TO THE DIAGNOSIS OF SKELETAL DYSPLASIAS

Our approach to the diagnosis of skeletal dysplasias follows an organized plan of examination of the fetal skeleton, performed in the following manner:

Long bones: All long bones should be measured in all extremities. Comparisons with other segments (Fig. 8.8) should be performed to establish whether the limb shortening is predominantly rhizomelic, mesomelic, or acromelic or involves all segments. Detailed examination of each bone is necessary to exclude the absence or hypoplasia of individual bones, which are frequently absent in certain conditions (fibula, scapula). An attempt should be made to characterize the degree of mineralization. This can be assessed by examining the acoustic shadow behind the bone and the echogenicity of the bone itself. It should be stressed that there are limitations in the sonographic evaluation of mineralization of long bones and that other structures, such as the skull, are perhaps better suited for this assessment. (Fig. 8.9). The degree of long bone curvature should be examined. No objective means of assessing this sign has been found; experience is the only means by which the operator can discern the boundary between normality and abnormality. Campomelia (excessive bowing) is characteristic of certain disorders (e.g., campomelic dys-

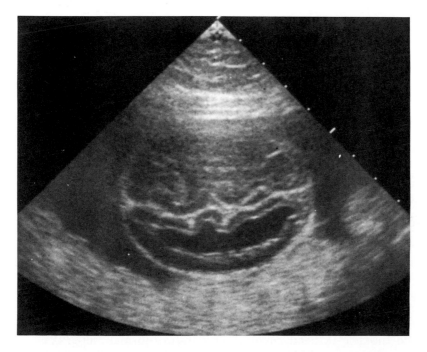

FIG. 8.9. Demineralization of the skull in a case of congenital hypophosphatasia.

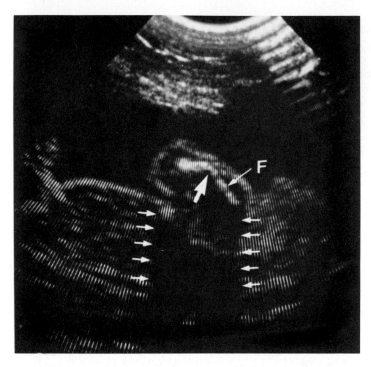

FIG. 8.10.   In utero fracture (large arrow) in a case of osteogenesis imperfecta. The small arrows outline the decreased shadowing cast by the bone. (F, femur.)

plasia). Finally, the possibility of fractures should also be considered, as they can be indicative of some conditions (e.g., osteogenesis imperfecta). The fractures may be extremely subtle or may lead to angulation and separation of the segments of the affected bone (Fig. 8.10 and 8.11).

Evaluation of thoracic dimensions: Several skeletal dysplasias are associated with a hypoplastic thorax. Such a finding is extremely important because chest restriction leads to pulmonary hypoplasia, a frequent cause of death in these conditions. The appropriateness of thoracic dimensions can be assessed by measuring the thoracic circumference at the level of the four-chamber view of the heart. The thoracic circumference can be measured or calculated using the formula

Thoracic circumference = (anteroposterior diameter + transverse diameter) × 1.57

The thoracic length is measured from the boundary between the neck and the chest and the diaphragm. Tables 8.7 and 8.8 illustrate nomograms with which to evaluate thoracic dimensions in fetuses with known gestational ages. When gestational age is uncertain, age-independent ratios can be used. The thoracic to abdominal circumference ratio (normal value: 0.77 to 1.01) and the thoracic to head circumference ratio (normal value: 0.56 to 1.04) permit evaluation of the transverse thoracic dimensions.[4]

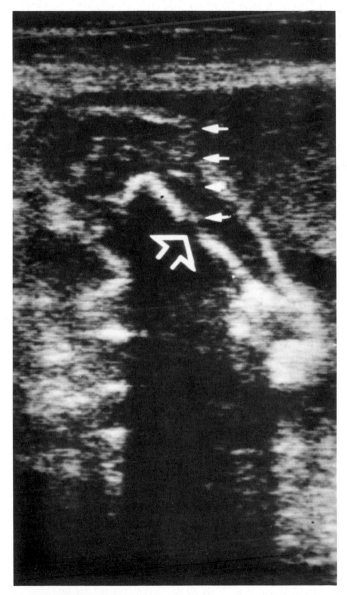

FIG. 8.11.   Potential pitfall. Shadowing from an upper extremity (arrows) creates
the false image of a femur fracture (open arrow).

TABLE 8.7.   Fetal thoracic circumference measurements[a]

Gestational Age (wk)	No.	Predictive Percentiles								
		2.5	5	10	25	50	75	90	95	97.5
16	6	5.9	6.4	7.0	8.0	9.1	10.3	11.3	11.9	12.4
17	22	6.8	7.3	7.9	8.9	10.0	11.2	12.2	12.8	13.3
18	31	7.7	8.2	8.8	9.8	11.0	12.1	13.1	13.7	14.2
19	21	8.6	9.1	9.7	10.7	11.9	13.0	14.0	14.6	15.1
20	20	9.5	10.0	10.6	11.7	12.8	13.9	15.0	15.5	16.0
21	30	10.4	11.0	11.6	12.6	13.7	14.8	15.8	16.4	16.9
22	18	11.3	11.9	12.5	13.5	14.6	15.7	16.7	17.3	17.8
23	21	12.2	12.8	13.4	14.4	15.5	16.6	17.6	18.2	18.8
24	27	13.2	13.7	14.3	15.3	16.4	17.5	18.5	19.1	19.7
25	20	14.1	14.6	15.2	16.2	17.3	18.4	19.4	20.0	20.6
26	25	15.0	15.5	16.1	17.1	18.2	19.3	20.3	21.0	21.5
27	24	15.9	16.4	17.0	18.0	19.1	20.2	21.3	21.9	22.4
28	24	16.8	17.3	17.9	18.9	20.0	21.2	22.2	22.8	23.3
29	24	17.7	18.2	18.8	19.8	21.0	22.1	23.1	23.7	24.2
30	27	18.6	19.1	19.7	20.7	21.9	23.0	24.0	24.6	25.1
31	24	19.5	20.0	20.6	21.6	22.8	23.9	24.9	25.5	26.0
32	28	20.4	20.9	21.5	22.6	23.7	24.8	25.8	26.4	26.9
33	27	21.3	21.8	22.5	23.5	24.6	25.7	26.7	27.3	27.8
34	25	22.2	22.8	23.4	24.4	25.5	26.6	27.6	28.2	28.7
35	20	23.1	23.7	24.3	25.3	26.4	27.5	28.5	29.1	29.6
36	23	4.0	24.6	25.2	26.2	27.3	28.4	29.4	30.0	30.6
37	22	24.9	25.5	26.1	27.1	28.2	29.3	30.3	30.9	31.5
38	21	25.9	26.4	27.0	28.0	29.1	30.2	31.2	31.9	32.4
39	7	26.8	27.3	27.9	28.9	30.0	31.1	32.2	32.8	33.3
40	6	27.7	28.2	28.8	29.8	30.9	32.1	33.1	33.7	34.2

[a] Measurements in centimeters (cm).
(From Chitkara et al.,[4] with permission.)

Evaluation of thoracic dimensions is a critical part of the workup because the cause of death in most lethal skeletal dysplasias is pulmonary hypoplasia secondary to an underdeveloped rib cage (Figs. 8.12 to 8.15). Table 8.9 displays skeletal dysplasias associated with alteration of thoracic dimensions.

Evaluation of hands and feet: Hands and feet should be examined to exclude polydactyly and syndactyly (Figs. 8.16 to 8.22) as well as extreme postural deformities such as those seen in diastrophic dwarfism. Table 8.10 displays disorders associated with hand and foot deformities.

TABLE 8.8. Fetal thoracic length measurements[a]

Gestational Age (wk)	No.	Predictive Percentiles								
		2.5	5	10	25	50	75	90	95	97.5
16	6	0.9	1.1	1.3	1.6	2.0	2.4	2.8	3.0	3.2
17	22	1.1	1.3	1.5	1.8	2.2	2.6	3.0	3.2	3.4
18	31	1.3	1.4	1.7	2.0	2.4	2.8	3.2	3.4	3.6
19	21	1.4	1.6	1.8	2.2	2.7	3.0	3.4	3.6	3.8
20	20	1.6	1.8	2.0	2.4	2.8	3.2	3.6	3.8	4.0
21	30	1.8	2.0	2.2	2.6	3.0	3.4	3.7	4.0	4.1
22	18	2.0	2.2	2.4	2.8	3.2	3.6	3.9	4.1	4.3
23	21	2.2	2.4	2.6	3.0	3.4	3.8	4.1	4.3	4.5
24	27	2.4	2.6	2.8	3.1	3.5	3.9	4.3	4.5	4.7
25	20	2.6	2.8	3.0	3.3	3.7	4.1	4.5	4.7	4.9
26	25	2.8	2.9	3.2	3.5	3.9	4.3	4.7	4.9	5.1
27	24	2.9	3.1	3.3	3.7	4.1	4.5	4.9	5.1	5.3
28	24	3.1	3.3	3.5	3.9	4.3	4.7	5.0	5.4	5.4
29	24	3.3	3.5	3.7	4.1	4.5	4.9	5.2	5.5	5.6
30	27	3.5	3.7	3.9	4.3	4.7	5.1	5.4	5.6	5.8
31	24	3.7	3.9	4.1	4.5	4.9	5.3	5.6	5.8	6.0
32	28	3.9	4.1	4.3	4.6	5.0	5.4	5.8	6.0	6.2
33	27	4.1	4.3	4.5	4.8	5.2	5.6	6.0	6.2	6.4
34	25	4.2	4.4	4.7	5.0	5.4	5.8	6.2	6.4	6.6
35	20	4.4	4.6	4.8	5.2	5.6	6.0	6.4	6.6	6.8
36	23	4.6	4.8	5.0	5.4	5.8	6.2	6.5	6.8	7.0
37	22	4.8	5.0	5.2	5.6	6.0	6.4	6.7	7.0	7.1
38	21	5.0	5.2	5.4	5.8	6.2	6.6	6.9	7.1	7.3
39	7	5.2	5.4	5.6	6.0	6.4	6.8	7.1	7.3	7.5
40	6	5.4	5.6	5.8	6.1	6.5	6.9	7.3	7.5	7.7

[a] Measurements in centimeters (cm).
(From Chitkara et al.,[4] with permission.)

Evaluation of the fetal cranium: Several skeletal dysplasias are associated with defects of membranous ossification and therefore affect skull bones. Orbits should be measured to exclude hypertelorism. Other findings that should be searched for are micrognathia, short upper lip, abnormally shaped ear, frontal bossing (Fig. 8.23), and cloverleaf skull deformity (Figs. 8.24 and 8.25). Table 8.11 presents abnormalities of the skull and face in the different skeletal dysplasias.

Despite all efforts to establish an accurate prenatal diagnosis, a careful study of the newborn will be required in all instances. The evaluation should

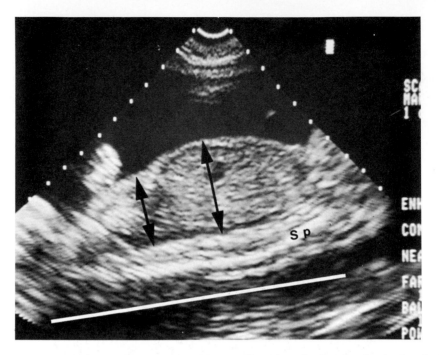

FIG. 8.12.   Longitudinal section of a fetus affected with thanatophoric dysplasia. Note the significant disproportion between the chest and the abdomen. (Sp, spine.) (From Jeanty and Romero,[7] with permission.)

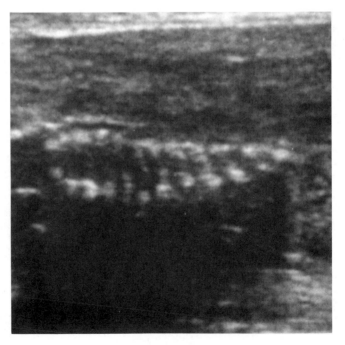

FIG. 8.13.   Longitudinal section of a fetus with short rib-polydactyly syndrome showing the very short ribs.

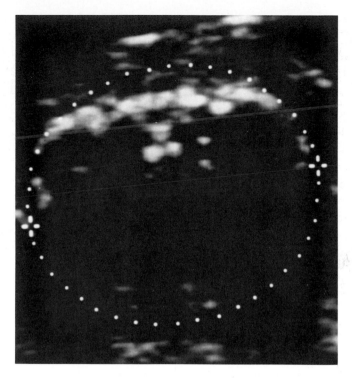

FIG. 8.14. Transverse section of the chest of the fetus shown in Figure 8.13. Note the short ribs.

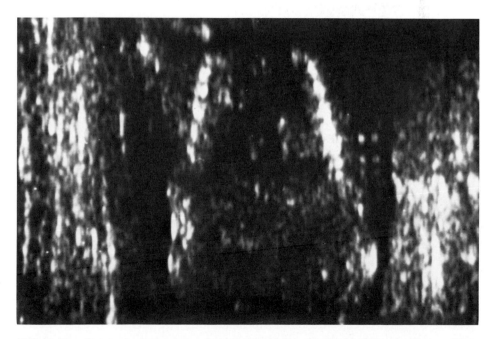

FIG. 8.15. Coronal section of a fetus with short rib-polydactyly syndrome. Note the disproportion between the thoracic and abdominal cavities.

TABLE 8.9.   Skeletal dysplasias associated with altered thoracic dimensions

---

Long, narrow thorax
   Asphyxiating thoracic dysplasia (Jeune)
   Chondroectodermal dysplasia (Ellis-van Creveld)
   Metatropic dysplasia
   Fibrochondrogenesis
   Atelosteogenesis
   Campomelic dysplasia
   Jarcho-Levin syndrome
   Achondrogenesis
   Osteogenesis Imperfecta congenita
   Hypophosphatasia
   Dyssegmental dysplasia
   Cleidocranial dysplasia

Short thorax
   Osteogenesis imperfecta (type II)
   Kniest dysplasia (metatropic dysplasia type II)
   Pena-Shokeir syndrome

Hypoplastic thorax
   Short rib-polydactyly syndrome (types I and II)
   Thanatophoric dysplasia
   Cerebro-costomandibular syndrome
   Cleidocranial dysostosis syndrome
   Homozygous achondroplasia
   Melnick-Needles syndrome (osteodysplasty)
   Fibrochondrogenesis
   Otopalatodigital syndrome (type II)

---

include a detailed physical examination performed by a geneticist or a physician with experience in the field of skeletal dysplasias and radiograms of the skeleton. The latter should include anterior, posterior, lateral, and Towne views of the skull, and anteroposterior views of the spine and extremities with separate films of hands and feet. Examination of the skeletal radiographs will permit precise diagnoses in the overwhelming majority of cases, since the classification of skeletal dysplasias is largely based on radiographic findings. In lethal skeletal dysplasias, histologic examination of the chondroosseous tissue should be included, as this information may help reach a specific diagnosis. Chromosomal studies should be included, as a specific group of constitutional bone disorders is associated with cytogenetic abnormalities. Biochemical studies are helpful in rare instances (e.g., hypophospha-

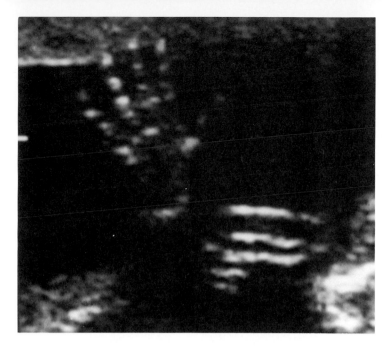

FIG. 8.16. Fetal hand in the second trimester. Metacarpal bones and phalanges can be visualized. Carpal bones cannot be imaged because they are not ossified.

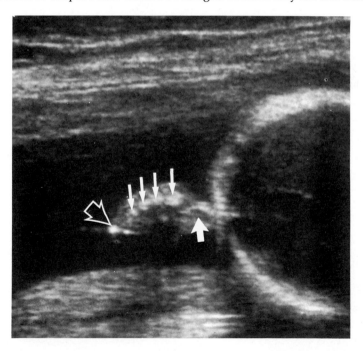

FIG. 8.17. Polydactyly in a fetus with short rib-polydactyly syndrome, showing six fingers. The large solid arrow points to the thumb. Small arrows indicate the next four fingers. The open arrow points to an extra digit. The presence of the extra digit on the ulnar side defines postaxial polydactyly.

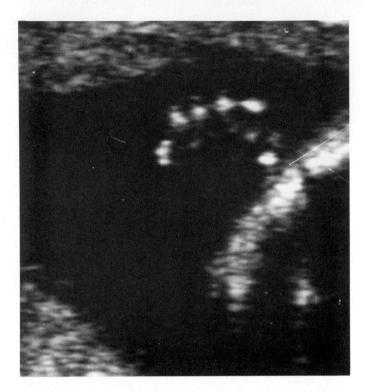

FIG. 8.18. Transverse section of a hand of a fetus with short rib-polydactyly syndrome showing postaxial polydactyly. Six digits are easily identified.

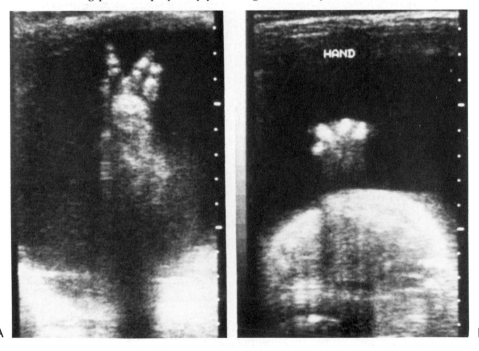

A

B

FIG. 8.19. Syndactyly. Only four fingers are visualized. (A) Long axis view of the hand; (B) Transverse section of the hand. (Courtesy of Dr. Carl Otto.)

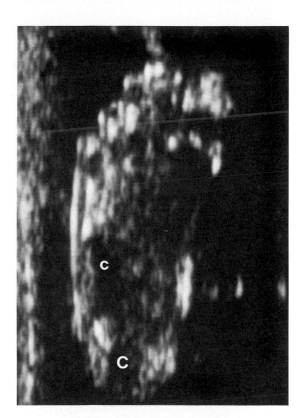

FIG. 8.20. Fetal foot at 28 weeks. The five toes and the fourth and fifth metatarsal bones are clearly visible. (C, cartilage of the calcaneal tuberosity; c, cartilage of the cuboid bone.)

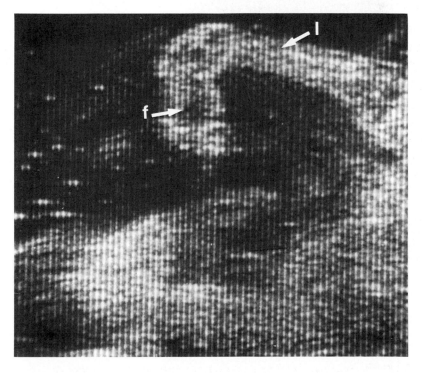

FIG. 8.21. Clubfoot. (l, leg; f, foot.) (From Jeanty and Romero,[7] with permission.)

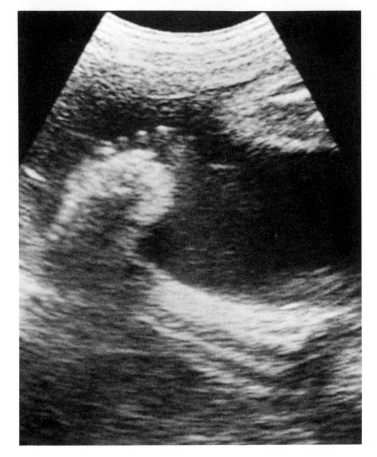

FIG. 8.22. Clubfoot.

tasia). DNA restrictions and enzymatic activity assays should be considered in those cases in which the phenotype suggests a metabolic disorder, such as a mucopolysaccharidosis. Although a full discussion about such disorders is beyond the scope of this text, they are well-known causes of constitutional bone diseases.

SKELETAL DYSPLASIAS DIAGNOSED IN UTERO

A growing number of skeletal dysplasias have been recognized in utero. A complete account of each disorder is beyond the scope of this chapter, and we refer the reader to texts on the subject for further details.[5] Table 8.12 provides a list of skeletal dysplasias diagnosed in utero and their most salient clinical features.

TABLE 8.10.   Skeletal dysplasias associated with polydactyly and
syndactyly

Postaxial polydactyly
　　Chondroectodermal dysplasia
　　Short rib-polydactyly syndrome (types I and II)
　　Asphyxiating thoracic dysplasia
　　Otopalatodigital syndrome
　　Mesomelic dysplasia, Werner type (associated with absence of thumbs)

Preaxial polydactyly
　　Chondroectodermal dysplasia
　　Short rib-polydactyly syndrome (type II)
　　Carpenter syndrome

Syndactyly
　　Poland syndrome
　　Acrocephalosyndactylies (Carpenter syndrome, Apert syndrome)
　　Otopalatodigital syndrome (type II)
　　Mesomelic dysplasia, Werner type
　　TAR syndrome
　　Jarcho-Levin syndrome
　　Roberts syndrome

Brachydactyly
　　Mesomelic dysplasia, Robinow type
　　Otopalatodigital syndrome

Hitchhiker thumbs
　　Diastrophic dysplasia

Clubfeet deformity
　　Diastrophic dysplasia
　　Osteogenesis imperfecta
　　Kniest dysplasia
　　Spondyloepiphyseal congenita
　　Metatropic dysplasia
　　Mesomelic dysplasia, Nievergelt type
　　Chondrodysplasia punctata
　　Larsen syndrome
　　Roberts syndrome
　　TAR syndrome
　　Pena-Shokeir syndrome

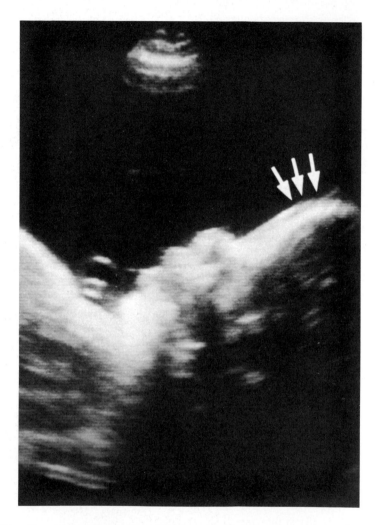

FIG. 8.23.   Frontal bossing in a sagittal scan. The arrows point to the prominent frontal bone.

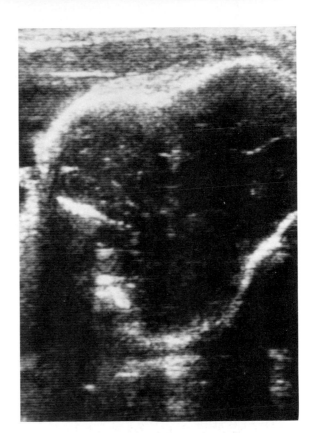

FIG. 8.24. Thanatophoric dysplasia. Coronal scan shows cloverleaf skull.

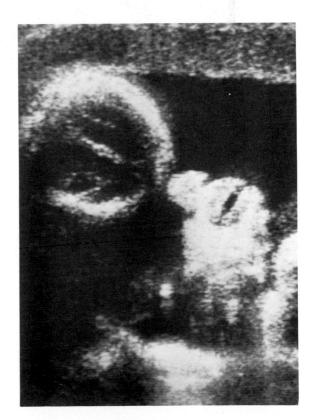

FIG. 8.25. Frontal bossing in a fetus with cloverleaf skull. Note the prominent forehead. Under normal circumstances, the forehead is not visible in a scan that permits imaging of the mouth and nose.

TABLE 8.11.   Skeletal dysplasias associated with skull and face deformities

Large head
    Achondroplasia
    Achondrogenesis
    Thanatophoric dysplasia
    Osteogenesis imperfecta
    Cleidocranial dysplasia
    Hypophosphatasia
    Campomelic dysplasia
    Short rib-polydactyly syndrome
      (type III)
    Robinow mesomelic dysplasia
    Otopalatodigital syndrome

    Spondyloepiphyseal dysplasia
    Campomelic syndrome
    Jarcho-Levin syndrome
    Ellis-van Creveld syndrome
    Short rib-polydactyly syndrome
      (type II)
    Metatropic dysplasia
    Dyssegmental dysplasia
    Otopalatodigital syndrome
      (type II)
    Roberts syndrome

Cloverleaf skull
    Thanatophoric dysplasia (rare
      variant)
    Campomelic syndrome

Short upper lip
    Chondroectodermal dysplasia

Other craniostenosis
    Apert syndrome
    Carpenter syndrome
    Hypophosphatasia

Swelling of the pinnae of the ear
    Diastrophic dysplasia

Micrognathia
    Campomelic dysplasia
    Diastrophic dysplasia

Congenital cataracts
    Chondrodysplasia punctata

    Weissenbacher-Zweymuller
      syndrome
    Otopalatodigital syndrome

Cleft palate
    Asphyxiating thoracic dysplasia
    Kniest dysplasia
    Diastrophic dysplasia

    Pena-Shokeir syndrome
    TAR syndrome
    Langer syndrome

(Table continues).

TABLE 8.12. Skeletal dysplasias diagnosed in utero

	Large Head	Small Thorax	Short Limbs	Spine Deformity	Short Hand	Foot Deformity	Polydactyly	Syndactyly	Distinguishing Features
Achondrogenesis	+	+	+						Gross micromelia, poor ossification
Achondroplasia	+	+	+	Kyphosis	+	+			Trident hand, large skull
Apert syndrome								+	Turricephaly, syndactyly
Asphyxiating thoracic dysplasia (Jeune syndrome)		+	+/−		+			+	Cleft lip and palate, bell-shaped thorax
Campomelic dysplasia	+	+	+			+			Bowed femora and tibia, micrognatia
Carpenter syndrome								+	Craniostenosis, syndactyly, preaxial polydactyly
Chondrodysplasia punctata		+	+	+	+				Assymetric limbs, hypertelorism
McKusik syndrome (cartilage-hair hypoplasia)		+	+	Lordosis	+	+			"Limp" hands and feet
Ellis-Van Creveld syndrome		+	+		+		+		Acromesomelic limb shortening
Diastrophic dysplasia		+	+	Kyphosis	+	+			Hitchhiker's thumb, ear blister, cleft palate
Dyssegmental dysplasia		+	+	+					Cleft palate, disorganization of vertebral bodies
Fibrochondrogenesis		+	+						Pear-shaped vertebral bcdy
Hypophosphatasia		+	+						Poor mineralization, fractures
Kniest dysplasia		+	+	Scoliosis/kyphosis					Cleft palate, dumbbell femur
Larsen syndrome				Kyphosis	+	+			Spinal deformity, cleft palate, hypertelorism, clubfeet

TABLE 8.12. (*Continued*).

	Large Head	Small Thorax	Short Limbs	Spine Deformity	Short Hand Deformity	Foot Deformity	Polydactyly Syndactyly	Distinguishing Features
Mesomelic dysplasia								
Langer type			+					Micrognatia, short radius with lateral and dorsal bowing
Robinow type	+		+	+	+	+		Abnormal face, hypertelorism, hemivertebra, mesomelic shortening of the upper extremities
Nievergelt type			+		±	+		Clubfeet, flexion deformities
Rheinhardt type			+		+			Limb bowing
Werner type			+				+	Absence of thumbs, extreme bilateral hypoplasia of tibia
Metatropic dysplasia			+	Scoliosis		+		Tail-like sacral appendage
Osteogenesis imperfecta								
Type I			+					Mild bowing of femur
Type II		+	+					Rib fractures, crumpled femora
Type III		+	+	+				Bowed limbs, fractures
Type IV								Bowed limbs, fractures
Otopalatodigital syndrome (type II)	+		+		+	+	+	Cleft palate, micrognatia, bowed long bones

Disorder	1	2	3	4	5	6	Findings
Pena-Shokeir syndrome	+					+	Micrognatia, hypertelorism, clubfeet, absence of body movement
Roberts syndrome		+			+	+	Clubfoot, cleft lip and palate, tetraphocomelia
Short rib-polydactyly							
Type I		+		+	+	+	Narrow thorax, postaxial polydactyly
Type II		+		+	+	+	Cleft palate, pre- or postaxial polydactyly
Type III		+		Scoliosis	+	+	Vertebral hypoplasia
Spondyloepiphyseal dysplasia (Atelosteogenesis)		+		+	+		Hypoplasia of distal segment of humerus and femur, enlargement of proximal portion, cleft palate, clubfeet
Spondylothoracic dysplasia (Jarcho-Levin syndrome)				Lordosis		+	Hemivertebra, fused vertebra, cleft palate, "crab-chest" deformity
Thanatophoric dysplasia			+		+		Bowed limbs, cloverleaf skull, "telephone receiver" femora
Thrombocytopenia with absent radius syndrome (TAR)					+	+	Bilateral absence of radius, clubfeet, micrognatia

ACKNOWLEDGMENT

These studies were partially supported by a grant from the Walter Scott Foundation for Medical Research. Dr. Roberto Romero is a recipient of a Physician Scientist Award from the National Institutes of Health.

REFERENCES

1. Camera G, Mastroiacovo P: Birth prevalence of skeletal dysplasias in the Italian multicentric monitoring system for birth defects. p. 441. In Papadatos, CJ, Bartsocas CE (eds): Skeletal Dysplasias. Alan R Liss, New York, 1982

2. Kurtz AB, Wapner RJ: Ultrasonographic diagnosis of second trimester skeletal dysplasias: A prospective analysis in a high-risk population. J Ultrasound Med 2:99, 1983

3. Benacerrf BR, Greene MF, Barss VA: Prenatal sonographic diagnosis of congenital hemivertebra. J Ultrasound Med 5:257, 1986

4. Chitkara U, Rosenberg J, Chervenak FA, et al: Prenatal sonographic assessment of the fetal thorax: Normal values. Am J Obstet Gynecol 156:1069, 1987

5. Romero R, Pilu G, Jeanty P, et al: Prenatal Diagnosis of Congenital Anomalies. p. 311. Appleton and Lange, E Norwalk, CT, 1987

6. Kozlowski K, Beighton P: Gamut Index of Skeletal Dysplasias. An Aid to Radiodiagnosis. Springer-Verlag, Berlin, 1986

7. Jeanty P, Romero R: Obstetrical Ultrasound. McGraw-Hill, New York, 1983

9 The Placenta

PETER A. T. GRANNUM

An ultrasound examination of the intrauterine environment must include an assessment of the fetus, the amniotic fluid, and the placenta. An understanding of the relationship of these three components will lead to a more astute clinical judgment concerning the state of the intrauterine environment. Ultrasound assessment of the placenta includes determining the position of the placenta (placenta previa), premature separation of the placenta (abruptio placenta), and the developmental ultrasound morphology of the placenta (placental grading). This chapter deals with the information, clinical inference, and application of the knowledge gained from the examination of the placenta.

ULTRASOUND DEVELOPMENT

Placental Grades

Prior to the tenth week of gestation, the chorion frondosum, from which the definitive placenta develops, appears as a conglomeration of high-level echoes (Figs. 9.1 and 9.2). By the twelfth week of gestation, the three main structures of the placenta are easily visible. These structures—the chorionic plate, the substance of the placenta, and the basal layer area—and the changes they undergo throughout the gestational period form the basis of placental grading.

On the basis of the ultrasound changes in the placenta through the gestational period, four grades have been described[1] (Fig. 9.3):

Grade 0: The chorionic plate is smooth, the substance of the placenta and the basal layer devoid of echogenic densities.
Grade 1: The chorionic plate may assume subtle indentations that may be difficult to see, if the fetus is closely approximated. The substance will contain linear echogenic densities with their long axis parallel to the long axis of the placenta. They are randomly dispersed in the substance of the placenta. The basal layer remains devoid of densities.

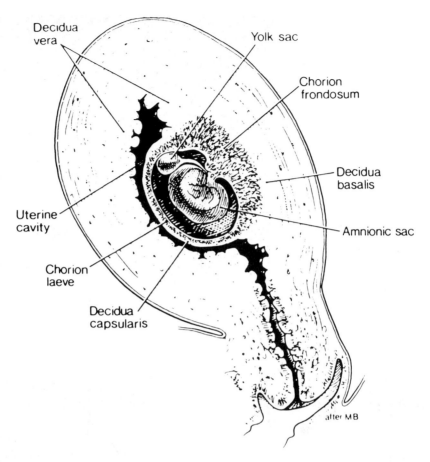

Decidua vera

Yolk sac

Chorion frondosum

Decidua basalis

Amnionic sac

Uterine cavity

Chorion laeve

Decidua capsularis

after M B

FIG. 9.1.   Chorion frondosum, chorion laeve. (From Pritchard et al.,[33] with permission.)

Grade 2: The chorionic plate may be more markedly indented. Extending from the chorionic plate are linear densities (coma densities) that travel from the chorionic plate toward the basal layer. In the grade 2 placenta, these extensions resemble a broken line. Most often they are seen extending from the chorionic plate. The densities present in the substance in the grade 1 placenta persist. The hallmark sign of the grade 2 placenta is the presence of basal echogenic densities. These densities are linear, are irregular in shape, and have their long axis parallel to the long axis of the placenta. They can be dense enough to cast acoustic shadows.

Grade 3: The hallmark sign of the grade 3 placenta is the presence of the linear echogenic densities extending from the chorionic plate to the basal layer area *without* a break. A solid line without a break is essential for the diagnosis of a grade 3 placenta. The chorionic plate may be markedly indented. The substance of the placenta will reflect the same densities seen in the grade 2 configuration. Occasionally, large echogenic densities

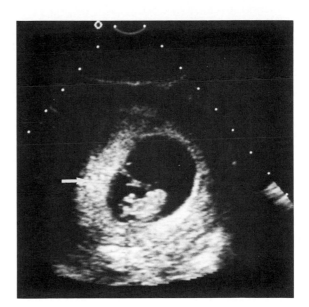

FIG. 9.2. Ultrasound at 8 weeks gestation showing the high level echoes of the developing placenta (arrow). (Courtesy of Jacqueline Green, RDMS, Perinatal Unit, Yale-New Haven Hospital.)

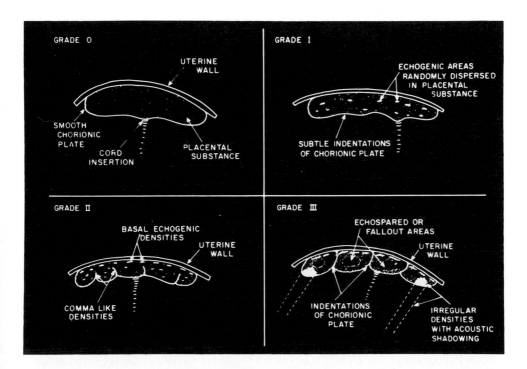

FIG. 9.3. Diagrammatic version of the grading classifications of the placenta grades 0 through 3. (From Grannum et al.,[1] with permission.)

that cast their own acoustic shadows can be seen near the chorionic plate. They most likely represent the white rubbery infarcts seen on the fetal surface of the placenta; they are of no clinical significance unless they are multiple. Often an echo-spared area can be seen at the central portion of a lobule. These spared areas represent the central portions of the cotyledons devoid of villi, presumably destroyed by the maternal arterial jet pressure.[2] The basal densities present in the grade 2 placenta also persist, but they may be larger, become confluent, and be dense enough to cast their own acoustic shadows.

How to Scan the Placenta in Reference to Placental Grading

The sound waves must travel perpendicular to the chorionic plate. Care must be exercised when examining a laterally positioned placenta. If the placenta is examined along its long axis, that is, parallel to the chorionic plate, the lobules will appear to be one on top of the other, which is anatomically incorrect (Fig. 9.4). It may then be impossible to distinguish between a grade 2 and grade 3 configuration.

For the anterior placenta, the near-gain settings should be carefully regulated so as to highlight the basal layer area. If the overall total gain control is turned up too high, it may be impossible to visualize the subtle echogenic densities within the placental substance or in the basal layer area.

Care should be taken to distinguish between a grade 2 and grade 3 placenta. In the grade 2 placenta, the linear densities between the chorionic plate and the basal layer area should be magnified to establish whether it is a solid or broken line. The solid line would indicate a grade 3 placenta. Reverberation from the anterior abdominal wall (rectus sheath) must be distinguished from basal echogenic densities. A summary of placental grading is presented in Table 9.1.

Placental Grading Changes During the Gestational Period

In normal pregnancies, the mean gestational age at which grade 1 appears is 31.1 weeks; grade 2, 36.6 weeks; and grade 3, 38 weeks.[3] At term (37 weeks or greater), the incidence of grade 1 is approximately 40 percent; grade 2, 45 percent; and grade 3, 5 to 15 percent.

Clinical Significance of Placental Grading

Postdatism

In an attempt to evaluate the use of placental grading in identifying the postmature fetus, 85 truly postdate pregnancies were reviewed.[4] The postdates fetus with the postmaturity syndrome was defined as having meconium staining of the skin, meconium in the amniotic fluid, long nails, peeling skin, hypoglycemia, and hypocalcemia. In this study, no grade 0 or grade

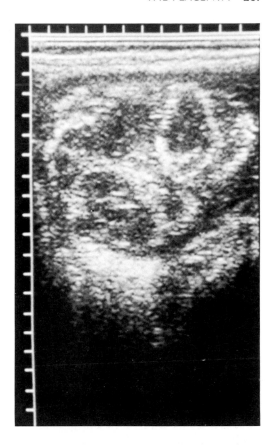

FIG. 9.4. Scan showing a laterally positioned placenta scanned with the soundwaves traveling parallel to the chorionic plate. Note that the lobules appear to be on top of each other.

1 placentas were noted, and both grade 2 and grade 3 placentas were found with similar frequency. Therefore, in the presence of a grade 0 or grade 1 placenta in a patient thought to be at 42 weeks, the gestational age of the fetus should be seriously questioned. The incidence of the postmaturity syndrome in this series was 12.9 percent, which was equally distributed between the grade 2 and grade 3 placentas. Thus, placental grading cannot be used to identify the postmature fetus. When the neonatal ponderal index of the fetuses were examined, the ponderal index was noted to be higher in the fetuses with grade 2 than with grade 3 placentas (Fig. 9.5). This finding suggests the possibility of mild malnutrition in fetuses with grade 3 placentas. In this study, 81.8 percent of postmature infants that underwent ultrasound had oligohydramnios, which remains an important heralding sign for the postmaturity syndrome in postdates pregnancies.

Acceleration of Placental Grading

In a study of 1,096 obstetric ultrasound examinations of 473 nondiabetic pregnancies, the appearance of a grade 1 placenta prior to 27 weeks, a grade 2 prior to 32 weeks, or a grade 3 prior to 34 weeks was found in pregnancies complicated with intrauterine growth retardation and pre-eclampsia.[5]

TABLE 9.1. Ultrasonic changes in the maturing placenta and their relationship to fetal pulmonic maturity

Region	0	I	II	III
			Grade	
Basal layer	No densities	No densities	Linear arrangement of small echogenic areas (basal stippling)	Larger and partially confluent echogenic areas
Placental substance	Finely homogeneous	Few scattered echogenic areas	Linear echogenic densities (comma-like densities)	Circular densities with central echopoor areas
Chorionic plate	Straight and well-defined	Subtle undulations	Early demarcation of cotyledons in the direction of the basal layer	Septation of cotyledons extending to the basal layer[a]

[a] The most important ultrasound finding of a grade III placenta.

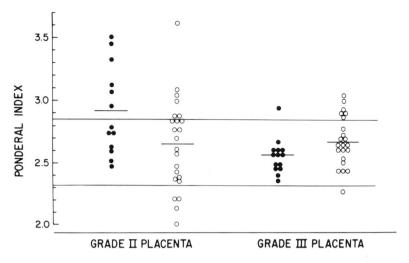

FIG. 9.5. Ponderal index with grade II or grade III placenta. (From Moya et al.,[4] with permission.)

In the examination of 1,468 patients by Proud and Grant,[6] the appearance of a grade 3 placenta at 34 to 36 weeks was seen in 15 percent of cases (223 patients). In this group of patients, there was an estimated two- to eightfold increased risk of meconium-stained liquor, Apgar scores of less than 7 at 5 minutes, low birth weight, perinatal death, and need for an emergency cesarean section for fetal distress during labor. Because the sensitivities were very low, it was concluded that definitive management cannot be dictated based on these findings, but increased antenatal surveillance was warranted.[6] Similar results were suggested by Quinlan et al.[7] in 1982. In addition, Proud and Grant[6] noted that 23 percent of their patients who smoked during pregnancy developed a grade 3 placenta between 34 and 36 weeks, as compared with 13 percent of the nonsmokers. In a clinical setting, the finding of an accelerated placental development on a routine ultrasound examination should alert the physician that the intrauterine environment may be deteriorating. With these findings in mind, antepartum surveillance should be established in these patients until delivery. The patients should be followed closely for the development of pre-eclampsia.

Delayed Placental Maturation

Unpublished data from my laboratory suggest that a delayed change from a grade 0 to grade 1 configuration (i.e., a grade 0 appearing after 32 to 33 weeks) may be associated with the onset of gestational diabetes. Similar results were reported by Hills et al.[8] In these patients, a glucose screen to rule out gestational diabetes is recommended.

Placental Grading and Fetal Pulmonic Maturity

In the initial study published in 1979,[1] the correlation of fetal pulmonic maturity and placental grades in normal patients 35 weeks to term demonstrated that a mature L/S ratio (>2) was found, 68 percent of the time with a grade 1 placenta, 88 percent with a grade 2 placenta, and 100 percent with a grade 3 placenta. In 1983, Clair et al.[9] examined 78 high-risk obstetric patients, including diabetics between 33 weeks and term. Of the 13 grade 3 placentas found, 23 percent of fetuses had immature lungs, but none of the neonates in this group developed respiratory distress syndrome (RDS).[9] In 1986, Shah and Graham[10] correlated ultrasound examinations of 215 patients between 26 and 42 weeks with the presence or absence of RDS and came to the same conclusion. Petrucha and Platt[11] stated that the combination of a biparietal diameter of greater than 9.2 cm and a grade 3 placenta was associated with fetal pulmonic maturity.

Contrary to the above studies, in a study of 563 patients, Harman et al.[12] demonstrated an incidence of 7 percent immature L/S ratio results with the grade 3 placenta. Similar results were reported in 1982 by Quinlan et al.[13] and by Tabsh[14] in 1983.

In 230 patients studied, Kazzi and associates[15] divided the placental appearance into three groups: (A) no grade 3 areas, (B) only a portion with grade 3 areas, and (C) grade 3 throughout. They found a 12 percent incidence of neonatal hyaline membrane disease in group A; 8 percent in group B; and no respiratory distress in group C.[15]

From these observations, there appears to be an association of placental maturation based on the grading classification[1] and fetal pulmonic maturity as established by biochemical markers or neonatal presence or absence of RDS. Some studies report a higher correlation than others. It should be borne in mind that this relationship is based on a gestational age correlation and is not sensitive enough to be used solely as a predictor of fetal pulmonic maturity. It should be used as an assessment of the overall fetal status. In general, the more mature the placenta and the more advanced the gestational age, the more likely the fetal lungs are to be mature. Estimation of phosphatidyl glycerol and the L/S ratio should remain the "gold standard" for determining fetal pulmonic maturity.

Intrauterine Growth Retardation

The presence of a grade 3 placenta may help differentiate the small for gestational age (SGA) fetus from a constitutionally small fetus. Kazzi et al.[15] tested this hypothesis in a study of 109 pregnancies resulting in birth weights of less than 2,700 g. In this group, 44 patients had a grade 3 placenta and 65 had a non-grade 3 (i.e., grade 0, 1, or 2). The presence of a grade 3 placenta was followed by the delivery of a SGA neonate 59 percent of the time. In patients less than 34 weeks, the grade 3 placenta was significantly related to the delivery of the SGA infant with a true positive rate of 62 percent and a sensitivity of 66 percent ($P < 0.008$).[16]

Grade 3 Placenta and Fetal Biophysical Profile

Vintzileos et al.[17] have included placental grading as part of their biophysical profile examination. Other parameters include an assessment of fetal breathing, tone, movement, amniotic fluid, and nonstress testing. These investigators established that the grade 3 placenta was associated with an abnormal fetal heart rate tracing (44.4 percent) and abruptio placenta (14.8 percent) during labor.[17] The use of placental grading as part of the biophysical profile is not widely accepted, however.

Placental Grading and Placental Thickness

As the placenta matures from a grade 0 to a grade 3, there is an associated "thinning" of the placenta. The mean thickness of a grade 1 placenta is 3.8 cm, grade 2 is 3.6 cm, and a grade 3 is 3.4 cm.[18] Placental thickness should be measured at a point between the cord insertion site and the edge of the placenta.

Clinically, placental thickness should be used along with an assessment of the clinical setting and the intrauterine environment as a whole. For example, a placental thickness of less than 2.5 cm is more likely to be associated with a poor intrauterine environment, as with intrauterine growth retardation. However, a thin placenta in the face of polyhydramnios may not have the same clinical significance, as it is being compressed. A placenta measuring greater than 4 cm in thickness may suggest the onset of gestational diabetes, especially if there is delayed maturation and increased amniotic fluid. In this situation, a glucose tolerance screen may be indicated. Although a placental thickness of greater than 4 cm may not always indicate a clinical problem, one must be aware of the findings of placentomegaly in immune and nonimmune hydrops, where placental thickness can be as great as 6 to 8 cm. The progress of the hydrops can be followed by assessment of placental thickness along with other ultrasound findings such as polyhydramnios, fetal ascites, pleural and pericardial effusions, and subcutaneous edema.

Placental Surface Area

Bleker et al.[19] in 1977 demonstrated that the surface area of the placenta increased linearly throughout the gestational period in 15 percent of cases; in the remaining 85 percent, a growth plateau was reached after 34 to 35 weeks.[19]

Hoogland[20] in 1980 used the surface area measurement of the placenta as a diagnostic screen for intrauterine growth retardation. In his study, he noted that if the surface area of the placenta was less than 187 cm^2 at 150 days of gestation, there was a 67 percent chance of existing or developing intrauterine growth retardation.[20] This method is tedious and has not been generally used in routine practice.

PLACENTAL LOCALIZATION

First Trimester

It is possible with high-resolution equipment to identify clearly the area of the chorion frondosum, the definitive placenta, at 7 to 12 weeks gestation. It appears as an area of high-level echoes (Fig. 9.2). The identification of the placenta at this stage of pregnancy has become particularly important in the procedure of chorion villous sampling. Here the chorion frondosum can be sampled successfully under ultrasound guidance, either vaginally via a catheter (Portex) or abdominally via an 18- to 20-gauge needle (see Ch. 11). Examination of the villi permits the prenatal diagnosis of certain chromosomal and enzyme defects in the fetus in the first trimester.

Second and Third Trimester

The cause of bleeding in the late second trimester and third trimester is most often due to placenta previa, until proved otherwise. Ultrasonography is the diagnostic modality of choice.[21-24]

In the mid-second trimester, the incidence of placenta previa is approximately 20 percent, whereas at term, the incidence is 0.5 percent.[21] King[25] described this apparent change of position and termed it placental migration. The diagnosis of placenta previa is determined by assessing the presence of the placenta in the lower uterine segment and its relationship to the internal os.

Differentiating of a low-lying placenta from marginal partial or complete (total) placenta previa is generally easy. When the placenta is posterior, it may sometimes be difficult to see the lower margins of the placenta, especially if the presenting part is shadowing the lower edge of the placenta. At 18 to 20 weeks, if the placenta barely touches or overlaps the os, but the major portion of the placenta extends along the long axis of the uterine wall, the chances are excellent that this placenta will migrate and be normally positioned at the time of delivery. Follow-up scans are indicated to make sure that the migration does occur. On the other hand, a placenta covering the os with portions equally placed on both sides is more likely to remain a placenta previa. Again, serial ultrasound scans are important throughout gestation, since the mode of delivery will be dictated by the final position of the placenta in relationship to the cervical os. Because changes in relative placental position can be noted well into the third trimester, clinical management regarding mode of delivery should not be based on an ultrasound examination made 2 weeks prior. The examination must be repeated prior to delivery.

Diagnosis of the anterior placenta previa in the second trimester is easily made and represents one of the few indications for a reasonably full bladder. The bladder acts as an acoustic window and permits clear visualization of the area of the internal os (Fig. 9.6). The bladder should not be overdistended, as it can cause approximation of the anterior and posterior uterine walls, making a low-lying placenta appear as a placenta previa (Fig. 9.7).

The posterior placenta can often be difficult to recognize due to acoustic shadowing from the fetal body. Lateral scanning or elevation of the fetal presenting part by an abdominal hand will permit visualization of the lower uterine segment area. In addition, if the measurement between the presenting part and the sacral promontory is more than 2 cm, the possibility of a posterior placenta previa must be entertained (Fig. 9.8). With a normally positioned placenta, the presenting part is usually closely approximated to the sacral promontory. Vaginal scanning facilitates visualization of the posterior placenta previa when the fetal head precludes adequate visualization of the placental tip.

PLACENTAL ABRUPTION

Abruptio placenta can be diagnosed by ultrasonography, but it should be noted that the absence of findings on an ultrasound examination should not preclude the diagnosis of abruptio placenta. There are two signs to look for: (1) retroplacental clot, and (2) the retromembranous clot. The retroplacental clot can be recognized as a sonolucent area between the placenta and the uterine wall. As the clot becomes organized, this area will become more echodense (Fig. 9.9). It must be distinguished from the large vessels of the placental bed often seen in the laterally positioned placenta (Fig. 9.10) or the posterior placenta. The retromembranous clot can be identified when the membranes are noted to be separated from the uterine wall by an enlarging clot. The progress of the abruption can be followed by measuring the size of both the retromembranous and retroplacental separation. The clinical and hematologic parameters are more important, however, than the ultrasound findings for determining clinical management.

MULTIPLE GESTATION

In the assessment of a pregnancy with multiple gestation, it is important to note the number of placentas and their morphology and to identify the dividing membranes. In the Caucasian population, 80 percent of twins will have a dichorionic placenta, while in Nigeria, 95 percent of the twin population will have a dichorionic placenta.

In the presence of a single-appearing placenta, with or without a dividing membrane (monochorionic diamnionic or monochorionic monoamnionic), the possibility of a twin–twin transfusion must be considered. The incidence of those vascular connections varies from 85 to 100 percent.[26,27] There are two types of vascular communications: superficial and deep. The superficial connections are found mostly on the fetal surface of the placenta and are between the chorionic arteriole of one fetus and the chorionic arteriole of the other. The deep anastomosis is usually of the arteriovenous type (Fig.

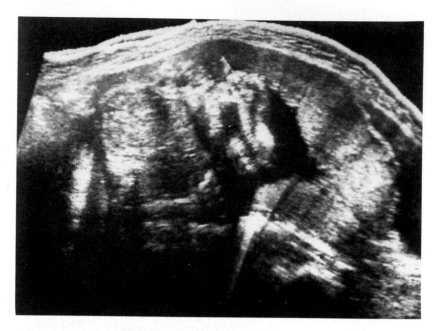

FIG. 9.6.   Anterior placenta previa.

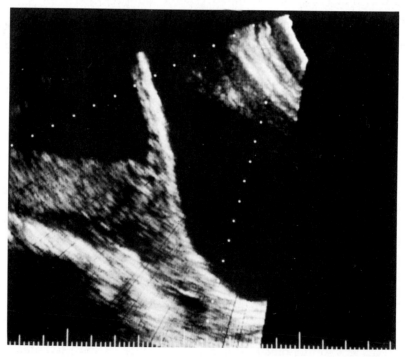

FIG. 9.7.   Overdistended bladder creating the appearance of a placenta previa, when in fact it is a low-lying placenta.

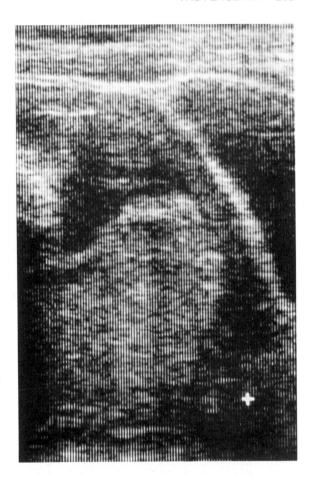

FIG. 9.8. Posterior placenta previa. The caliper marks the area of the internal os, which in this figure cannot be definitively recognized. Nevertheless, it is completely covered by the placenta.

9.11) and is of greater consequence to fetal growth. In the twin–twin transfusion syndrome, one fetus (the donor) develops intrauterine growth retardation, while the recipient fetus develops polycythemia. Although hydrops is not a frequent finding, it can occasionally be found. Vascular connections between dichorionic fused placentas are rare, although there are a few reports in the literature.[28] Erskine et al.[29] used Doppler ultrasound to assist in the diagnosis of twin–twin transfusions. Doppler may be used to identify the vessels, especially if they are on the surface of the placenta. In a study using pulsed Doppler, evaluation of the umbilical artery found concordant waveforms in 44 of 45 normal sets of twins and correctly identified discordant growth in 9 of 11 such sets. In the nine abnormal sets, Doppler discordance before the biometric changes in six sets.[30]

Although discordant growth of twins is more common in a single placenta with anastomotic vascular channels, two separate nonfused placentas do not preclude this possibility. Local factors in one of the placentas (as in a singleton pregnancy) can lead to intrauterine growth retardation in that fetus. Vascular connections are not implicated in this type of discordant growth.

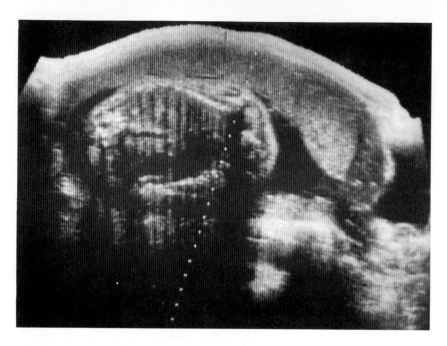

FIG. 9.9. Placental abruptio showing organized retroplacental clot. (From Grannum,[34] with permission.)

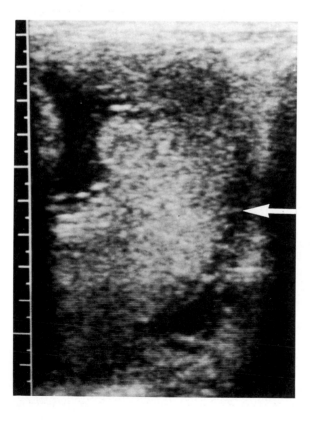

FIG. 9.10. The large sinuses of the placental bed in a laterally positioned placenta (arrow) must not be confused with an abruptio placenta.

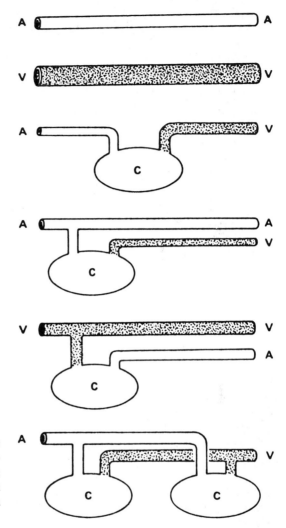

FIG. 9.11. Various anastomotic channels, found in the monochorionic twin placentae. (A, artery; V, vein; C, shared lobule with capillary anastomosis.) (From Fox,[35] with permission.)

Ultrasound evaluation of the twin pregnancy with discordant growth may sometimes be reflected in the difference in appearance of placentas. Often the growth-retarded donor twin may demonstrate an accelerated placental maturation.

Identification of the dividing membranes should be a mandatory part of the ultrasound examination. If it appears that there is only one placenta, without evidence of a dividing membrane, a monochorionic monoamnionic placentation must be seriously considered. In this type of placentation, there is increased perinatal morbidity due to premature labor (usually secondary to polyhydramnios), the possibility of cord entanglement, 30 percent risk of twin–twin transfusion,[27] and an increased risk of congenital anomalies. This increase is due mostly to an increase in structural anomalies in the monozygotic twins.[31] Another complication, although not common, involves twin–twin transfusion whereby the thromboplastic material from the dead twin passed into the circulation of the living twin, precipitating the onset of disseminated intravascular coagulation.[32]

CONCLUSION

The developing placenta as seen sonographically from the early first trimester to the end of the third trimester holds important clues to the fetal condition. Identification of the chorion frondosum and the ability to sample it under ultrasound guidance during the first trimester are useful in obtaining important genetic information of the fetus. The development of the placenta, as evidenced by placental grading in the second and third trimester, offers additional information concerning the intrauterine environment. It is not sensitive enough to be used to determine fetal pulmonic maturity. Ultrasound assessment to determine placental position remains an important clinical tool. Vaginal ultrasound may, in the future, enable sonographers and sonologists to be more precise in determining the relationship of the placenta and the internal os, further reducing the cesarean section rate for this entity. Doppler ultrasound of the fetoplacental circulation itself holds promise in its ability to determine fetal well-being.

REFERENCES

1. Grannum PAT, Berkowitz RL, Hobbins JC: The ultrasonic changes in the maturing placenta and their relation to fetal pulmonic maturity. Am J Obstet Gynecol 133:915, 1979

2. Crawford JM: Vascular anatomy of the human placenta. Am J Obstet Gynecol 84:1543, 1962

3. Levine L: Placenta grades and gestational age. Doctoral thesis, Yale University School of Medicine, March 1981

4. Moya F, Grannum P, Pinto K, et al: Ultrasound assessment of the postmature pregnancy. Obstet Gynecol 65:319, 1985

5. Hooper KD, Komppa GH, Bice P, et al: A reevaluation of placental grading and its clinical significance. J Ultrasound Med 3:261, 1984

6. Proud J, Grant AM: Third trimester placental grading by ultrasonography as a test of fetal wellbeing. Br Med J 294:1641, 1987

7. Quinlan RW, Cruz AC, Buhi WC, Martin M: Changes in placental ultrasonic appearance. II. Pathologic significance of Grade III placental changes. Am J Obstet Gynecol 144:471, 1982

8. Hills D, Irwin GA, Tuck S, Baim R: Distribution of placental grade in high risk gravidas. AJR 143:1011, 1984

9. Clair MR, Rosenberg E, Tempkin D, Andreotti RF, Bowie JD: Placental grading in the complicated or high-risk pregnancy. J Ultrasound Med 2:297, 1983

10. Shah YG, Graham D: Relationship of placental grade to fetal pulmonary maturity and respiratory distress syndrome. Am J Perinatol 3:53, 1986

11. Petrucha RA, Platt LD: Relationship of placental grade to gestational age. Am J Obstet Gynecol 144:733, 1982

12. Harman CR, Manning FA, Stearns E, Morrison I: The correlation of ultrasonic placental grading and fetal pulmonary maturation in five hundred sixty-three pregnancies. Am J Obstet Gynecol 143:941, 1982

13. Quinlan RW, Cruz AC, Buhi WC, Martin M: Changes in placental ultrasonic appearance. I. Incidence of Grade III changes in the placenta in correlation to fetal pulmonary maturity. Am J Obstet Gynecol 144:468, 1982

14. Tabsh KM: Correlation of real-time ultrasonic placental grading with amniotic fluid lecithin/sphingomyelin ratio. Am J Obstet Gynecol 145:504, 1983

15. Kazzi GM, Gross TL, Sokol RJ, Kazzi SN: Noninvasive prediction of hyaline membrane disease: An optimized classification of sonographic placental maturation. Am J Obstet Gynecol 152:213, 1985

16. Kazzi GM, Gross TL, Sokol RJ, Kazzi SN: Detection of intrauterine growth retardation: A new use for sonographic placental grading. Am J Obstet Gynecol 145:733, 1983

17. Vintzileos AM, Campbell WA, Ingardia CJ, et al: The fetal biophysical profile and its predictive value. Obstet Gynecol 62:271, 1983

18. Grannum PAT, Hobbins JC: The placenta. Radiol Clin North Am 20:353, 1982

19. Bleker OP, Kloosterman GJ, Breur W, Mieras DJ: The volumetric growth of the human placenta: A longitudinal ultrasonic study. Am J Obstet Gynecol 127:655, 1977

20. Hoogland HJ: Ultrasonographic aspects of the placenta. Nijmegen, Alphen a/d Rijn: The Netherlands, Koninkijke Drukkerij GJ Thieme, BV

21. Wexler P, Gottesfield KR: Second trimester placenta previa: An apparently normal placentation. Obstet Gynecol 50:706, 1977

22. Kohorn EI, Walker RHS, Morrison J, Campbell S: Placental localization. Am J Obstet Gynecol 103:868, 1969

23. Kobayashi M, Hellman LM, Fillisti L: Placental localization by ultrasound. Am J Obstet Gynecol 106:279, 1970

24. Williamson D, Bjorgen J, Barer B, Wormann M: The ultrasonic diagnosis of placenta previa: Value of the post-void scan. J Clin Ultrasound 6:58, 1978

25. King DL: Placental migration demonstrated by ultrasonography. Radiology 109:167, 1973

26. Bernirschke K: Accurate recording of twin placentation—A plea to the obstetrician. Obstet Gynecol 18:334, 1961

27. Strong SJ, Corney G: The placenta in twin pregnancy. Pergamon Press, Oxford, 1967

28. Bhargava I, Chakravarty A: Vascular anastomoses in twin placentae and their recognition. Acta Anat 95:471, 1975

29. Erskine RLA, Ritchie JWK, Murnaghan GA: Antenatal diagnosis of placental anastomosis in a twin pregnancy using Doppler ultrasound. Br J Obstet Gynaecol 93:955, 1986

30. Gerson AG, Wallace DM, Bridgens NK, et al: Duplex Doppler ultrasound in the evaluation of growth in twin pregnancies. Obstet Gynecol 70:419, 1987

31. Schnizel AAGL, Smith DW, Miller JR: Monozygotic twinning and structural defects. J Pediatr 95:921, 1979

32. Moore CM, McAdams AJ, Sutherland JM: Intrauterine disseminated intravascular coagulation: A syndrome of multiple pregnancy with a dead twin fetus. J Pediatr 74:523, 1969

33. Pritchard J, McDonald P, Gant N (eds): Williams Obstetrics. 17th Ed. Appleton & Lange, E Norwalk, CT, 1985

34. Grannum PAT: p 469. In Campbells (ed): Clinical Obstetrics and Gynecology. Vol. 10. WB Saunders, Philadelphia, 1983

35. Fox H: Major Problems in Pathology. Vol. 7. WB Saunders, Philadelphia, 1978

10 Sonography of the Fetal Cranium

GIANLUIGI PILU AND LUCIANO BOVICELLI

Congenital anomalies of the central nervous system (CNS) account for 10 to 20 percent of all malformations detected at birth. Epidemiologic studies indicate an overall incidence of about 1 in 100 births.[1,2] The frequency appears to be even higher in spontaneous abortions,[3-5] suggesting that these defects have a very high intrauterine fatality rate.

The CNS was probably the first fetal system to be investigated in utero by diagnostic ultrasound. Anencephaly was the first congenital anomaly to be recognized by this technique before viability.[6] CNS anomalies are among the fetal malformations most frequently encountered by obstetric sonographers. From 1976 to 1986 at the Prenatal Pathophysiology Unit of the University of Bologna, CNS anomalies accounted for 35 percent of all fetal anomalies recognized with ultrasonography. Nevertheless, the accuracy of sonography in predicting fetal CNS defects has not yet been assessed. Modern high-resolution ultrasound equipment yields a unique potential in evaluating normal and abnormal fetal neuroanatomy since the very early stages of development.[7-18] Our experience indicates that both the sensitivity and specificity of targeted examinations in at-risk pregnancies are very high. Conversely, the accuracy of level 1 nontargeted examinations is indeed quite low. During 1982 to 1985, 127 infants with CNS anomalies included mainly anencephaly, spina bifida, and hydrocephalus. Although 94 percent of pregnancies underwent routine sonographic evaluation of the fetal anatomy at a point in gestation at which identification of the lesion was theoretically possible, a prenatal diagnosis was made in only 62 percent of cases. Furthermore, the diagnosis was made prior to fetal viability only in about 10 percent of cases.[19] These discouraging data seem to indicate that most obstetric sonographers are still scarcely familiar with even the basic elements of the investigation of fetal cranium. The purpose of this chapter is to review the current experience in the intrauterine interpretation of normal cerebral anatomy and to provide guidelines for the recognition of anomalies either arising from or involving this area.

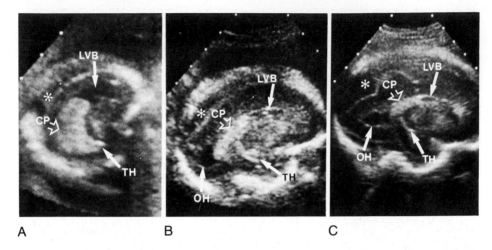

A   B   C

FIG. 10.1. Parasagittal scans of the fetal head, demonstrating the intrauterine development of the lateral ventricle. The modifications in size and shape of the body (LVB), temporal horn (TH), and occipital horn (OH) throughout gestation can be readily appreciated. (A) At 16 weeks, the brightly echogenic choroid plexus occupies most of the ventricular lumen. (B) At 23 weeks, the beginning of the development of the occipital horn (OH) can be seen. (C) At 30 weeks, the ventricle has assumed its definitive configuration. The subarachnoid space (*) overlying the cerebral convexity is normally generous. (From Romero et al.,[158] with permission.)

NORMAL INTRACRANIAL ANATOMY OF THE FETUS

The lateral ventricles and the corresponding choroid plexuses are the first cerebral structures that can be identified with sonography in the fetus. In the late first trimester, the lateral ventricles occupy most of the intracranial cavity and are almost entirely filled by the echogenic choroid plexuses.[20] Major developmental changes occur in the architecture of the fetal brain during the following weeks. The size of the lateral ventricles, compared with the mass of the hemispheres, decreases steadily throughout the first half of pregnancy (Fig. 10.1). The optimal fetal age for a proper sonographic investigation of intracranial structures is probably at 18 to 25 weeks. At this time, a detailed evaluation of the entire ventricular system, subarachnoid spaces (Fig. 10.2), and diencephalic and rhombencephalic structures (Fig. 10.3) is possible.

The clinical role of the sonographic biometry of the fetal cranium is well established. Measurement of the biparietal diameter[21–23] and head circumference[23,24] is currently used both for assessing gestational age and fetal growth and for identifying cranial abnormalities. Measurement of the cerebellar transverse diameter was recently suggested for similar purposes.[25–27] Table 10.1 presents a nomogram of the normal values of these three biometric parameters throughout gestation.

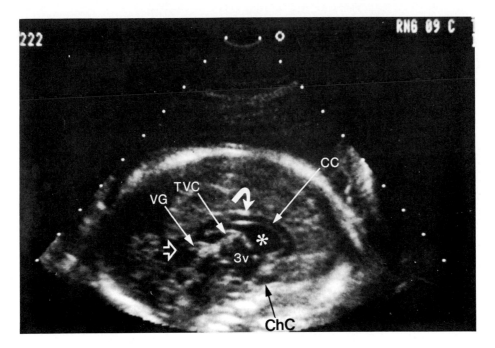

FIG. 10.2.   Mid-sagittal scan of the brain of a normal mid-trimester fetus. The corpus callosum is seen as a sonolucent band interposed between the patent cavum septi pellucidi (*) and the echogenic pericallosal cistern (curved arrow). The sonolucent area demarcated superiorly by the cavum septi pellucidi and inferiorly by the roof of the third ventricle (3v) is the triangular velum cistern (TVC), which is inferiorly continuous with the cistern of the vein of Galen (open arrow). Within the latter, the vein of Galen (VG) is seen. The sonolucent area which is seen anteriorly and inferiorly to the third ventricle is the chiasmatic cistern (ChC). (From Pilu et al.,[46] with permission.)

HYDROCEPHALUS

The incidence of congenital hydrocephalus ranges between 0.3 and 1.5 in 1,000 births in different epidemiologic surveys.[2] In the vast majority of cases, this lesion arises as a consequence of an obstruction to cerebrospinal fluid (CSF) circulation.

The first attempts to diagnose hydrocephalus in utero with sonography were made by demonstrating a gross enlargement of the head.[28] Head measurements are obviously unreliable for an early diagnosis, as macrocrania usually does not develop until late in fetal life. It was recently demonstrated that in many cases of fetal ventriculomegaly the BPD is within normal limits, even in the late third trimester.[29] Sonographic identification of fetal hydrocephalus depends on the direct demonstration of the enlargement of the ventricular system. Confusion may arise at times, as the relative size of ventricles and cortex undergoes important modifications throughout gestation. No-

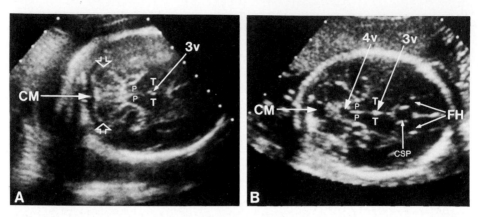

FIG. 10.3. Suboccipitobregmatic view of the fetal brain. The sonolucent thalami (T) and cerebral peduncles (P), the frontal horns (FH), cavum septi pellucidi (CSP), and third ventricle (3v) are seen. The prominent cisterna magna (CM) outlines the cerebellum. (A) The superior cerebellar vermis is seen bridging between the cerebellar hemispheres. This scanning plane is commonly used for the measurement of the cerebellar transverse diameter (open arrows). (B) A slight posterior angulation of the transducer permits visualization of the fourth ventricle (4v), which is separated from the cisterna magna by the echogenic inferior cerebellar vermis. (From Pilu et al.,[50] with permission.)

mograms of the normal size of cerebral ventricles against gestation are now available. The normal values of the measurements of the frontal horns,[30,31] bodies,[7,10,30] temporal horns,[30] and atria[31] of the lateral ventricles have been established.

Biometry facilitates immediate recognition of moderate to severe ventriculomegaly since mid-gestation. However, several investigators have pointed out that the size of both frontal horns and bodies of lateral ventricles may be within the normal range in cases of mild or early hydrocephalus.[10,31,32] A qualitative evaluation has been suggested to be more sensitive than biometry in these cases. Chinn and associates[33] observed that throughout gestation, the large fetal choroid plexus fills the lumen of the lateral ventricle at the level of the atrium almost entirely, being closely apposed to both the medial and lateral wall. In early hydrocephalus, the choroid plexus is shrunken and anteriorly displaced, thus being clearly detached from the medial wall of the ventricle (Fig. 10.4).

Ventricular enlargement can result from many pathologic entities differing in both etiology and clinical course. In a pediatric series, aqueductal stenosis was found in 43 percent of cases, communicating hydrocephalus in 38 percent, and Dandy-Walker malformation (DWM) in 13 percent.[34] The recognition of fetal hydrocephalus should prompt an attempt to identify the specific anatomic lesion.

Simultaneous distention of both lateral ventricles and third ventricle in the presence of a normal posterior fossa may indicate either aqueductal steno-

TABLE 10.1. Nomogram of the biparietal diameter (BPD), head circumference (HC), and cerebellar transverse diameter (CTD) according to percentile distribution

Gestational Age (Weeks)	BPD (mm) Percentiles			HC (mm) Percentiles			CTD (mm) Percentiles		
	10	50	90	10	50	90	10	50	90
15	30	33	35	120	126	128	10	14	16
16	34	35	38	123	125	141	14	16	17
17	36	38	43	134	138	160	16	17	18
18	38	42	44	142	154	169	17	18	19
19	42	45	48	145	159	178	18	19	22
20	45	47	53	146	173	190	18	20	22
21	48	50	57	185	191	211	19	22	24
22	50	53	55	193	193	203	21	23	24
23	53	56	60	203	206	222	22	24	26
24	56	60	64	219	224	230	22	25	28
25	61	63	68	219	234	251	23	28	29
26	63	65	67	235	241	246	26	29	32
27	64	68	70	237	243	246	26	30	32
28	68	70	72	246	253	264	27	30	34
29	71	74	79	254	274	301	29	34	38
30	72	75	79	253	277	298	31	35	40
31	75	76	83	274	291	303	32	38	42
32	75	80	84	275	288	208	33	38	42
33	80	81	87	292	297	322	32	40	44
34	81	84	91	326	326	327	33	40	44
35	78	87	93	300	301	303	31	40	47
36	84	88	91	309	313	318	36	43	55
37	87	89	92	303	313	324	37	45	55
38	87	90	94	—	—	—	40	48	55
39	92	92	92	—	—	—	52	52	55

(Modified from Goldstein et al.,[26] with permission.)

sis or communicating hydrocephalus. Aqueductal stenosis may arise from both genetic and environmental factors. An X-linked recessive pattern of transmission is thought to account for 25 percent of cases occurring in males.[34] A multifactorial etiology, with a recurrence risk of about 1 to 2 percent, is probably responsible for most of the remaining cases.[34]

Aqueductal stenosis carries a rather severe prognosis. The mortality rate of treated infants ranges between 10 and 30 percent.[35,36] In one study, only

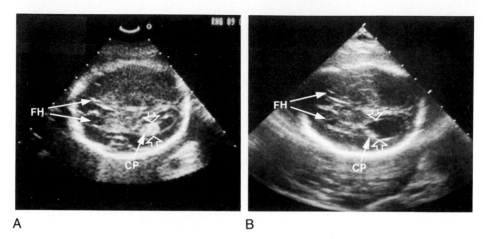

A   B

FIG. 10.4. Axial views of the fetal brain passing through the frontal horns (FH) and atria in a normal fetus (A) and in a fetus with ventriculomegaly (B) at the same gestational age (24 weeks). Normalcy is indicated by the brightly echogenic choroid plexus (CP) that fills the atrium entirely, being closely apposed to both the medial and lateral wall (open arrows). Hydrocephalus is attested by the anterior displacement of the shrunken choroid plexus that appears clearly detached from the medial wall of the ventricle.

50 percent of treated infants developed normal intelligence.[36] In another study, the mean IQ following shunting was 71.[35] The X-linked type aqueductal stenosis seems to have an even worse outcome. A mortality rate as high as 80 percent and the presence of intellectual impairment in almost all treated survivors have been reported.[37,38]

Communicating hydrocephalus results from either an obstruction along the normal pathway of the CSF outside the ventricular system or from failure of fluid reabsorption. It has been reported in association with subarachnoid hemorrhage,[39] agenesis of arachnoid granulation,[40] thrombosis of cerebral venous sinuses,[41] and overproduction of CSF due to a papilloma of the choroid plexus.[42] A multifactorial etiology with a recurrence risk of 1 to 2 percent has been suggested.[34] Communicating hydrocephalus is also commonly associated with spina bifida.[43]

A confident diagnosis of communicating hydrocephalus may be made in the presence of tetraventricular hydrocephalus associated with enlargement of the cerebral cisterns (Fig. 10.5). This finding has been reported to have limited sensitivity in newborns, as it could be documented in only 30 percent of cases.[44] However, the natural history of this anomaly, as outlined by neuroradiologic studies in children,[45] seems to encompass three different successive stages: (1) distention of the subarachnoid spaces; (2) both enlargement of the cerebral ventricles and subarachnoid spaces are visible; and (3) only triventricular hydrocephalus is seen. Such observations may suggest that in the fetus, during early stages of development of communicating hydrocephalus, distention of the subarachnoid spaces is seen more frequently than in newborns, permitting a specific diagnosis in a larger number of cases.[46]

Communicating hydrocephalus is associated with a much better prognosis than the internal obstructive forms. A mortality rate of 11 percent and a normal intellectual development in 84 percent of cases was reported in one study.[36] More recently, a survival rate of 100 percent and a normal intellectual development in all treated cases has been reported.[35]

Several familial cases of DWM have been reported, suggesting that this lesion can be inherited, in at least some cases, as an autosomal-recessive trait.[47–49] However, a multifactorial etiology with a recurrence risk of 1 to 5 percent accounts for the vast majority of cases.[49] DWM may also be a part of a number of genetic and nongenetic syndromes.[49]

Dandy-Walker malformation is featured by the association of hydrocephalus, a retrocerebellar cyst, and a defect in the cerebellar vermis through which the posterior fossa cyst communicates with the fourth ventricle. In spite of this classic definition, it has been recently demonstrated that hydrocephalus is an inconsistent finding in newborn infants. In the largest pediatric series now available,[48] it was found that in 80 percent of cases ventriculomegaly was absent at birth, developing only after months or even years of life. Our experience with the prenatal diagnosis of DWM supports this observation. In two cases of DWM recognized in utero, ventriculomegaly made its comparison only during the first weeks after birth. The mechanism responsible for the postnatal onset of hydrocephalus is unknown. Bleeding of the retrocerebellar cyst following traumatic vaginal delivery has been suggested.[48] However, it may be of note that in both of our previously mentioned cases, atraumatic delivery by cesarean section had occurred.

As hydrocephalus may be absent in the fetus, prenatal diagnosis of DWM relies mainly on the demonstration of the typical posterior fossa abnormality[50] (Fig. 10.6). We have found that in most cases of DWM, lateral separation of the cerebellar hemispheres results in an abnormally increased transverse cerebellar diameter. However, the sonographic appearance of the vermian defect and retrocerebellar cyst is striking, and biometry is rarely if ever necessary to identify this lesion. DWM is frequently associated with other nervous and non-nervous malformations, including agenesis of the corpus callosum, heterotopia, polymicrogyria, agyria, macrogyria, polydactylism-syndactylism, congenital heart disease, polycystic kidneys, and cleft palate.[48,51] The association with agenesis of corpus callosum is relevant, as it has been suggested as representing an adverse prognostic factor for intellectual development.[52] Recent series of treated infants indicate an overall mortality rate ranging from 12 to 26 percent and a normal IQ in 30 to 60 percent of cases.[48,52]

It should be stressed that with any of the previously mentioned forms of congenital hydrocephalus, there is a chance for a normal intellectual development. Despite the common belief, there is not a strict correlation between the severity of ventricular enlargement and the outcome of affected infants.[235,53–56]

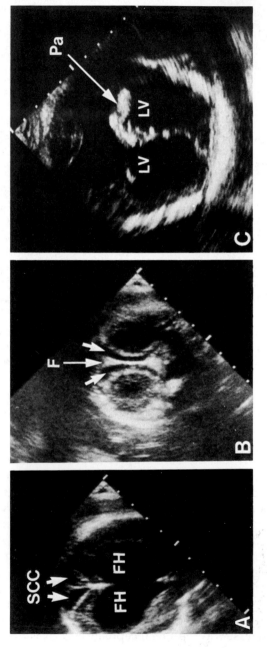

FIG. 10.5. Distention of the subarachnoid cisterns is attested by the enlarged supracortical cisterns (SCC) overlying the cerebral convexity (A) and by the prominent interhemispheric fissure (arrowheads) (B). Choroid plexus papilloma (Pa) associated with communicating hydrocephalus (C) (F, falx cerebrii; LV, atria of lateral ventricles). (From Pilu et al.,[46] with permission.)

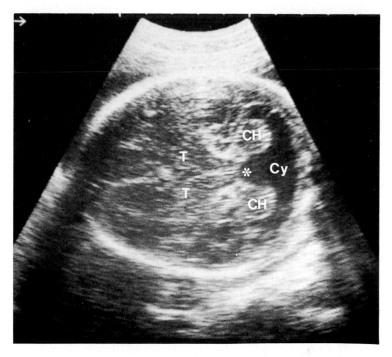

FIG. 10.6. Fetal Dandy-Walker malformation. The defect of the cerebellar vermis connecting the area of the fourth ventricle (·) to the posterior fossa cyst (Cy) is demonstrated. The cerebellar hemispheres (CH) are laterally separated. T-thalami.

Infants with a cerebral mantle thickness of a few millimeters can develop a normal and even superior intelligence, if adequately treated.[53] The prognosis seems to depend more on the anatomic type of hydrocephalus than on the degree of ventriculomegaly.[35,36] The optimal obstetric management of congenital hydrocephalus is still controversial. In the vase majority of cases diagnosed prior to viability, the parents will probably elect termination of pregnancy. In continuing pregnancies, exclusion of associated anomalies is mandatory, as they are reported to occur with an incidence ranging between 30[16] to 60 percent.[15] Maternal screening for group TORCH infections, fetal karyotyping, and a detailed sonographic evaluation of the entire fetal anatomy, including echocardiography should be performed in each case. Many authorities believe that in cases of isolated hydrocephalus, atraumatic delivery by cesarean section as soon as pulmonic maturity is achieved, as well as early neurosurgical care, maximize the chances of survival and normal development for affected infants.[35,57–59] As fetal cephalocentesis is associated with major complications, this procedure is contraindicated, unless severe life-threatening associated anomalies are found.[60]

Intrauterine decompression of congenital obstructive hydrocephalus by ventriculoamniotic shunting has recently been suggested.[61] Experimental studies on animal models hold promise.[62] The preliminary experience on human fetuses is less encouraging. The Registry of the International Society of Fetal Medicine and Surgery indicates that out of a total of 44 fetuses who underwent shunting between 1982 and 1985, the procedure-related death rate was 10 percent. Fifty-three percent of survivors had a severe handicap and 12 percent a mild handicap; only 35 percent were developing normally at the time of follow-up.

NEURAL TUBE DEFECTS

The nervous system derives from the neural plate, a dorsal thickening of the ectoderm that can be recognized as early as the fourteenth day of gestation. The faster growth rate of the lateral portions of the neural plate results in the formation of two longitudinal folds demarcating an internal groove. The folds fuse with each other in the midline, starting the transformation of the groove into a tube at about the midportion of the embryo. Closure then proceeds cephalad and caudad. From 20 to 24 days gestation, the neural tube is almost entirely closed, with the only exception of the two openings at the extremities—the anterior and posterior neuropore. The anterior neuropore undergoes obliteration at about 24 days, followed by the posterior neuropore at about 26 days.

Two pathogenetic theories of neural tube defects (NTD) have been postulated. Failure of closure of the anterior neuropore (anencephaly) or posterior neuropore (spina bifida) is the most widely accepted. Gardner[63] suggested secondary rupture of the already fused neural tube following embryonic hydrocephalus.

The average incidence of NTD is 1 to 2 per 1,000 birth. The incidence rises to almost 7 in 1,000 in South Wales.[64,65] The etiology of NTD is multifactorial, with a recurrence risk after the birth of one affected child of 3 to 5 percent. The interested reader is referred to the extensive review compiled by Blocklehurst.[66]

Anencephaly

Anencephaly is featured by the absence of the cranial vault, cerebral hemispheres, and diencephalic structures. The head is covered by a vascular membrane (area cerebrovasculosa). Associated anomalies, including spina bifida, cleft lip and palate, and omphalocele are commonly found. Polyhydramnios is almost the rule. Sonographic prenatal diagnosis is easy. As the fetal head can be consistently identified with modern ultrasound equipment starting from 10 to 11 weeks gestation, it is likely that anencephaly can be recognized from this period. Anencephaly is an invariably fatal lesion. In the United

States, termination of pregnancy can be offered to couples whenever the diagnosis is made.[67]

Spina Bifida

The prenatal identification of spinal disraphism is considered elsewhere in this book. This chapter deals with the intracranial abnormalities found with this condition. The association among spina bifida aperta, ventriculomegaly, and varying degrees of hypoplasia of the posterior fossa structures is attested by both autoptic[68–70] and diagnostic imaging studies.[71–76] Cerebral anomalies associated with spina bifida are thought to derive mainly from the displacement of part of the brain stem and cerebellum through the foramen magnum and cervical canal, an anomaly commonly referred to as either Chiari II or Arnold-Chiari malformation. In the early stages, the ventriculomegaly that accompanies spina bifida belongs to the communicating type, and it is thought to derive from a distal block at the level of the foramen magnum.[77] At birth in 60 to 70 percent of cases, a secondary stenosis at the level of the acqueduct is formed.[43] As the fetal head is easily accessible to sonographic examination, identifying alterations of the cerebral architecture predictive of spina bifida would greatly assist the sonographer in the difficult task of detecting this anomaly. Nicolaides and associates[78] recently reported a retrospective study of the intracranial anatomy in fetuses with spina bifida. These workers described a typical abnormality of the cerebellum, which appeared on sonography as a crescent with the concavity pointing anteriorly (the so-called "banana sign"). They also found that fetuses with spina bifida usually have enlarged atria of lateral ventricles and frontal bossing (the "lemon sign"). In our own experience with 18 fetuses with spina bifida prospectively examined, we have found that abnormalities of the posterior fossa and/or lateral ventricles were present in all, starting from as early as 18 weeks gestation. In 16 cases (88.8 percent), it was either impossible to visualize the cerebellum or the cerebellar transverse diameter was abnormally small (Figs. 10.7 and 10.8). In only 14 cases (77.7 percent), there was overt ventriculomegaly attested by biometry. However, 17 fetuses (94.4 percent) had a disproportion between the atrial lumen and the corresponding choroid plexus. In none of our 18 cases could we document the presence of the "banana sign." Conversely, frontal bossing was found in all our cases.

The peculiarity of the ventricular distention seen in infants with Arnold-Chiari malformation has been described in depth both in computed tomography (CT)[74] and in sonographic studies.[75] The prominent caudate nucleus determines a typical alterations in the shape of the frontal horns (Figs. 10.9 and 10.10).

The association between spina bifida and severe hydrocephalus has been regarded in the past as a poor prognostic factor for intellectual development.[79] More recent experience seems to indicate that in many cases control of hydrocephalus by shunting results in normal intelligence.[80]

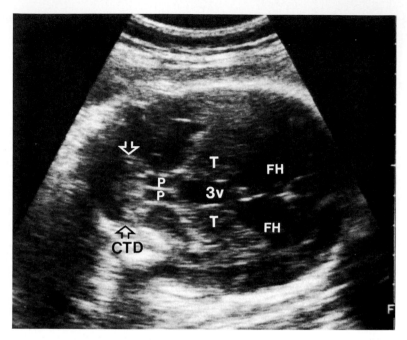

FIG. 10.7. Suboccipitobregmatic view of the brain of a fetus with Arnold-Chiari malformation. The frontal horns (FH) and third ventricle (3v) are enlarged. The cerebral peduncles (P) appear elongated. The posterior fossa is poorly visualized. The cisterna magna cannot be demonstrated, and the cerebellum is impacted among the petrous ridges of the temporal bone. The cerebellar transverse diameter (CTD) is abnormally small. (T, thalami, 3V, third ventricle.)

Cephaloceles

The observation that cephaloceles may occur in families with a history of either anencephaly or spina bifida, or both, suggests an etiologic relationship among these defects.[81] The term cephalocele indicates a protrusion of the intracranial contents through a bony defect of the skull. True encephaloceles are characterized by the presence of brain tissue inside the lesion. When only meninges protrude, the term cranial meningocele is more appropriate. Cephaloceles arise most often from the midline at the level of the occipital bone and less frequently from the frontal and parietal bones and from the base of the skull. Impairment of CSF circulation as well as hydrocephalus are frequently found. True encephaloceles with massive protrusion of brain tissue may be associated with microcephaly. Cephaloceles may occur either as isolated lesions or as a part of a number of genetic and non genetic syndromes,[82] such as Meckel syndrome[83] and the amniotic band syndrome.[84]

The prenatal sonographic identification of a true encephalocele is easy, as the presence of brain tissue within the meningeal sac is striking (Fig.

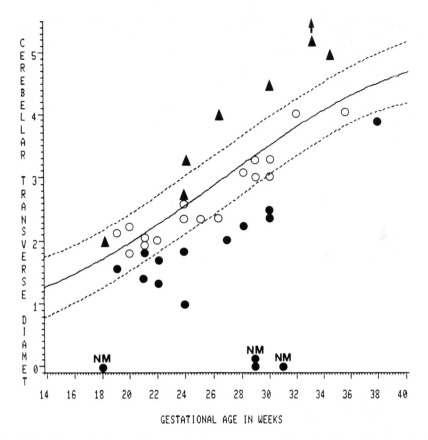

FIG. 10.8. Normal values of the cerebellar transverse diameter throughout gestation. (●) Cases of fetal spina bifida. (○) Fetuses with isolated obstructive hydrocephalus. Not surprisingly, most fetuses with Dandy-Walker malformation (▲) were found to have abnormally large values of cerebellar transverse diameter.

10.11). Differentiation of a cranial meningocele from soft tissue edema or a cystic hygroma of the neck is notoriously difficult.[85] Recognition of the bony defect permits a specific diagnosis.[31] However, many defects are only a few millimeters in size and fall easily below the resolution power of current ultrasound equipment. Some clues may assist in making a proper diagnosis. Cranial cephaloceles are often associated with hydrocephalus. Cystic hygromas arise from the region of the neck, have multiple internal septations and a thick wall, and are often associated with hydrops.[86] Cephaloceles protruding from the base of the skull inside the orbits, nasopharyns, or oropharynx are obviously rather inaccessible to prenatal ultrasound investigation. As cephaloceles are often associated with a number of genetic and nongenetic defects or syndromes, a careful search for other deformities is recommended.

The outcome depends on the type of cephalocele. Infants with pure meningocele develop a normal intelligence in 60 percent of cases following treat-

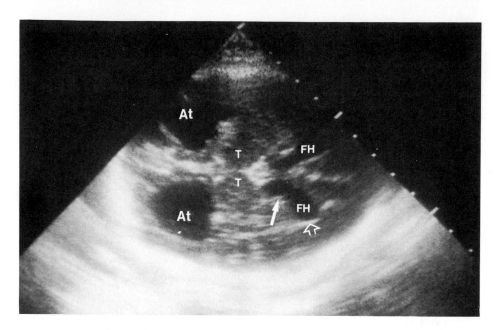

FIG. 10.9.   Axial scan of the head of a third-trimester fetus with Arnold-Chiari malfor-mation. Note the squared-off frontal horns (open arrow) and the indentation due to the prominent caudate nucleus (solid arrow). (FH, frontal horns; T, thalami; At, atria.)

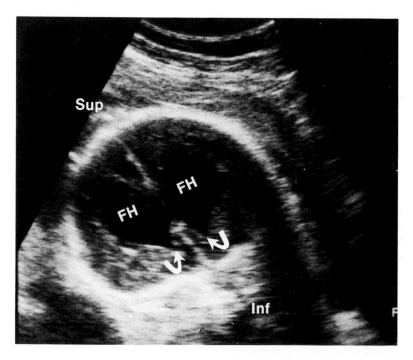

FIG. 10.10.   Coronal view of the brain of a fetus with Arnold-Chiari malformation, demonstrating the typical inferior pointing (curved arrows) of the frontal horns (FH).

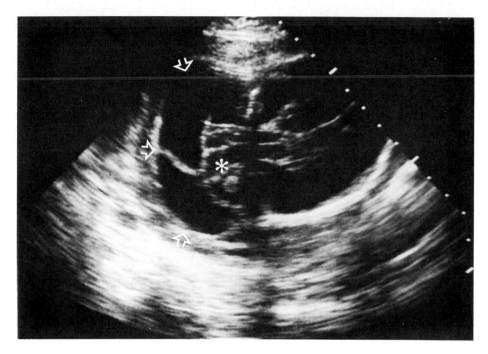

FIG. 10.11. Occipital encephalocele (open arrows). Most of the cerebellum (*) protrudes inside the meningeal sac. The infant had associated microcephaly.

ment. True encephaloceles carry a mortality rate of 40 percent and a high incidence of intellectual impairment and neurologic sequelae.[87] Termination of pregnancy can be offered prior to viability. A cesarean delivery is recommended in cases of cranial meningocele. Massive encephaloceles associated with microcephaly have a dismal prognosis, and conservative management may be offered to the couple.[13]

DISORDERS OF VENTRAL INDUCTION

The term ventral induction refers to the interrelated developmental events occurring in the embryonic forebrain from the fifth to the sixth week of gestation that lead to the formation of the cerebral hemispheres, optic thalami, and diencephalic derivatives (optic bulbs, hypophysis, and pineal body). These events are probably influenced by the prechordal mesenchyma, which is thought to induce the development of part of the splanchnocranium and facial structures as well. Disorders of ventral induction include a group of midline cerebral defects that encompass a wide spectrum of severity: holoprosencephaly, septo-optic dysplasia, and agenesis of the corpus callosum[88] (Fig. 10.12). These anomalies are frequently associated with craniofacial malformations.

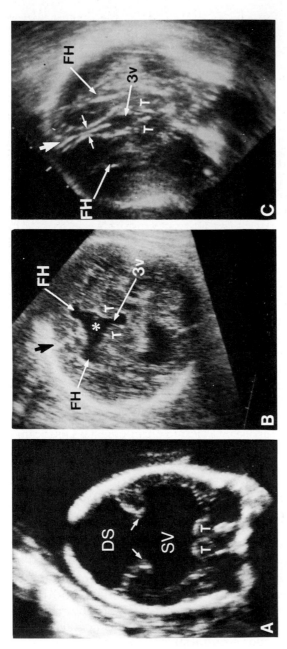

FIG. 10.12. The spectrum of disorders of ventral induction. (A) Alobar holoprosencephaly. A coronal scan of the fetal head reveals a single primitive ventricular cavity (SV). The cerebral cortex (thin arrows) is only partially enfolded above the ventricle that balloons out to form a large dorsal sac (DS). The bulblike fused thalami (T) can be seen on the floor of the ventricle. (From Pilu et al.,[97] with permission.) (B) Lobar holoprosencephaly. A coronal scan shows the flattened roof of the fused (*) frontal horns (FH) that amply communicate with the inferior third ventricle. The thalami (T) appear unusually round. A well-formed interhemispheric fissure (black arrow) is seen. However, the falx was found to be absent at birth. (C) Agenesis of the corpus callosum. A coronal scan shows that the third ventricle (3v) is enlarged and upwardly displaced in the position normally occupied by the corpus callosum. The interhemispheric fissure (thin arrows) is typically prominent and the falx cerebrii (arrowhead) comes in close contact with the roof of the third ventricle. The frontal horns (FH) are widely separated.

Holoprosencephaly

Holoprosencephaly is the consequence of a disorder in the diverticulation of the embryonic prosencephalon. Early failure of the ventral induction provided by the prechordal mesenchyma also leads to maldevelopment of the median facial structures.[89] The association between brain anomalies and facial dysmorphism is typical of the holoprosencephalic sequence.[90] Failure of the forebrain to undergo paired symmetric division and diverticulation results in varying degrees of fusion of the cerebral structures. In the most severe form of holoprosencephaly, the alobar variety, the interhemispheric fissure, and falx cerebri are absent; there is a single primitive ventricle (holoventricle); the thalami are fused on the midline; and there is absence of the third ventricle, neurohypophysis, olfactory bulbs, and tracts. In semilobar holoprosencephaly, the two cerebral hemispheres are partially separated posteriorly, but there is still a single ventricular cavity. In both the alobar and semilobar forms, the roof of the primitive ventricular cavity, the thela choroidea, which is normally enfolded within the brain, may balloon out between the cerebral convexity and the skull to form a cyst of variable size (the dorsal sac). Alobar and semilobar holoprosencephaly are often associated with microcephaly, less frequently with macrocephaly. In the lobar variety, the interhemispheric fissure is well developed anteriorly and posteriorly, but there is a variable degree of fusion of the cyngulate gyrus and of the frontal horns of lateral ventricles.

The incidence of holoprosencephaly is unclear. Cyclopia and cebocephaly, two subtypes of this anomaly, occur in 1 in 40,000 and 1 in 16,000 births, respectively.[91] The incidence of holoprosencephaly in abortions has been reported to be as high as 4 in 1000.[92]

The etiology is heterogeneous. In most cases, the anomaly is isolated and sporadic. The association with chromosomal aberrations is well documented. Holoprosencephaly is found in 62 percent of infants with trisomy 13.[93] A familial tendency with autosomal-dominant transmission has also been described.[91] The influence of various teratogens, maternal diabetes, congenital infections, and drug ingestion in pregnancy has been suggested but never clearly proved. The overall recurrence risk is 6 percent.[94]

Prenatal diagnosis of the alobar variety of holoprosencephaly is easy. The single primitive ventricle, absence of the third ventricle, fusion of the thalami (which have a typical bulblike appearance), and the cystic dorsal sac can be easily demonstrated in the fetus by sonography from the second trimester.[95–97] The pleomorphic facial anomalies typically associated with alobar holoprosencephaly have all been correctly identified in fetuses by sonography.[95–101] Figs. 10.13 to 10.15). Only one case of prenatal diagnosis of semilobar holoprosencephaly has been reported thus far.[102] Cerebral findings were very similar to those described in cases of alobar holoprosencephaly. In two fetuses with ventriculomegaly, lobar holoprosencephaly was identified by the demonstration of fusion and squaring of the roof of the frontal horns.[103] We suspected this condition in a ventriculomegalic fetus due to both the

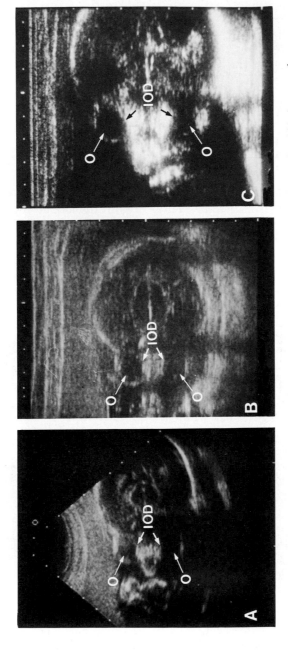

FIG. 10.13. Axial scans of the upper fetal face demonstrating the orbits (O). (A) A normal interorbital distance (IOD) is shown. (B) Hypotelorism. (C) Hypertelorism. Although hypotelorism is the most typical craniofacial malformation found in cases of holoprosencephaly, hypertelorism has also been documented.[89] (B from Pilu et al.,[101] with permission.)

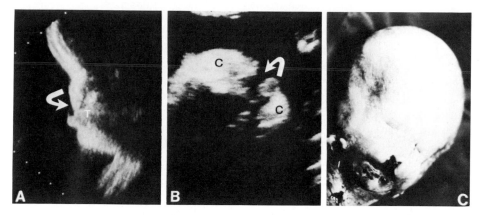

FIG. 10.14.   Holoprosencephaly associated with median cleft lip. (A) Arhinia (curved arrow) is demonstrated in a profile of the fetal face. (B) Typical median cleft of the lip and anterior palate. (C) View of the stillborn fetus, shown for comparison. (From Pilu et al., [101] with permission.)

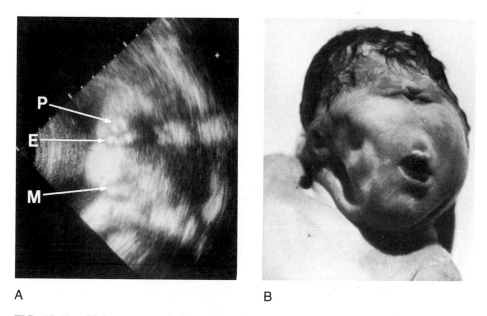

FIG. 10.15.   Holoprosencephaly with cyclopia. (A) A coronal scan of the fetal face demonstrates the proboscis (P) and the single median eyelid (E). (B) A view of the stillborn infant is shown for comparison. (M, mouth).

presence of fusion of the frontal horns and third ventricle and to the striking bulblike appearance of the thalami, closely resembling the one previously described in cases of alobar holoprosencephaly (Fig. 10.12). Obstructive hydrocephalus, particularly if associated with Arnold-Chiari malformation, may result in disruption of the septum pellucidum, giving rise to an ample communication between the frontal horns. However, under these conditions, the roof of the frontal horns is not flattened but appears indented at the level of the interhemispheric fissure.[103] It is also generally possible to demonstrate that, at a lower level than the one normally occupied by the septum pellucidum, the frontal horns are separated from each other and communicate with the third ventricle through the well-defined foramina of Monro (Fig. 10.16).

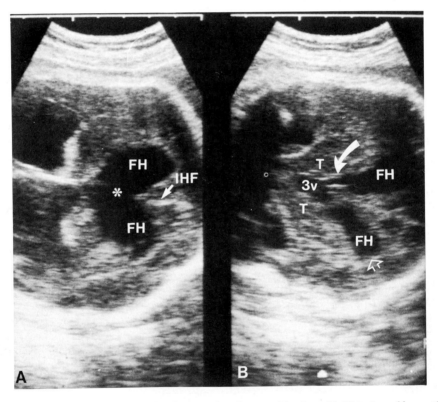

FIG. 10.16. Axial scans of the brain of a fetus with Arnold-Chiari malformation and ventriculomegaly. (A) An ample communication (*) between the enlarged frontal horns (FH). A disruption of the septum pellucidum is inferred by the demonstration of the indented roof of frontal horns at the level of the interhemispheric fissure (IHF). (B) At a slightly lower level, the frontal horns appear separated and are seen to communicate with the third ventricle (3v) through paired foramina of Monro (curved arrow). Note the typical squaring off of the lateral walls of frontal horns (open arrow). (T, thalami).

Alobar holoprosencephaly is fatal within the very first days or weeks of life. Semilobar holoprosencephaly may be compatible with longer survival, but infants are virtually amented.[91] If these conditions are recognized prior to viability, termination of pregnancy can be offered to the couple. If the diagnosis is made later in pregnancy, conservative management is strongly recommended.[95] Infants with lobar holoprosencephaly frequently suffer from mental retardation, but they may be totally asymptomatic.[104] A careful search for associated anomalies, including karyotyping, is certainly indicated. Isolated lobar holoprosencephaly does not seem to require any alteration of standard obstetric management. A cesarean delivery may be indicated in those cases with associated hydrocephalus and macrocrania.

Septo-optic Dysplasia

Septo-optic dysplasia (De Morsier syndrome) is a rare cerebral anomaly featured by absence of the septum pellucidum and optic disc hypoplasia. Affected persons have visual impairment and pituitary-hypothalamic axis disfunction.[105] Occasional findings include ventriculomegaly, mental retardation, hemiparesis, and craniofacial abnormalities such as hypotelorism and cleft lip-cleft palate. The etiology is unknown.

Computed tomography[106,107] and transfontanellar sonographic findings[108] in septo-optic dysplasia have a striking similarity to those of lobar holoprosencephaly. We have experience with one case. A sonographic examination performed at 25 weeks gestation in a pregnant patient referred because of a suspicious level 1 scan revealed fetal ventriculomegaly with atypical findings that included absence of the septum pellucidum, flattening of the roof and mild inferior pointing of the fused frontal horns, a small dysmorphic third ventricle, normal thalami and posterior fossa, and enlarged subarachnoid spaces. The fetus was also found to have bilateral cleft lip and palate (Fig. 10.17). Our experience indicates that mild disorders of ventral induction, such as lobar holoprosencephaly and septo-optic dysplasia, can be identified in utero. However, it is uncertain whether these two conditions can be differentiated with sonography prior to birth. The diagnosis of septo-optic dysplasia in infants depends on the clinical data and the CT visualization of small optic nerves and optic canals and malrotation of the optic chiasm.[106–108] The demonstration of these findings in the fetus does not seem possible at present.

Agenesis of the Corpus Callosum

Connecting fibers bridging between the two cerebral hemispheres appear at about the third month of gestation. They arise from the massa commisuralis, an embryologic structure formed by the fusion of the lateral margins of the groove, which separates the two primitive hemispheric vesicles. The rostrad portion of the corpus callosum is the first to be formed. Growth

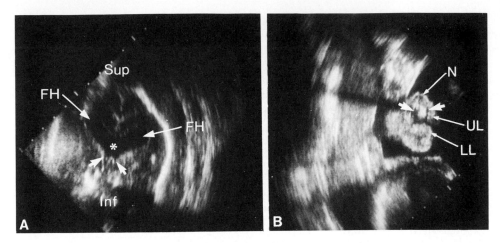

FIG. 10.17.   Septo-optic dysplasia. (A) The enlarged and fused (*) frontal horns (FH) have a flattened roof, and there is mild inferior pointing. (B) Anterior coronal scan of the fetal face, demonstrating bilateral cleft lip (arrowheads). (Sup, superior; Inf, inferior; N, nose; UL, LL, upper and lower lip.)

then proceeds caudally, the definitive configuration of the corpus callosum being assumed only by the fifth month. Agenesis of the corpus callosum (ACC) may be either complete or partial. In the latter condition, aplasia affects the posterior portion that is ontogenetically the last one to be formed.

The incidence of ACC is controversial. Figures ranging from almost 1 in 100 to 1 in 19,000 have been reported.[109] The etiology is unclear. ACC may be found in association with chromosomal aberrations such as trisomy 18. A Mendelian inheritance with autosomal-dominant, autosomal-recessive, and sex-linked transmission as well has been documented on several occasions.[100] ACC is also a part of several genetic syndromes, including Aicardi,[111] Andermann,[112,] acrocallosal,[113] and F.G. syndrome.[114] Anatomic anomalies including CNS malformations (abnormal convolutional patterns, DWM, microce phaly, aplasia, or hypoplasia of pyramidal tracts) and a wide variety of non-nervous deformities are very frequently found, suggesting that ACC may be a part of a widespread developmental disturbance.[115]

Agenesis of the corpus callosum is invariably associated with a typical alteration of the intracranial architecture that includes a marked lateral separation of the bodies of lateral ventricles and enlargement of the atria and occipital horns. Such rearrangement of ventricular morphology is commonly refer red to as colpocephaly. The third ventricle is frequently enlarged and displaced upward in the position normally occupied by the corpus callosum.[109,116]

Criteria for the diagnosis of ACC after birth have been well established in both radiologic[117,118] and sonographic studies,[119,120] and include mainly the recognition of the previously mentioned deformations of the ventricular system. Neonatal transfontanellar sonography permits a specific diagnosis by directly demonstrating the absence of the corpus callosum. ACC was also recently identified with sonography in the fetus since mid-gestation.[121] In our own experience of seven cases identified in utero, colpocephaly could be easily demonstrated in all (Fig. 10.18). Upward displacement of the third ventricle proved to be an inconsistent finding, as it was seen only in 45 percent of cases (see Figs. 10.12, and 10.18).

Recognition of ACC in the fetus should always prompt a careful search for associated anomalies. A detailed investigation of the entire fetal anatomy by high-resolution ultrasound, echocardiography, and karyotyping is indicated.

Many patients with ACC suffer from mental retardation and neurologic abnormalities and are psychologically abnormal. However, the condition may be entirely asymptomatic.[109] No specific risk figures are available. Association with other anomalies increases the likelihood of a poor outcome. However, many severe deformities frequently associated with ACC, such as anomalies of the pyramidal tracts, are not predictable with prenatal ultrasound. Drawing

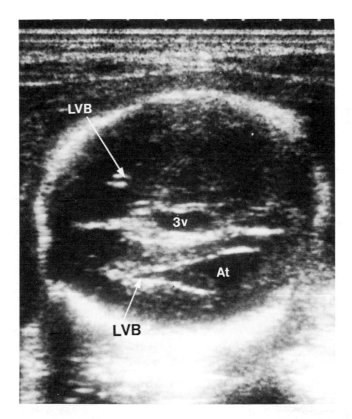

FIG. 10.18. Typical ventricular configuration of agenesis of the corpus callosum: colpocephaly and upward displacement of the enlarged third ventricle (3v). Note the enlarged atria (At) and laterally separated bodies of lateral ventricles (LVB).

guidelines for parental counseling and for obstetric management is difficult. Prior to viability, we believe that termination of pregnancy can be offered to the couple. In continuing pregnancies, it would seem that no specific management is required. ACC may be associated with macrocephaly. In these cases, a cesarean delivery may be required.

CEREBRAL DISRUPTIONS: PORENCEPHALY AND HYDRANENCEPHALY

Congenital porencephaly is defined as the presence of cystic cavities within the cerebral matter. The cavities may communicate with either the ventricular system or subarachnoid space, or both. Loss of cerebral tissue may derive from either a destructive process, usually on an anoxic basis (encephaloclastic porencephaly), or from primary maldevelopment of the brain (schizencephaly).[122,123] The former condition is more frequenlty observed. The lesions are usually irregular and unilateral. Impairment of CSF circulation and hydrocephalus are often seen. Conversely, schizencephaly is characterized by clefts within the cerebral substance that are frequently bilateral and symmetric. Hydranencephaly may be regarded as an extreme form of en-

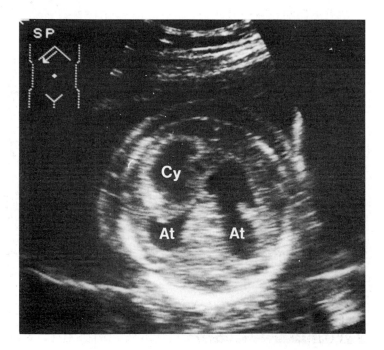

FIG. 10.19. Porencephaly in a fetus with multiple congenital anomalies. The atria of lateral ventricles (At) are dilated, and a large cyst (Cy) is seen within the cerebral parenchyma. (From Grannum and Pilu,[18] with permission.)

cephaloclastic porencephaly. It is characterized by absence of most of the cerebral hemispheres. The brain stem and rhombencephalic structures are usually spared, and the cranial cavity is filled with CSF.[124] Hydrancephaly has been reported in association with congenital infections, including toxoplasmosis and cytomegalovirus and intrauterine occlusion or atresia of the internal carotid arteries.[124–128]

Cystic cavities within the fetal brain are easily demonstrated with ultrasonography[11,16] (Fig. 10.19), but it is unclear whether a differential diagnosis between porencephaly and intracranial cysts of different nature, such as arachnoid cysts and congenital cystic tumors, is possible. The fluid-filled cranial cavity typical of hydrancephaly is easily detected by antenatal ultrasonography. However, a specific identification of this condition may be difficult. The differential diagnosis includes severe hydrocephalus and holoprosencephaly. One of the most valuable sonographic findings in hydranencephaly is the demonstration of the intact brain stem, which, in the absence of the surrounding cortex, bulges inside the fluid-filled intracranial cavity[16] (Fig. 10.20). This finding somewhat resembles the bulblike appearance of the hypoplastic thalami that can be seen in alobar and semilobar holoprosencephaly. However, in the latter condition, it is usually possible to demonstrate the pancaked frontal cortex. The outcome for infants with congenital brain disruptions is dictated by the size and location of the lesion. Extensive porencephaly and hydranencephaly have a dismal prognosis.[129,130]

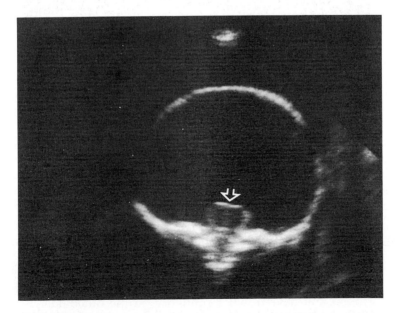

FIG. 10.20. Fetal hydranencephaly. The brain stem (arrow) protrudes within the fluid-filled intracranial cavity. (From Pilu et al.,[16] with permission.)

DISORDERS OF NERVE CELL PROLIFERATION
Microcephaly

The association between decreased head size and reduction of both brain mass and total cell number is well established.[131] However, there is disagreement with regard to the clinical threshold of abnormality. Some authors have suggested using as a diagnostic criterion a head circumference below −2 SD from the mean.[132] Others prefer to consider abnormal head circumference below −3 SD.[133] The incidence of microcephaly obviously varies in different surveys depending on the definition used to identify the lesion.

Microcephaly should not be considered as a separate clinical entity but rather as a symptom of many etiologic disturbances. Etiology includes both genetic and environmental factors.[134,135] The clinical subdivision suggested by Book and associates[133] distinguishes between those cases resulting from nongenetic insults (e.g., anoxia, infections, radiation) and genetic microcephaly, which includes all cases in which microcephaly is transmitted as a Mendelian trait either by itself or as a part of any of a number of syndromes.

Microcephaly is featured by a typical disproportion between the skull and the face. The forehead is sloping. The brain is small (microcephaly), the cerebral hemispheres being affected to a major extent than the diencephalic and rhombencephalic structures. Abnormal convolutional patterns including macrogyria, microgyria, and agyria are frequently found. The ventricles may be dilated. Microcephaly is frequently seen in cases of porencephaly, lissencephaly, and holoprosencephaly.

Many difficulties arise in attempting to identify fetal microcephaly. The value of head measurements alone may be hampered by incorrect dating or intrauterine growth retardation. Furthermore, the natural history of fetal microcephaly is largely unknown. Progressive intrauterine development of the lesion interfering with early recognition has been described.[136] A comparison of biometric parameters, such as the head circumference to abdominal circumference ratio[137] and the femur length to biparietal diameter ratio,[138] has been suggested. Chervenak and associates[139] have provided most useful nomograms. Nevertheless, both false-positive and false-negative diagnoses have been reported.[139] It is clear that the predictive value of ultrasonography has some limitations and that further investigation is required. A qualitative evaluation of the intracranial anatomy is a very useful adjunct to biometry, as many cases of microcephaly are associated with morphologic derangement. The demonstration of a sloping forehead increases the index of suspicion (Fig. 10.21).

Establishing a reliable prognosis for fetuses affected by microcephaly is difficult. Associated anomalies should be accurately ruled out, as they are frequently found and have a major influence on the outcome. The clinical data regarding isolated microcephaly are controversial. In one series of 134 infants with a head circumference below −2 SD from the mean, only one had normal intelligence.[132] More recent studies are in disagreement with

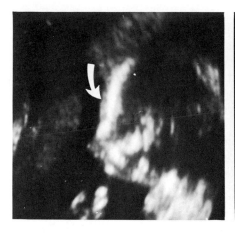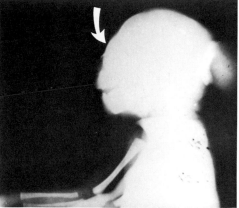

FIG. 10.21.   Sagittal scan of the face demonstrating the sloping forehead of a second-trimester fetus with microcephaly and an occipital cephalocele. A radiograph of the abortus is provided for comparison.

these observations. In a group of 28 infants with head circumference below −2 SD from the mean, only 50 percent were found to have mental retardation.[140] In another study, infants with a head circumference between −2 and −3 SD from the mean were mentally retarded in 18 percent of cases, and infants with a head circumference below −3 SD from the mean were mentally retarded in 72 percent of cases.[141] It is hard to derive precise prognostic figures from these data. However, it is clear that a small head does not necessarily imply intellectual impairment.

Megalencephaly

The clinical significance of megalencephaly[142] is unclear. People with abnormally large brains are usually of normal or even superior intelligence, but an abnormally large brain may be associated with mental retardation and neurologic impairment.[142] Megalencephaly is also a part of congenital anomalies and syndromes, such as Beckwith-Wiedemann syndrome, achondroplasia,[143] neurofibromatosis,[144] and tuberous sclerosis. Obstetric and pediatric sonographers are not infrequently challenged by the problem of megalencephaly, a condition that should be suspected in the presence of abnormally large head measurements without evidence of hydrocephalus or intracranial masses. In these cases, examination of the couple may be of help, as asymptomatic megalencephaly is frequently familial.

Unilateral megalencephaly is a rare anomaly characterized by overgrowth of one lobe or an entire hemisphere. As of 1968, 50 cases had been reported in the literature.[145] The etiology is unknown. Unilateral megalencephaly has been reported in association with hemigigantism of the body.[146] In most cases, both macroscopic and microscopic abnormalities are found in the affected portion of the brain,[145] including aberrant convolutional patterns (micropolygyria, pachygyria, agyria), and ectopic nodules of gray matter. Mild to moderate enlargement of the corresponding lateral ventricle is usually found. Histologic studies of the affected brains have revealed a diffuse increase in neuronal size. CT findings include enlargement of one cerebral hemisphere in the absence of mass effect, a shift of the midline structures, and mild ipsilateral ventriculomegaly.[147]

We recently identified unilateral megalencephaly in a third-trimester fetus (Fig. 10.22). Albeit a rare condition, unilateral megalencephaly should be considered in the differential diagnosis of conditions associated with a shift of the midline, which also includes porencephaly and congenital brain tumors.

It is difficult to establish a reliable prognosis for infants affected by this condition. In most cases, mental retardation and uncontrollable seizures are

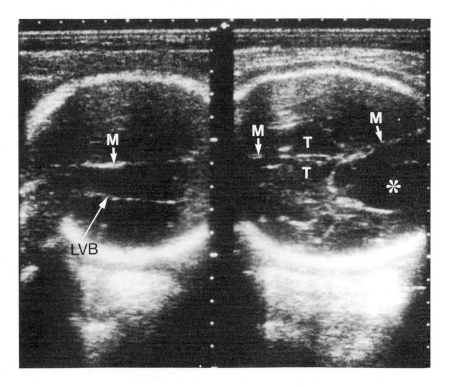

FIG. 10.22. Unilateral megalencephaly in a third-trimester fetus. The diagnosis was prompted by the shift of the midline (M) and by the gross asymmetry of the cerebral hemispheres, in the absence of obvious intracerebral masses. The hemisphere distal to the transducer appears unusually prominent, particularly at the level of the occipital lobe. The ipsilateral body of the lateral ventricle is almost normal, but a striking enlargement of the occipital horn (*) is seen. (T, thalami). This fetus had significant associated macrocrania.

present.[148] Further experience is needed to establish the optimal obstetric management of fetal unilateral megalencephaly. In our own case, a cesarean delivery was performed because of severe macrocrania. It is unclear whether unilateral megalencephaly is predictable prior to viability.

ABNORMALITIES OF THE CHOROID PLEXUS

Choroid Plexus Papillomas

Choroid plexus papillomas (CPP) are neuroectodermal neoplasms that are very frequently congenital in occurrence. With the exception of malignant cases, CPP are histologically identical to the normal choroid plexus. They are most frequenlty found within the lateral ventricles, at the level of the atria, but they have been described within the third and fourth ventricle as well. CPP are frequently associated with hydrocephalus, which may arise by one of two mechanisms: intraventricular obstruction, or overproduction of CSF.[149] Prenatal diagnosis of CPP associated with communicating hydrocephalus has been reported[46] (see Fig. 10.5).

Choroid plexus papillomas carry a rather severe prognosis. In the two largest available series of treated children, the mortality rate ranged between 27 to 37 percent. The survivors developed normal intelligence in approximately 60 percent of cases.[150,151]

The obstetric management should not differ from that outlined for other forms of congenital hydrocephalus. CPP have a high vascular content, and injury to the lesion carries a high risk of a fatal intraventricular bleeding. Therefore, we believe that intrauterine shunting procedures are contraindicated.

Cysts of the Choroid Plexus

Prenatal identification of cysts within the choroid plexus of lateral ventricles was first reported by Chudleigh and associates.[152] In the five cases described in their original report, the cysts were detected at 17 to 19 weeks of pregnancy and spontaneously disappeared between 20 and 23 weeks. The infants were neurologically normal at birth. This report prompted a more extensive review of this condition,[153] in which it was stressed that choroid plexus cysts are commonly found in asymptomatic infants by transfontanellar sonography and have been documented in more than 50 percent of serial autopsy surveys.[154] However, large cysts, with diameters ranging between 2 and 8 cm, have been reported to cause symptoms of intracranial hypertension.[155] More recently, four cases of choroid plexus cysts associated with trisomy 18 were reported.[156,157]

We have seen 12 cases of fetal cysts of the choroid plexus between 1983 and 1987. The cysts were unilateral in eight cases (Fig. 10.23) and bilateral in four (Fig. 10.24). In 11 cases, the cysts were small and did not cause any

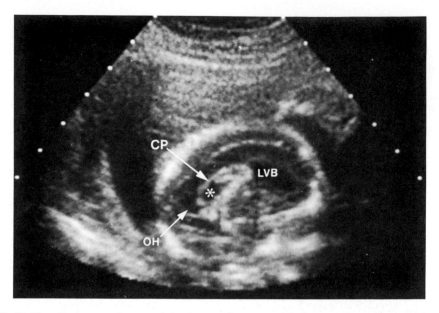

FIG. 10.23. Parasagittal scan of the brain of an 18-week fetus with a choroid plexus cyst (*). The cyst does not distort the architecture of the ventricle. (CP, choroid plexus; LVB, OH, body and occipital horn of lateral ventricle.) (From Grannum and Pilu,[17] with permission.)

distortion of the ventricular architecture. In one case, a large unilateral cyst was found at 22 weeks gestation, in association with mild enlargement of the corresponding lateral ventricle. The couple requested termination of pregnancy. Dissection of the abortion specimen confirmed ventriculomegaly and a large cyst lined by a thin layer of normal choroid plexus tissue. The karyotype was normal. In all the remaining cases, the cysts were seen to decrease in size with advancing gestation. A complete disappearance occurred in nine cases, while in two cases small cystic remnants could be seen until the late third trimester. The fetal karyotype was determined in 10 cases, and one fetus was found to have trisomy 18.

On the basis of this scanty experience, it is hard to draw guidelines for parental counseling and obstetric management. Although the pediatric literature indicates that small choroid plexus cysts have no clinical significance, it would seem that their detection in utero may increase the risk of chromosomal aberrations, and specifically of trisomy 18. We believe that determination of fetal karyotype should be recommended. In the presence of normal chromosomes, those cysts not causing distortion of ventricular morphology should be considered benign. Serial examinations are suggested, but the parents should be reassured. Large cysts, associated with enlargement of the lateral ventricles may represent a different clinical entity. If ventriculomegaly is found, the principles of counseling and management do not differ from those previously outlined for the other forms of this condition.

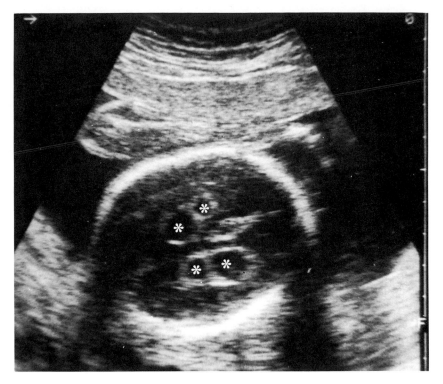

FIG. 10.24.   Axial scan of the head of a second-trimester fetus with worrisome multiple choroid plexus cysts (*). The karyotype of the fetus was normal, and the cyst entirely disappeared in the following weeks. The infant was neurologically normal at birth.

REFERENCES

1. McIntosh R, Merritt KK, Richards MR, et al: The incidence of congenital anomalies: A study of 5,964 pregnancies. Pediatrics 14:505, 1954

2. Myrianthopoulos NC: Epidemiology of central nervous system malformations. p. 139. In Vinken PJ, Bruyn GW (eds): Handbook of Clinical Neurology. Elsevier, Amsterdam, 1977

3. Singh RP, Carr DH: Anatomic findings in human abortions of known chromosome constitution. Obstet Gynecol 29:806, 1967

4. Nishimura H: Incidence of malformations in abortions. p. 275. In Fraser FC, McKusick VA (eds): Congenital Malformations. Excerpta Medica, New York, 1970

5. Creasy MC, Alberman ED: Congenital malformations of the central nervous system in spontaneous abortions. J Med Genet 13:9, 1976

6. Campbell S, Johnstone FD, Holt EMT, et al: Anencephaly: Early ultrasound diagnosis and active management. Lancet 2:1226, 1972

7. Johnson ML, Dunne MG, Mack LA, et al: Evaluation of fetal intracranial anatomy by static and real-time ultrasound. J Clin Ultrasound 8:311, 1980

8. Fiske CE, Filly RA: Ultrasound evaluation of the normal and abnormal fetal neural axis. Radiol Clin North Am 20:285, 1982

9. Hidalgo H, Bowie J, Rosenberg ER, et al: In utero sonographic diagnosis of fetal cerebral anomalies. AJR 139:143, 1982

10. Jeanty P, Dramaix-Wilmet M, Delbeke D, et al: Ultrasonic evaluation of fetal ventricular growth. Neuroradiology 21:127, 1981

11. Chervenak FA, Berkowitz RL, Romero R, et al: The diagnosis of fetal hydrocephalus. Am J Obstet Gynecol 147:703, 1983

12. Chervenak FA, Berkowitz RL, Tortora M, et al: The diagnosis of ventriculomegaly prior to fetal viability. Obstet Gynecol 64:652, 1984

13. Chervenak FA, Isaacson G, Mahoney MJ, et al: Diagnosis and management of fetal cephalocele. Obstet Gynecol 64:86, 1984

14. Chervenak FA, Duncan C, Ment LR, et al: Perinatal management of myelomeningocele. Obstet Gynecol 63:376, 1984

15. Chervenak FA, Duncan C, Ment LR, et al: Outcome of fetal ventriculomegaly. Lancet 2:179, 1984

16. Pilu G, Rizzo N, Orsini LF, et al: Antenatal recognition of fetal cerebral anomalies. Ultrasound Med Biol 12:319, 1986

17. Grannum P, Pilu G: In utero neurosonography—The normal fetus and variations in cranial size. Semin Perinatol 11:85, 1987

18. Grannum P, Pilu G: In utero neurosonography—Neuroembryologic and encephaloclastic lesions. Semin Perinatol 11:98, 1987

19. Cocchi G, Morini MS, Calzolari E, et al: Sensitivity of ultrasound in detection of central nervous system malformations. Eur J Epidemiol 2:329, 1986

20. Crade M, Patel J, McQuown D: Sonographic imaging of the glycogen stage of the fetal choroid plexus. Am J Neuroradiol 2:345, 1981

21. Kurtz AB, Wagner RJW, Kurtz RJ: Analysis of biparietal diameter as an accurate indicator of gestational age. J Clin Ultrasound 8:319, 1980

22. Hadlock FP, Deter RL, Harrist RB: Fetal biparietal diameter: A critical re-evaluation of the relation to menstrual age by means of real-time ultrasound. J Ultrasound Med 2:97, 1982

23. Jeanty P, Cousaert E, Hobbins JC, et al: A longitudinal study of fetal head biometry. Am J Perinatol 1:118, 1984

24. Campbell S, Thoms A: Ultrasound measurement of the fetal head to abdomen circumference ratio in the assessment of growth retardation. Br J Obstet Gynaecol 89:165, 1982

25. MacLeary RD, Kuhus LR, Bozz MJ: Ultrasonography of the fetal cerebellum. Radiology 151:439, 1984

26. Goldstein I, Reece EA, Pilu G, et al: Cerebellar measurements using sonography in the evaluation of fetal growth and development. Am J Obstet Gynecol, 1987

27. Reece EA, Goldstein I, Pilu G, et al: Fetal cerebellar growth unaffected by intrauterine growth retardation: A new parameter for prenatal diagnosis. Am J Obstet Gynecol, 1987

28. Freeman RK, McQuown DS, Secrist LJ, et al: The diagnosis of fetal hydrocephalus before viability. Obstet Gynecol 49:109, 1977

29. Callen PW, Chooljian D: The effect of ventricular dilatation upon biometry of the head. J Ultrasound Med 5:17, 1986

30. Denkhaus H, Winsberg F: Ultrasonic measurement of the fetal ventricular system. Radiology 131:781, 1979

31. Pearce JM, Little D, Campbell S: The diagnosis of abnormalities of the fetal central nervous system. p. 243. In Sanders RC, James AE (eds): The Principles and Practice of Ultrasound in Obstetrics and Gynecology. Appleton and Lange, E Norwalk, CT, 1985

32. Fiske CE, Filly RA, Callen PW: Sonographic measurement of lateral ventricular width in early ventricular dilation. J Clin Ultrasound 9:303, 1980

33. Chinn DH, Callen PW, Filly RA: The lateral cerebral ventricle in early second trimester. Radiology 148:529, 1983

34. Burton BK: Recurrence risks in congenital hydrocephalus. Clin Genet 16:47, 1979

35. McCullough DC, Balzer-Martin LA: Current prognosis in overt neonatal hydrocephalus. J Neurosurg 57:378, 1982

36. Guthkelch AN, Riley NA: Influence of aetiology on prognosis in surgically treated infantile hydrocephalus. Arch Dis Child 44:29, 1969

37. Edwards JH, Norman RM, Roberts JM: Sex-linked hydrocephalus: Report of a family with 15 affected members. Arch Dis Child 36:481, 1961

38. Howard FM, Till K, Carer CO: A family study of hydrocephalus resulting from aqueduct stenosis. J Med Genet 18:252, 1981

39. Ellington G, Margolis G: Block of arachnoid villus by subarachnoid hemorrhage. J Neurosurg 30:651, 1969

40. Gutierrez Y, Friede RL, Kaliney WJ: Agenesis of arachnoid granulations and its relationship to communicating hydrocephalus. J Neurosurg 43:553, 1975

41. Kalbag RM, Woolf AL: Cerebral Venous Thrombosis. Oxford University Press, London, 1967

42. Gradin WC, Taylor C, Fruin AH: Choroid plexus papilloma: Report of a case and review of the literature. Neurosurgery 12:217, 1983

43. Mori K: Anomalies of the Central Nervous System. Neuroradiology and Neurosurgery. Thieme Stratton, New York, 1985

44. Raybaud C, Bamberger Bozo C, Laffont J, et al: Investigations of nontumoral hydrocephalus in children. Neuroradiology 16:24, 1978

45. Robertson WC, Gomez MR: External hydrocephalus: Early findings in congenital communicating hydrocephalus. Arch Neurol 35:541, 1978

46. Pilu G, De Palma L, Romero R, et al: The fetal subarachnoid cisterns: An ultrasound study with report of a case of congenital communicating hydrocephalus. J Ultrasound Med 5:365, 1986

47. Brown JR: The Dandy-Walker syndrome. In Vinken PJ, Bruyn GW (eds): p. 623. Handbook of Clinical Neurology. Vol. 30. Elsevier, Amsterdam, 1977

48. Hirsch JF, Pierre Kahn A, Reiner D, et al: The Dandy-Walker malformation: A review of 40 cases. J Neurosurg 61:515, 1984

49. Murray JC, Johnson JA, Bird TD: Dandy-Walker malformation: Etiologic heterogeneity and empiric recurrence risks. Clin Genet 28:272, 1985

50. Pilu G, Romero R, De Palma L, et al: Antenatal diagnosis and obstetrical management of Dandy-Walker syndrome. J Reprod Med 31:1017, 1986

51. Hart MN, Malamud N, Ellis WG: The Dandy-Walker syndrome: A clinico-pathological study based on 28 cases. Neurology (NY) 22:771, 1972

52. Sawaja R, McLaurin RL: Dandy-Walker syndrome: Clinical analysis of 23 cases. J Neurosurg 55:89, 1981

53. Lorber J: Medical and surgical aspects in the treatment of congenital hydrocephalus. Neuropaediatric 2:239, 1970

54. Yashon D, Jane JA, Sugar O: The course of severe untreated infantile hydrocephalus: Prognostic significance of the cerebral mantle. J Neurosurg 23:509, 1965

55. Young HF, Nulsen FE, Weiss MH, et al: The relationship of intelligence and cerebral mantle in treated infantile hydrocephalus. Pediatrics 52:38, 1973

56. Shurtleff DB, Foltz EL, Loeser JD: Hydrocephalus: A definition of its progression and relationship to intellectual function, diagnosis and complication. Am J Dis Child 125:688, 1973

57. Cochrane DD, Myles ST: Management of intrauterine hydrocephalus. J Neurosurg 57:590, 1982

58. Vintzileos AM, Ingardia CJ, Nochimson DJ: Congenital hydrocephalus: A review and protocol for perinatal management. Obstet Gynecol 62:539, 1983

59. Chervenak FA, Berkowitz RL, Tortora M, et al: The management of fetal hydrocephalus. Am J Obstet Gynecol 151:933, 1985

60. Chervenak FA, Romero R: Is there a role for fetal cephalocentesis in modern obstetrics? Am J Perinatol 1:170, 1984

61. Clewell WH, Johnson ML, Meier PR et al: A surgical approach to the treatment of fetal hydrocephalus. N Engl J Med 306:1320, 1982

62. Michejda M, Hodgen GD: In utero diagnosis and treatment of nonhuman primate fetal skeletal anomalies. I. Hydrocephalus. JAMA 246:1093, 1981

63. Gardner WJ: Myelocele: Rupture of the neural tube? Clin Neurosurg 15:57, 1968

64. Laurence KM, Carter CO, David PA: Major central nervous system malformations in South Wales. I. Incidence, local variations and geographical factors. Br J Prev Soc Med 22:146, 1968

65. Laurence KM, Carter CO, David PA: Major central nervous system malformations in South Wales. II. Pregnancy factors, seasonal variation, and social class effects. Br J Prev Soc Med 22:212, 1968

66. Brocklehurst G: Spina bifida. p. 519. In Vinken PJ, Bruyn GW (eds): Handbood of Clinical Neurology. Vol. 30. Elsevier, Amsterdam, 1978

67. Chervenak FA, Farley MA, Walters L, et al: When is termination of pregnancy during the third trimester morally justifiable? N Engl J Med 310:501, 1984

68. Emery JL, Mackenzie N: Medullo-cervical dislocation deformity (Chiari II deformity) related to neurospinal dysraphism (meningomyelocele). Brain 96:155, 1973

69. Variend S, Emery JL: The weight of cerebellum in children with myelomeningocele. Dev Med Child Neurol 15(suppl 29):77, 1973

70. Emery JL: Deformity of the aqueduct of Sylvius in children with hydrocephalus and myelomeningocele. Dev Med Child Neurol 17(suppl 32):40, 1974

71. Lorber J: Systematic ventriculographic studies in infants born with meningomyelocele and encephalocele. The incidence and development of hydrocephalus. Arch Dis Child 36:381, 1961

72. Naidich TP, Pudlowski RM, Naidich JB, et al: Computed tomographic signs of Chiari II malformation. Part I. Skull and dural partitions. Radiology 134:65, 1980

73. Naidich TP, Pudlowski RM, Naidich JB: Computed tomographic signs of Chiari II malformation. Part II. Midbrain and cerebellum. Radiology 134:391, 1980

74. Naidich TP, Pudlowski RM, Naidich JB: Computed tomographic signs of the Chiari II malformation. Part III. Ventricles and cisterns. Radiology 134:657, 1980

75. Babcock DS, Han BK: Cranial sonographic findings in meningomyelocele. AJR 135:563, 1981

76. Goodwin L, Quisling RG: The neonatal cisterna magna: ultrasonic evaluation. Radiology 149:691, 1983

77. Russell DS, Donald C: The mechanism of internal hydrocephalus in spina bifida. Brain 58:203, 1935

78. Nicolaides KH, Campbell S, Gabbe SG, et al: Ultrasound screening for spina bifida: Cranial and cerebellar signs. Lancet 2:72, 1986

79. Lorber J: Results of treatment of myelomeningocele. Dev Med Child Neurol 13:279, 1971

80. Mapstone TB, Rekate HL, Nulsen FE et al: Relationship of CSF shunting and IQ in children with myelomeningocele: A retrospective analysis. Childs Brain 11:112, 1984

81. Warkany J; Congenital Malformations. Notes and Comments. Year Book Medical Publishers, Chicago, 1971

82. Cohen MM, Lemire RJ: Syndromes with cephaloceles. Teratology 25:161, 1982

83. Mecke S, Passarge E: Encephalocele, polycystic kidneys and polydactyly as an autosomal recessive trait simulating certain other disorders. The Meckel syndrome. Ann Genet 14:97, 1971

84. Seeds JW, Cefalo RC, Herbert WP: Amniotic band syndrome. Am J Obstet Gynecol 144:243, 1982

85. Nicolini U, Ferrazzi E, Minonzio M et al: Prenatal diagnosis of cranial masses by ultrasound: Report of five cases. J Clin Ultrasound 11:170, 1983

86. Chervenak FA, Isaacson G, Blakemore KJ et al: Fetal cystic hygroma. Cause and natural history. N Engl J Med 309:822, 1983

87. Lorber J: The prognosis of occipital encephalocele. Dev Med Child Neurol 13:279, 1971

88. Leech RW, Shuman RM: Holoprosencephaly and related midline cerebral anomalies. A review. J Child Neurol 1:3, 1986

89. DeMyer W: Holoprosencephaly. p. 431. In Vinken PJ, Bruyn GW (eds): Handbook of Clinical Neurology. Vol. 30. Elsevier, Amsterdam, 1977

90. DeMyer W, Zeman W, Palmer CG: The face predicts the brain. Diagnostic significance of median facial anomalies for holoprosencephaly (arhinencephaly). Pediatrics 34:256, 1964

91. Roach E, DeMyer W, Palmer K, et al: Holoprosencephaly: birth data, genetic and demographic analysis of 30 families. Birth Defects 11:294, 1975

92. Matsunaga E, Shiota Y: Holoprosencephaly in human embryos: Epidemiological studies of 150 cases. Teratology 16:261, 1977

93. Battin JJ: Congenital malformations and chromosomal abnormalities. Fetal Ther 1:68, 1986

94. Cohen MM: An update on the holoprosencephalic disorders. J Pediatr 101:865, 1982

95. Chervenak FA, Isaacson G, Mahoney MJ, et al: The obstetric significance of holoprosencephaly. Obstet Gynecol 63:114, 1984

96. Filly RA, Chinn DH, Callen PW: Alobar holoprosencephaly. Ultrasonographic prenatal diagnosis. Radiology 151:455, 1984

97. Pilu G, Romero R, Rizzo N, et al: Criteria for the antenatal diagnosis of holoprosencephaly. Am J Perinatol 4:41, 1987

98. Blackwell DE, Spinnato JA, Horsch G, et al: Prenatal diagnosis of cyclopia. Am J Obstet Gynecol 143:848, 1982

99. Lev-Gur M, Maklad NF, Patel S: Ultrasonic findings in fetal cyclopia. A case report. J Reprod Med 28:554, 1983

100. Benacerraf BR, Frigoletto FD, Bieber FR: The fetal face. Ultrasound examination. Radiology 153:495, 1984

101. Pilu G, Reece EA, Romero R, et al: Prenatal diagnosis of cranio-facial malformations with sonography. Am J Obstet Gynecol 155:45, 1986

102. Cayea PD, Balcar I, Alberti O, et al: Prenatal diagnosis of semilobar holoprosencephaly. AJR 142:455, 1984

103. Hoffman-Tretin JC, Horoupian DS, Koenigsberg M, et al: Lobar holoprosencephaly with hydrocephalus: Antenatal demonstration and differential diagnosis. J Ultrasound Med 5:691, 1986

104. Osaka K, Matsumoto S: Holoprosencephaly in neurosurgical practice. J Neurosurg 48:787, 1978

105. de Morsier G: Etudes sur le dysraphies cranioencephaliques. III. Agénésie du septum pellucidum avec malformations du tractus optique: la dysplasie septo-optique. Schweiz Arch Neurol Neurochir Psychiatry 77:267, 1956

106. Menelfe C, Rocchioli P: CT of septo-optic dysplasia. AJR 133:1157, 1979

107. Fitz CR: Midline anomalies of the brain and spine. Radiol Clin North Am 20:95, 1982

108. Williams JL, Faerber EN: Septooptic dysplasia (De Morsier syndrome). J Ultrasound Med 4:265, 1985

109. Ettlinger G: Agenesis of the corpus callosum. p. 285. In Vinken PJ, Bruyn GW (eds): Handbook of Clinical Neurology. Vol. 30. Elsevier, Amsterdam, 1977

110. Young ID, Trounce JQ, Levene MI, et al: Agenesis of the corpus callosum and macrocephaly in siblings. Clin Genet 28:225, 1985

111. Aicardi J, Lefebvre J, Lerique-Koechlin A: A new syndrome: Spasms in flexion, callosal agenesis, ocular abnormalities. Electroencephalogr Clin Neurophysiol 19:609, 1965

112. Andermann F, Andermann E, Joubert M, et al: Familial agenesis of the corpus callosum with anterior horn cell disease. A syndrome of mental retardation, areflexia and paraplegia. Trans Am Neurol Ass 97:242, 1972

113. Schinzel A: Four patients including two sisters with the acrocallosal syndrome (agenesis of the corpus callosum in combination with preaxial hexadactily). Hum Genet 62:382, 1982

114. Opitz JM, Kaveggia EG: The F.G. syndrome. An X-linked recessive syndrome of multiple congenital anomalies and mental retardation. Z Kinderheilkd 117:1, 1974

115. Parrish M, Roessman U, Levinsohn M: Agenesis of the corpus callosum: A study of the frequency of associated malformations. Ann Neurol 6:349, 1979

116. Loeser JD, Alvord EC: Agenesis of the corpus callosum. Brain 91:553, 1968

117. Davidoff LM, Dyke CG: Agenesis of the corpus callosum. Its diagnosis by encephalography. Report of 3 cases. AJR 32:1, 1934

118. Byrd SE, Harwood-Nash DC, Fitz CR: Absence of the corpus callosum: Computed tomographic evaluation in infants and children. J Can Assoc Radiol 29:108, 1978

119. Gebarski SS, Gebarski KS, Bowerman RA, et al: Agenesis of the corpus callosum: Sonographic features. Radiology 151:443, 1984

120. Babcock DS: The normal, absent and abnormal corpus callosum: Sonographic findings. Radiology 151:449, 1984

121. Comstock CH, Culp D, Gonzalez J, et al: Agenesis of the corpus callosum in the fetus: Its evolution and significance. J Ultrasound Med 4:613, 1985

122. Yakovlev PI, Wadsworth RC: Schizencephalies; a study of the congenital clefts in the cerebral mantle. I. Clefts with fused lips. J Neuropathol Exp Neurol 5:116, 1946

123. Yakovlev PI, Wadsworth RC: Schizencephalies; a study of the congenital clefts in the cerebral mantle. I. Clefts with hydrocephalus and lips separated. J Neuropathol Exp Neurol 5:169, 1946

124. Halsey JH, Allen N, Chamberlin HR: Hydanencephaly. p. 661. In Vinken PJ, Bruyn JW (eds): Handbook of Clinical Neurology. Vol 30. Elsevier, Amsterdam, 1977

125. Lange-Cossack R: Die Hydranencephalie (Blasehirn) als sanderform der Grobhirnlosigkeit. Arch Psychiatr Nervenkr 1:117, 1944

126. Johnson EE, Warner M, Simonds JP: Total absence of the cerebral hemispheres. J Pediatr 38:69, 1951

127. Norman RM: Malformation of the nervous system, birth injury and diseases in early life. p. 23. In Greenfield JG (ed): Neuropathology. Arnold, London, 1958

128. Aicardi J, Goutieres F, Deverbois AH: Multicystic encephalomalacia of infants and its relation to abnormal gestation and hydranencephaly. J Neurol Sci 15:357, 1972

129. Gross H, Simanyi M: Porencephaly. p. 681. In Vinken PJ, Bruyn GW (eds): Handbook of Clinical Neurology. Vol. 30. Elsevier, Amsterdam, 1977

130. Halsey JH, Allen N, Chamberlin HR: The chronic decerebrate state of infancy. Arch Neurol 19:339, 1968

131. Winick M, Rosso P: Head circumference and cellular growth of the brain in normal and marasmic children. J Pediatr 74:774, 1969

132. O'Connell EJ, Feldt RH, Stickler GB: Head circumference, mental retardation and growth failure. Pediatrics 36:62, 1965

133. Book JA, Schut JW, Reed SC: A clinical and genetical study of microcephaly. Am J Ment Defic 57:637, 1953

134. Winsmuller HF, Koch G: Microzephalie. Palm and Enke, Erlangen, 1975

135. Ross JH, Frias JL: Microcephaly. p. 507. In Vinken PJ, Bruyn GW (eds): Handbook of Clinical Neurology. Vol. 30. Elsevier, Amsterdam, 1977

136. Campbell S, Allan L, Griffin D, et al: The early diagnosis of fetal structural abnormalities. p. 547. In Lerski RA, Morley P (eds): Ultrasound '82. Pergamon, Oxford, 1983

137. Kurtz AB, Wapner RJ, Rubin CS et al: Ultrasound criteria for in utero diagnosis of microcephaly. J Clin Ultrasound 8:11, 1980

138. Hohler CW, Quetel TA: Comparison of ultrasound femur length and biparietal diameter in late pregnancy. Am J Obstet Gynecol 141:759, 1981

139. Chervenak FA, Jeanty P, Cantraine F, et al: The diagnosis of fetal microcephaly. Am J Obstet Gynecol 149:512, 1984

140. Avery GB, Meneses L, Lodge A: The clinical significance of "measurement microcephaly." Am J Dis Child 123:214, 1972

141. Martin HP: Microcephaly and mental retardation. Am J Dis Child 119:128, 1970

142. DeMyer W: Megalencephaly in children: clinical syndromes, genetic patterns and differential diagnosis from other causes of megalencephaly. Neurology (NY) 22:634, 1972

143. Dennis JP, Rosenberg HS, Ellsworth CA: Megalencephaly, internal hydrocephalus and other neurological aspects of achondroplasia. Brain 84:427, 1961

144. Holt JF, Kuhns LR: Macrocranium and macrencephaly in neurofibromatosis. Skel Radiol 125:1976

145. Bignami A, Palladini G, Zappella M: Unilateral megalencephaly with nerve cell hypertrophy. An anatomical and quantitative histochemical study. Brain Res 9:103, 1968

146. Rugel SJ: Congenital hemihypertrophy. Report of a case with postmortem observations. Am J Dis Child 71:530, 1946

147. Fitz CR, Harwood-Nash DC, Boldt DW: The radiographic features of unilateral megalencephaly. Neuroradiology 15:145, 1978

148. Tijam AT, Stefanko S, Schenk VWD et al: Infantile spasms associated with hemihypsarrhythmia and hemimegalencephaly. Dev Child Neurol 20:779, 1978

149. Gradin WC, Taylor C, Fruin AH: Choroid plexus papilloma: Report of a case and review of the literature. Neurosurgery 12:217, 1983

150. Matson DD, Crofton FDL: Papilloma of the choroid plexus in childhood. J Neurosurg 17:1002, 1960

151. Hawkins JC: Treatment of choroid plexus papilloma in children: Brief analysis of twenty years' experience. Neurosurgery 6:380, 1980

152. Chudleigh P, Pearce MJ, Campbell S: The prenatal diagnosis of transient cysts of the fetal choroid plexus. Prenat Diagn 4:135, 1984

153. Fakhry J, Schechter A, Tenner MS, et al: Cysts of the choroid plexus in neonates: Documentation and review of the literature. J Ultrasound Med 4:561, 1985

154. Shuangsoti S, Netsky MG: Neuroepithelial (colloidal) cysts of the nervous system. Neurology (NY) 16:887, 1966

155. Neblett CR, Robertson JW: Symptomatic cysts of the telencephalic choroid plexus. J Neurol Neurosurg Psychiatry 34:324, 1971

156. Nicolaides KH, Rodeck CH, Gosden CM: Rapid karyotyping in non lethal fetal malformations. Lancet 1:283, 1986

157. Bundy AL, Saltzman DH, Pober B, et al: Antenatal sonographic findings in trisomy 18. J Ultrasound Med 5:361, 1986

158. Romero R, Pilu G, Jeanty P, et al: Prenatal Diagnosis of Congenital Anomalies. Appleton & Lange, E Norwalk, CT, 1987

11 Invasive Fetal Therapy

KAREN E. MEHALEK
LAUREN LYNCH
RICHARD L. BERKOWITZ

The recent impact of ultrasound on perinatal management includes not only the increase in diagnostic acumen, but also in utero treatment of correctable fetal disorders. Ultrasound assessment of the natural history of fetal disease has permitted identification of conditions that, if left untreated, worsen in utero, leading to perinatal morbidity and mortality. Although the list of potentially treatable fetal conditions is long, the diseases that have generally been treated in utero under sonographic guidance are limited to erythroblastosis fetalis, obstructive uropathy, and hydrocephalus.

INTRAUTERINE TRANSFUSIONS

The primary problem in erythroblastosis fetalis is hemolysis of fetal red blood cells (RBCs) by maternal immunoglobin G (IgG) antibodies that have crossed the placenta. This results in fetal anemia with secondary extramedullary hematopoiesis, primarily in the liver and spleen. Distortion and enlargement of the hepatic parenchyma by this process results in portal hypertension and decreased ability of the liver to synthetize albumin. These factors lead to the development of fetal ascites and edema, a condition referred to as hydrops fetalis (Fig. 11.1). Although congestive heart failure may develop terminally, it does not seem to be the primary cause of hydrops. Fetal death or premature delivery can be prevented by the administration of blood in utero. Transfused blood compatible with that of the mother and that will not be destroyed by her antibodies corrects the fetal anemia and consequently improves tissue oxygenation. In utero transfusion also reduces the production of fetal erythropoietin and extramedullary erythropoiesis. This leads to a drop in portal and umbilical venous pressure and improves hepatic circulation and hepatocellular function.

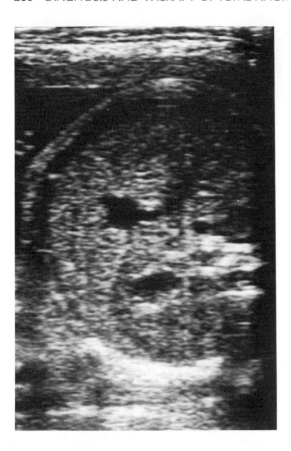

FIG. 11.1. Cross section of fetal abdomen with ascites in a 30-week hydropic fetus with a hematocrit of 12 percent.

INTRAPERITONEAL TRANSFUSIONS

Serial amniocentesis followed by intraperitoneal transfusions when indicated has been the traditional way of following and treating pregnancies at risk for erythroblastosis fetalis. The extent of fetal hemolysis can be estimated by spectrophometric analysis for bilirubin pigment in amniotic fluid. This determination is performed by measuring the deviation of the fluid sample at 450 μm from the linear projection of the spectral absorption curve and is referred to as the delta OD_{450}. Observations by Liley [1] on a series of patients at various gestational ages after 28 weeks led to the correlation between delta OD_{450} at a given gestational age and fetal outcome. Liley developed a curve in which delta OD_{450} was plotted against gestational age and proposed three zones: zone I, an unaffected or mildly affected fetus; zone II, a moderately to severely affected fetus, and zone III, a severely affected fetus. This curve has subsequently been extrapolated linearly back into the second trimester, but work by Nicolaides et al.[2] suggests that this may not be valid for fetuses at 26 weeks or earlier.

In utero transfusion is indicated once the delta OD_{450} falls in high zone II or III and the fetus is too immature to be delivered. Intervention is also indicated if there is any evidence of hydrops regardless of the delta OD_{450}. If the fetus is hydropic, the hematocrit is usually less than 15 percent.[2,3] With modern ultrasound equiment, very early hydropic changes can be sought before the development of overt hydrops has developed. Benacerraf and Frigoletto [4] described demarcation of fetal bowel preceding the development of frank ascites (Fig. 11.2). Normally a single layer of bowel wall is seen, but both serosal and mucosal layers of the fetal bowel can be visualized when a thin layer of ascites fluid separates the loops. In many cases, hydramnios may be the earliest predictor of anemia in isoimmunized pregnancies[3] (Fig. 11.3).

After a transfusion in utero has been performed, amniotic fluid delta OD_{450} levels cannot be relied on for diagnostic purposes because of the interference of blood breakdown products. Thus, once intraperitoneal transfusions are initiated, they should be continued on schedule until delivery.

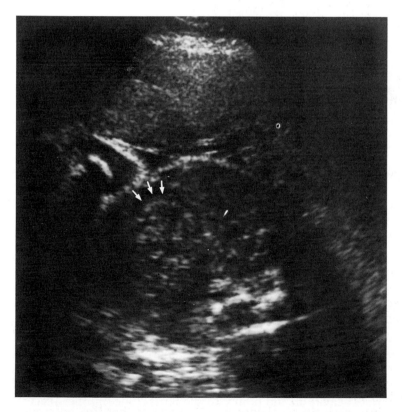

FIG. 11.2. Demarcation of the bowel wall (arrows) in a fetus with early ascites. (Courtesy of Dr. B. Benacerraf, Boston, MA.)

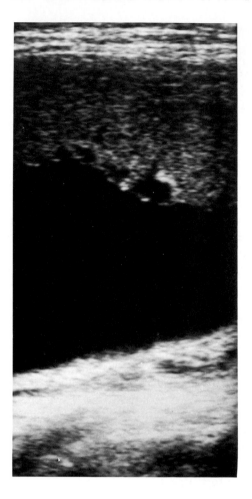

FIG. 11.3. Hydramnios was the only ultrasound finding in this 28-week Rh-sensitized fetus with a hematocrit of 23 percent.

Techniques

The technique for intraperitoneal transfusion varies somewhat among institutions but is typically as follows: the mother is sedated and, after aseptic and local anesthetic preparations, a 16- or 18-gauge Touhy needle is inserted into the fetal abdominal cavity under ultrasound guidance. A recently reported modificiation is the use of a 20-gauge spinal needle.[5] The ideal site of entry into the fetus is below the umbilical vein but above the bladder, as this minimizes the risk of traumatizing an enlarged liver. Proper needle placement is verified by aspirating ascitic fluid in the hydropic fetus or by injecting a small amount of sterile saline solution and observing layering of fluid in the peritoneal cavity in the nonhydropic fetus. Once proper placement has been verified, the transfusion can be accomplished directly through the needle, or a polyvinyl catheter can be threaded into the fetal abdomen and the needle removed.

The amount of blood transfused into the peritoneal cavity is usually estimated by the following formula[6]:

$$\text{Gestation (in weeks)} - 20 \times 10 \text{ ml}$$

If ultrasonography demonstrates a large amount of ascites, most of it should be removed before transfusing and the RBC volume should not exceed the volume of fluid removed. The type of blood for transfusion is O-Rh negative packed RBCs crossed-matched against the mother's blood.

Outcome

Earlier series show poorer results after intraperitoneal transfusion than those reported later because of improved techniques and the greater experience of operators. In 1978 Bowman[7] published the results of the 14-year experience at his institution, which included 611 transfusions in 257 infants. The overall neonatal survival rate was 59 percent, with 68 percent of the nonhydropic fetuses and 36 percent of those with hydrops surviving. When the final 8 years of the study were considered independently, the overall survival was 70 percent, with 78 percent of the nonhydropic fetuses and 50 percent of those with hydrops surviving the neonatal period. In 1983, the same group published impressive outcome data following the institution of real-time ultrasound surveillance during and after the transfusions.[7a] Overall survival for the interval from 1980 to 1982 was 92 percent (22 of 24 fetuses transfused), with 75 percent good outcomes in the hydropic fetuses. These are by far the best survival rates reported for fetuses treated with intraperitoneal transfusions. A more extensive review has been published by Berkowitz.[8]

INTRAVASCULAR TRANSFUSIONS

Although intraperitoneal transfusion has been the traditional technique used in the treatment of erythroblastosis fetalis, a more direct approach to the fetal circulation has recently been advocated. There are several major advantages to the intravascular approach. One is the ability to document that the fetal RBCs carry the antigen of concern. This information is of vital importance in cases in which the father is a heterozygote for the antigen involved. If the fetus did not inherit the antigen, unnecessary subsequent intervention is avoided.

Measurements of the fetal hematocrit permits more accurate assessment of the degree of hemolysis, especially during the second trimester when amniotic fluid delta OD_{450} determinations have a high false-negative rate.[2] In addition, measurements of the hematocrit before the transfusion permits a more exact estimation of the amount of blood required and the post-transfusion hematocrit verifies that an optimal amount of blood has been administered. This information together with a post-transfusion fetal Kleihauer-Betke test provides a more accurate guide for timing of the next transfusion or delivery. Intraperitoneal placement of RBCs relies on absorption through the subdiaphragmatic lymphatics into the circulation, which may be particularly erratic in hydropic fetuses. Intravascular transfusion eliminates this problem.

Although intravascular transfusion offers several advantages over the intraperitoneal approach, there are cases in which the fetal circulation is unaccessible for technical reasons. In these cases, the intraperitoneal route should be used.

Technique

Preprocedure preparation varies from one institution to another. At the Mount Sinai Medical Center, the patient is premedicated with a combination of a narcotic and a sedative. A single dose of an antibiotic is also given for prophylaxis.

The technique we use to perform intravascular transfusions in utero is

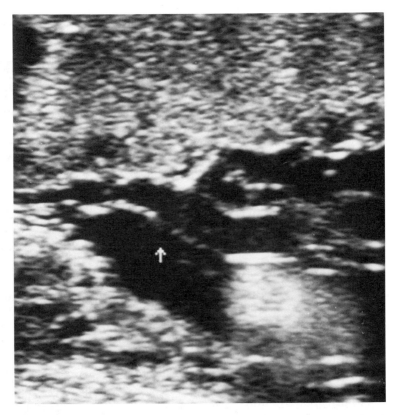

FIG. 11.4.   Cord insertion into an anterior placenta visualized with a 3.5-MHz linear transducer.

similar to the method described by Jeanty et al.[9] for amniocentesis. With use of a linear-array real-time transducer, a view of the long axis of the umbilical cord is obtained at its insertion site into the placenta (Fig. 11.4). Holding the transducer in one hand and the transfusion needle in the other, the operator guides the needle tip into the lumen of an umbilical vessel at the placental insertion site (Fig. 11.5). If a sector scanner is used, the same technique applies except that the transducer is held by the operator or an assistant several centimeters away from the needle insertion site in order to visualize the entire length of the needle. If the cord cannot be accessed at its insertion site into the placenta, the needle can be directed into the umbilical vein within the fetal liver or into a cord vessel at the site of entry into the fetal abdomen. A 20- or 22-gauge spinal needle is generally used. A sample of blood is withdrawn into a heparinized syringe and the RBCs are analyzed with an electronic cell sizer to confirm that the withdrawn sample is fetal in origin. Also, at the time of the first sampling, the fetal blood type is determined. The hematocrit is measured and if less than 30 percent, an immediate transfusion is performed. Washed and irradiated group O-Rh negative packed cells crossed-matched against the mother's blood are trans-

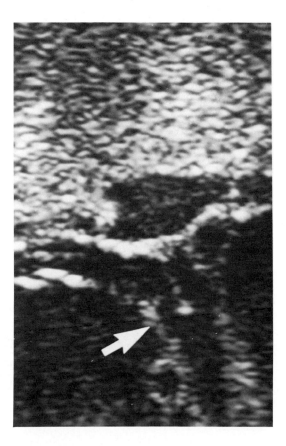

FIG. 11.5. Echogenic needle tip in the umbilical vein at the placental cord insertion.

fused at a rate of 2 to 5 ml/min directly into the umbilical vessel. The fetal heart is visually monitored throughout the procedure. The volume of packed RBCs to be transfused is estimated, and this is titrated by checking the hematocrit after two-thirds of this amount has been administered. After completion of the transfusion, a final sample is aspirated for analysis. The goal is to obtain a post-procedure hematocrit of 35 to 45 percent. A Kleihauer-Betke test is also performed on the final aspirate in order to determine the proportion of adult (i.e., transfused) cells in the fetal circulation. Ideally, the first fetal blood sample should be obtained when the fetus is already anemic but before hydrops has developed. At our institution, the first fetal blood sampling is empirically performed at 20 to 26 weeks, depending on the previous obstetric history and antibody titers. The timing of the next transfusion is individualized in each case, depending on the post-transfusion hematocrit and the Kleihauer-Betke test. In general, the intervals range between 1 to 3 weeks. The final transfusion is given at 32 to 34 weeks, depending on lung maturity.

Outcome

Although experience with intravascular transfusions is still limited, several small series have been reported. In 1984 Rodeck and Nicolaides[10,10a] described their experience with the fetoscopically guided intravascular approach in 25 severely Rh sensitized fetuses who underwent a total of 77 intrauterine transfusions. The overall survival rate in this series was 72 percent. Furthermore, in fetuses who received their first transfusion before 25 weeks the survival rate was 84 percent, including 11 of 13 fetuses with hydrops.

In 1986, Grannum et al.[10b] reported on nine percutaneous intravascular transfusions in four patients, six of which were exchange transfusions. The outcome was successful in three of the patients. Simultaneously, our group published a series of eight patients who underwent 16 intravascular transfusions.[11] A successful outcome was achieved in six of the eight cases (75 percent). We have since expanded our experience with this technique. Up to January 1987, 43 intravascular transfusions have been attemped, 38 (88 percent) of which have been technically successful. These procedures have been performed on a total of 17 patients. There have been three losses before 26 weeks and none after this gestational age. Of 14 completed pregnancies, 11 infants have survived (79 percent). The survival rate for hydropic fetuses has been 2 in 4 (50 percent).

Problems with Intravascular Transfusion

Although transfusing directly into the fetal circulation clearly has several advantages, it is a more technically demanding procedure than the intraperitoneal. Guiding the tip of a 20- or 22-gauge needle into the lumen of a vessel measuring 4 to 10 mm in diameter can be difficult.

Sometimes a greater problem is the inaccessibility of a cord vessel because of intervening fetal parts. This situation requires patience and often manipulation of the fetus to create access to the vessel. Furthermore, when dealing with a posterior placenta, very long needles may be difficult to guide with precision. The problem of fetal movement can be a significant one, especially when working within the liver or with a posterior placenta. In these cases, a muscle blocker can be administered to the fetus intramuscularly or directly into an umbilical vessel.

Finally, although the experience with the intravascular approach has been rewarding, there are still several unanswered questions such as the optimal timing of the transfusions and how much blood should be transfused. The latter is particularly relevant in cases of fetal hydrops, in which overtransfusion could conceivably aggravate pre-existing cardiac failure. Issues requiring further study include the use of exchange transfusions in utero and the performance of frequent transfusions of small amounts of blood versus the administration of blood sufficient to normalize the hematocrit. As more experience is gained in the use of this technique, it is hoped that the answer to these and other questions will be obtained.

INTRAUTERINE SHUNTING PROCEDURES

With intrauterine transfusion setting the foundation for successful in utero therapy, attention has turned to other conditions detectable in utero that often lead to neonatal morbidity and mortality. Improved sonographic resolution has enabled identification of structural defects that may be amenable to in utero therapy. The objective of such therapy is to reverse or arrest a pathologic process in order to prevent damage, while permitting normal development to proceed in utero. Increased pressure caused by abnormal fluid collections in the fetus can cause damage to adjacent organs or tissues while prohibiting normal development. Antenatal shunting and drainage procedures have already been used to decompress hydronephrosis, hydrocephalus, and fluid collections in the thorax. Other potentially correctable defects include diaphragmatic hernia and neural tube defects.

For a disorder to be amenable to in utero therapy, several conditions need to be satisfied. The sonographic diagnosis of the condition should be reasonably accurate. The natural history of the disease should be known, with evidence to suggest that intervention can alter outcome. Fetal surgery is only indicated for conditions likely to be fatal or to lead to severe handicap in the absence of treatment.

In 1982 members of the Fetal Medicine and Surgical Society set guidelines and selection criteria for therapy of obstructive uropathy and hydrocephalus.[12] The fetus under consideration for therapy should be a singleton, so as not to jeopardize a normal twin. Coexisting anomalies that might worsen prognosis should be excluded by performing high-resolution sonography and amniocentesis for karyotype and α-fetoprotein (AFP). The fetus should be less than 32 weeks or have documented lung immaturity, as delivery with neonatal therapy is preferable to in utero therapy unless the neonate is unlikely to survive due to prematurity. The patient must understand the risks and benefits of the treatment and be willing to return for follow-up study. The participants agreed that treatment should be provided by a multidisciplinary team, including a perinatal obstetrician, level II ultrasonographer, neonatologist, and pediatric surgeon with access to a level III high-risk obstetric service and intensive care nursery.

Detection of a significant structural or chromosomal abnormality enables the parents to consider termination of the pregnancy (within local legal limits). Since invasive procedures on the fetus have maternal risks, surgery in utero is not indicated at any gestational age in a fetus with severe associated anomalies. Karyotyping is valuable even in the third-trimester fetus, as knowledge of a chromosomally abnormal fetus may influence decisions regarding shunt placement, timing of delivery, and cesarean section.

In 1982, an International Fetal Surgery Registry was established to record cases of fetal surgery for obstructive uropathy or hydrocephalus. While reporting to the Registry may be biased, analysis of the cases helps provide an evaluation of the efficacy of in utero therapy.

Obstructive Uropathy

Obstructive uropathy resulting in hydronephrosis and oligohydramnios can have a severe effect on the developing renal and pulmonary systems of the fetus. Theoretically, diversion of urine from the dilated portion of the urinary tract into the amniotic fluid cavity should prevent both renal insufficiency and pulmonary hypoplasia and should permit normal development to occur.

Diagnosis

Accurate diagnosis is crucial before treatment can be considered. Routine visualization of the fetal kidneys is possible after 16 weeks. Located below the level of the stomach on either side of the spine, the kidneys are hypoechogenic and contain a central echo, the renal pelvis (Fig. 11.6). Later in gestation, the capsule and collecting system are strongly echogenic, while the parenchyma remains hypoechogenic. In the presence of obstruction, the kidneys may demonstrate either hydronephrotic changes with a dilated calyceal system and thin cortex, or increased renal parenchymal echogenicity with or without pelvic and calyceal distention (Fig. 11.7).

The bladder can be identified as early as 14 to 15 weeks. Micturition generally occurs at intervals of approximatley 40 minutes.[13] Failure to identify the bladder after 1 hour of scanning is highly suggestive of fetal renal failure, absent kidneys, or bilateral ureteral obstruction. The presence of megacystis, a dilated bladder that fails to empty over time, suggests obstruction at or distal to the urethrovesical junction.

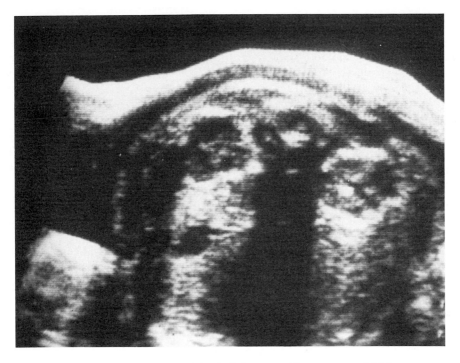

FIG. 11.6. Cross section of fetal abdomen with two normal kidneys.

Obstructive uropathy is identified as unilateral or bilateral and can be divided according to anatomic level[14]:

High: dilated renal pelvis only, seen in ureteropelvic junction obstruction (UPJ), or ureteral atresia

Mid: ureteral dilatation with or without a dilated renal pelvis, seen in ureterovesical junction obstruction (UVJ), bladder atresia, or transient hydroureter

Low: dilated bladder and proximal urinary tract, seen on posterior urethral valves, or urethral atresia.

Unilateral obstruction usually shows a normal-size bladder with a dilated ureter and/or renal pelvis in association with a normal contralateral kidney and renal pelvis.

Once a renal anomaly is detected, a thorough search for other anomalies is indicated. According to Potter and Craig,[15] up to 50 percent of these fetuses may have cardiovascular, gastrointestinal, skeletal, or central nervous system (CNS) anomalies. Recent series of fetal obstructive uropathy have demonstrated a 23 to 33 percent incidence of associated anatomic defects.[14–17] Fetuses with low-level obstruction seem to have the highest incidence of other anomalies. Reported anomalies include caudal regression syndrome ranging from

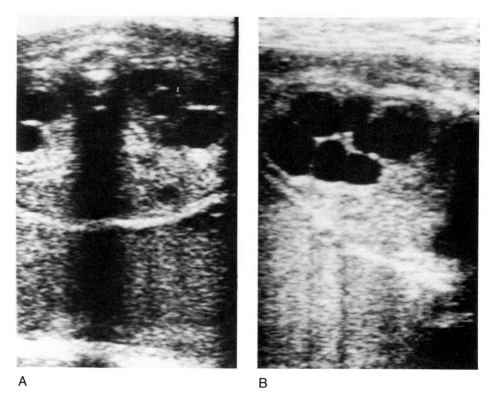

A   B

FIG. 11.7.   Transverse (A) and longitudinal (B) views of fetal abdomen with bilateral hydronephrosis.

imperforate anus to sirenomelia, malrotation of the large or small bowel, cloacal anomalies, cardiac defects, omphalocele, hydrocephalus, esophageal atresia, and diaphragmatic hernia.

Karyotype should be performed on fetal cells obtained from amniotic fluid, blood, or urine. Low-level obstruction has been associated with trisomy 18.[18,19] Rodeck and Nicolaides[10] report a 23 percent incidence of chromosomal abnormalities in fetuses with obstructive uropathy for whom rapid karyotyping was performed. The 1985 report from the International Fetal Surgery Registry reported six abnormal karyotypes in 73 shunted patients. All patients terminated their pregnancies once the abnormality was known. Reported chromosomal abnormalities associated with obstructive uropathy include trisomies 13, 18, and 21; tetraploidy; triploidy; deletions; and 47,XXY.[10,17,20]

Natural History

The prognosis of the fetus with urinary tract obstruction depends on the level, severity, and duration of obstruction. At one end of the spectrum is the fetus with severe bilateral obstruction and oligohydramnios who dies an early neonatal death from renal failure and pulmonary hypoplasia. At the other end is the fetus with mild obstruction and normal amniotic fluid volume who is born with normal renal and pulmonary function and who only requires neonatal urinary tract decompression.

Unilateral obstruction with a normal amount of amniotic fluid and a normal-appearing contralateral kidney carries a favorable prognosis for the fetus and therefore does not require intrauterine therapy.[14,21] The prognosis is more varied and can be quite poor, with bilateral obstruction. Partial bilateral obstruction producing hydronephrosis may be reversible following decompression during the neonatal period, and renal function may be normal. By contrast, complete obstruction of longstanding duration may result in cystic dysplasia with nonfunctioning kidneys at birth. The outcome is difficult to predict in fetuses with varying degrees of obstruction between these two extremes.

The most important nonrenal sequelae of obstruction is oligohydramnios, which can lead to pulmonary hypoplasia and neonatal death from respiratory insufficiency. The existence or development of oligohydramnios in a fetus with urinary tract obstruction is a poor prognostic factor.[14,21]

While absence of oligohydramnios implies normal pulmonary development, it does not always mean normal renal function. Harrison's 1982 series included seven fetuses thought to have equivocal renal function, since the amniotic fluid volume was not markedly decreased. The only neonatal death was in a fetus with other anomalies. Of the six remaining neonates, one-half had normal renal function, while the other half had abnormal tubular function or developed chronic renal failure.

Before prognosis can be determined, serial observations are necessary to determine whether the obstruction is progressive. Spontaneous in utero resolution of both upper and lower tract obstruction has been reported.[14,21–23]

Shunt Procedure

Most intrauterine fetal shunting procedures have used ultrasound-guided percutaneous placement of a vesicoamniotic catheter. A polyethylene catheter with a memory coil at one or both ends is loaded on a needle. A pigtail coil placed in the bladder helps prevent the catheter from falling out of the bladder, while a second pigtail or bend at the amniotic end of the shunt prevents the catheter from being drawn into the fetus (Figs. 11.8 and 11.9). Under ultrasonic visualization, the catheter-loaded needle is placed through the maternal abdomen and uterus and then directed into the site of obstruction (usually the bladder). Once the needle tip is visualized within the bladder, a separate piece of preloaded tubing seated on the needle above the catheter is used to push the shunt far enough off the needle so that the coil is constituted in the bladder. The needle is then withdrawn while the catheter is held in place with the pusher (Fig. 11.10).

In cases of oligohydramnios, catheter placement can be facilitated by prior infusion of warmed normal saline solution into the amniotic cavity. This

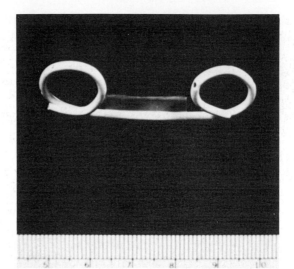

FIG. 11.8.   Double-pigtail bladder shunt.

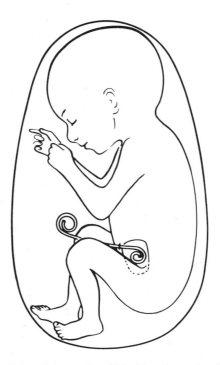

FIG. 11.9.   Schematic of bladder shunt in place.

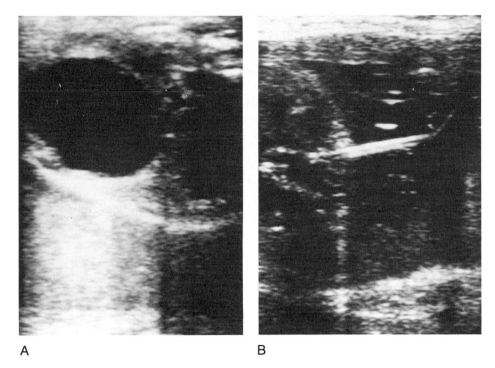

A   B

FIG. 11.10.   (A) Lower fetal abdomen with dilated bladder. (B) Decompressed bladder with echogenic shunt in place.

ensures an adequate pocket of fluid external to the fetal abdominal wall for placement of the distal end of the catheter. Correct placement of the catheter is verified by a decrease in size of the dilated bladder. Weekly assessment of amniotic fluid volume, urinary tract dilation, and catheter location should be made, as it is not uncommon for the catheter to stop functioning. The side holes of the catheter can become clogged or, as the fetus grows, the catheter can be pulled out of the bladder or withdrawn into either the abdominal cavity or the bladder. A second catheter can then be placed if continued in utero development of the fetus is considered desirable.

International Fetal Surgery Registry

From 1982 to 1986, 79 cases of catheter shunts for obstructive uropathy were reported to the registry, kept at the University of Manitoba[20] (Manning FA: personal communication, 1987). Eleven of the 79 fetuses were electively terminated subsequent to catheter placement, six for abnormal karyotype, five others for suspected severe renal disease. Of the 68 cases in which the pregnancy was continued, the survival rate was 50 percent. Survival was 100 percent for prune belly syndrome; all three cases showed no anatomic evidence of urethral obstruction. Lowest survival was seen with urethral atresia; all three fetuses died.

The most common diagnosis was posterior urethral valve, which had a survival of 74 percent. The mortality of untreated posterior urethral valve syndrome detected at birth is about 45 percent.[23a] While the number of patients in both series are small, this suggests that in utero therapy for posterior urethral valves may be of benefit.

Sixty-three of the fetuses with ongoing pregnancies were male, while only five were female. This is not surprising, as posterior urethral valves, the most common diagnosis in the treated series, is almost exclusively a male disease.[25] Overall survival for males was 50.9 percent, while only 20 percent of females survived. Three female fetuses had isolated urethral atresia, and two had urethral atresia with persistent cloacal syndrome. One of the latter survived.

Procedure-related mortality in ongoing pregnancies was 4.8 percent. Two deaths occurred at the time of shunt placement and were presumed attributable to trauma. The other procedure related loss occurred in a premature neonate born as a result of premature labor 48 hours after shunt placement. Pulmonary hypoplasia was the major cause of death in the remaining fetuses. Twenty-seven neonates died from respiratory insufficiency, while only one died of chronic renal failure. The quality of life in the survivors was good, as only two of the 34 survivors have chronic illness.

The Registry data illustrate the feasibility and possible value of in utero shunting for obstructive uropathy but also highlights the problem of our inability to diagnose pulmonary hypoplasia in the fetus. Harrison's group showed that in animals, pulmonary hypoplasia can be improved, or partially prevented, by decompression of the urinary tract in utero.[24] The critical period and amount of amniotic fluid necessary for normal lung development in the human fetus have not been determined. The critical periods and duration of obstruction resulting in renal dysplasia also require elucidation, as normal pulmonary function at birth does not guarantee normal renal function.

Management of Fetal Obstructive Uropathy

Patients with a suspected fetal urinary tract obstruction should undergo high-resolution sonography at a center experienced in the diagnosis and management of this disorder. Serial examinations may be required to determine the level, degree, and progression of obstruction. Special attention should be given to the appearance of the fetal kidneys, amount of amniotic fluid, and presence of nonrenal anomalies. Chromosomal analysis is mandatory.

Expectant management should be selected for fetuses with a normal amount of amniotic fluid, regardless of whether the obstruction is unilateral or bilateral. These fetuses are expected to have a good prognosis but require serial follow-up ultrasound examinations to look for worsening upper tract dilation and decrease in amniotic fluid volume. If the fluid volume decreases in a premature fetus who has no other anomalies, shunt placement is recommended.

Fetuses with severe bilateral obstruction (bilateral hydronephrosis and/or megacystis) associated with marked oligohydramnios are suspected to have a poor prognosis. Even with shunt placement, prolonged severe oligohydramnios prior to 20 weeks gestation usually leads to perinatal death from respiratory failure, often with dysplastic kidneys.[14,26-28] Bladder-amniotic shunts can be placed in gestations less than 24 weeks to achieve decompression and assess renal function. If amniotic fluid does not reaccumulate, prognosis for normal renal function and normal lung development is poor. In those cases, pregnancy termination can be elected.

When oligohydramnios develops later in gestation, lung development may be normal, but renal function may be permanently impaired and will not be corrected by drainage of the urinary tract.[21,29] It is therefore desirable to assess renal function prior to shunt placement. Failure of bladder refilling after aspiration or of amniotic fluid reaccululation after shunt placement has a poor prognosis. Sonographic appearance of the kidneys can be helpful, as cortical cysts or increased ecthogenicity of the renal parenchyma is highly specific for dysplasia.[30] Measurement of urinary electrolytes, specifically isotonic urine with high sodium and chloride concentrations, has been predictive of poor renal function.[31-33] Unfortunately, the presence of normal fluid reaccumulation, normal-appearing renal parenchyma, and normal urinary electrolytes does not always guarantee normal neonatal renal function.

Treatment may improve the prognosis in those fetuses with bilateral obstruction, no associated abnormalities and progressive decrease in amniotic fluid quantity. If evaluation of renal function suggests a good prognosis, intrauterine therapy should be considered for fetuses who have documented lung immaturity.

Improved success with shunting for obstructive uropathy will require better selection of fetuses as well as improvements in shunt technique. Accurate antenatal assessment of adequate pulmonary and renal function would improve selection. Ability to maintain shunt patency would decrease morbidity by requiring fewer procedures. Further study is required to determine whether open surgical techniques as opposed to percutaneous needle technique of shunt placement would yield superior results.

Hydrocephalus

Most children born with severe congenital obstructive hydrocephalus die or are left severely retarded. Milder cases treated with early neonatal shunting can have a favorable prognosis. It became logical to question whether in utero shunting of mild yet progressive hydrocephalus could prevent ongoing damage and permit normal brain development to proceed. The results of intrauterine shunting procedures have not yet met these expectations, primarily due to a failure to identify those fetuses that would benefit from decompression. The diverse etiologies of hydrocephalus, lack of information on their natural histories, and the inability to exclude other major anomalies accurately have contributed to suboptimal selection.

Diagnosis

By the twelfth week of gestation, the lateral ventricles of the fetus can be recognized filling the cranial vault, while the ventricles are filled in turn with the highly echogenic choriod plexes. At 15 to 17 weeks, the lateral wall of the ventricles can clearly be distinguished from the calvarium and the intervening mantle identified. As gestation advances, the ventricles appear to shrink as rapid proliferation and growth of the cerebral hemispheres occur. The diagnosis of early hydrocephalus is made by an elevated lateral ventricular width to hemispheric width ratio (LVW/HW).[9,34] At 15 weeks gestation, the LVW/HW averages 56 percent but ranges from 40 to 71 percent, while at term it should not be greater than 35 percent and usually averages 28 percent.[34] As a general rule, the lateral ventricle extends about two-thirds the distance from the midline to the inner edge of the skull at 15 weeks, then decreases to one-half, one-third, and one-fourth the distance by 18, 22, and 40 weeks, respectively.

The diagnosis of early hydrocephalus should be confirmed by evidence of progressive ventricular enlargement. As pointed out by Chervenak et al.,[35] approximately 2.5 percent of the normal population will have an abnormally elevated LVW/HW as defined by the nomograms of Johnson or Jeanty. Persistent elevation of LVW/HW ratio has been shown to be a reliable predictor of ventriculomegaly.[35,36] Enlargement of the skull seen in late hydrocephaly usually does not occur until after 28 weeks. In severe cases, cortical echoes are replaced by cystic areas extending laterally to the inner surface of the calvarium.

Etiology

Hydrocephalus is a morphologic finding that can result from a variety of causes. Once hydrocephalus is identified, an attempt to determine etiology should be made, as the clinical course and the prognosis will differ depending on etiology. The two mechanisms responsible for ventricular enlargement are (1) elevation of intracranial pressure (ICP) due to obstruction of fluid flow or to increased rate of fluid production, and (2) decrease in brain substance. Ventriculoamniotic shunts are useful only in cases resulting from the first mechanism in which a high ventricular/amniotic fluid pressure gradient will result in passive flow out of the ventricles. Most cases of prenatally diagnosed ventriculomegaly are due to elevation in ICP, either from blockage within the ventricular system (obstructive) or from lack of reabsorption due to blockade in the subarachnoid pathways (communicating). Choroid plexus papilloma, a tumor that secretes cerebrospinal fluid and causes elevated ICP, has not yet been reported in a fetus.[37]

Environmental and genetic causes of hydrocephalus have been identified in some cases, while other cases are identified only by their structural abnormalities. Intrauterine infections can cause inflammation or hemorrhage resulting in scarring and obstruction at the aqueduct of Sylvius or at the subarachnoid granulations. Toxoplasmosis, cytomegalovirus, syphilis, and rubella may cause ventriculomegaly by either obstruction or degeneration of brain substance. Sonographic identification of cerebral calcifications may be suggestive of an infectious etiology.

Genetic causes of hydrocephalus range from those with multifactorial inheritance with a low recurrence risk to autosomal-recessive syndromes with a 25 percent risk of recurrence. X-linked aqueductal stenosis accounts for 2 percent of all cases of isolated hydrocephalus but may be responsible for up to 25 percent of aqueductal stenosis in males.[38] Dandy-Walker syndrome, congenital atresia of the foramina of the fourth ventricle, may be of autosomal-recessive inheritance in some cases.[38] Ultrasonographic findings include a large cystic structure in the posterior fossa continuous with the fourth ventricle. Cerebellar agenesis, which may show an X-linked inheritance, has a poor prognosis and should be distinguished from Dandy-Walker syndrome.[39] Chromosomal anomalies, such as trisomy 18 or 13, may cause brain malformation with obstruction at the cerebral aqueduct or fourth ventricle.

The presence or absence of associated anomalies may aid in determining the etiology and prognosis of the ventriculomegaly. Recent series have shown major malformations occurring in 70 to 83 percent of fetuses with hydrocephalus, with only a small percentage of these attributable to chromosomal aberrations.[40–42] Spina bifida, the most common associated abnormality, is present in 25 to 30 percent of cases of fetal hydrocephalus. The Arnold-Chiari malformation, obstruction at the foramen magnum or fourth ventricle caused by downward displacement of the medulla oblongata and of the cerebellum, causes hydrocephalus in approximately 80 percent of cases of spina bifida. Thirty-seven percent of the hydrocephalic fetuses in Chervenak's 1985 series had intracranial anomalies, including microcephaly, agenesis of the corpus callosum, encephalocele, arteriovenous malformation, arachnoid cyst, and cebocephaly.

Anomalies have also been reported in the cardiovascular, renal, gastrointestinal, skeletal, respiratory, and reproductive systems. Severe anomalies are important to diagnose as their poor prognosis would preclude intervention for hydrocephalus. Of concern is the failure to detect these malformations before birth. Combining the experience of three recent series of fetal hydrocephalus, failure to diagnose a severe associated anomaly before birth occurred in 26 of the 95 (27 percent) cases.[37,40,41] Major malformations not identified before delivery included spina bifida, cardiac malformations, esophageal atresia, tracheoesophageal fistula, eventration of the diaphragm, sirenomelia, agenesis of the corpus callosum, alobar holoprosencephaly, AV malformation of the thalamus, cerebellar cyst, porencephalic cyst, polymicro-gyria, and congenital toxoplasmosis.

Ultrasonography can diagnose fetal ventriculomegaly accurately, even in the early second trimester, but the reported accuracy in diagnosing associated anomalies is suboptimal. Accuracy is likely to improve with experience, improving resolution of sonography, and adjuvant use of other modalities such as echocardiography, computed tomography (CT), and magnetic resonance imaging (MRI) in selected cases.

Natural History of Fetal Hydrocephalus

The natural history of ventriculomegaly in the fetus, particularly if found in the second trimester, is unclear. It is therefore difficult to determine prognosis for the fetus with isolated hydrocephalus and difficult to determine the effect of in utero treatment.

Several series have reported the outcome of fetuses with ventriculomegaly who were managed expectantly in utero.[37,41,43,44] Of the 26 fetuses with isolated ventriculomegaly at birth, 16 (61.5 percent) neonates survived and 13 (81 percent) of the survivors were normal at follow-up evaluation. Since this is a small series that only includes infants found to have no associated anomolies at birth, the true incidence of normal outcome for fetuses thought to have isolated ventriculomegaly requires larger series with longer follow-up management.

Shunt Procedure

Most of the shunts placed in human fetuses to date have been similar to that used by the Denver group,[45] with or without a valve. The Denver shunt is made of silicon rubber tubing and contains a valve to avoid sudden decompression of the ventricle and to prevent backflow of amniotic fluid into the ventricle. The amniotic end of the shunt has a thickened collar to prevent the shunt from being pushed into the fetal head. Modification of the original shunt has included placement of two rubber flanges that fold flat along the shunt during placement and then expand to keep the shunt anchored in the fetal skull.

Following maternal sedation and/or local anesthesia, a 13-gauge needle with a sharp stylet is inserted through the maternal abdomen and uterus into the fetal lateral ventricle. Entry through fetal calvaria is usually through the posterior parietal region above the level of the trigone. As a ventriculoamniotic shunt will be of benefit only in cases of elevated intracranial pressure, measurements of pressure within the amniotic fluid and the fetal ventricle are taken during placement of the needle. Once the needle is in place within the ventricle, the shunt is pushed through the needle and held in position with a blunt stylet as the needle is withdrawn.

Proper shunt placement can be determined by sonographic location of the catheter ends and confirmed by the gradual decrease in the LVW/HW ratio. Malfunction due to obstruction or migration from proper location is diagnosed by a rapid increase in the LVH/HW ratio.

Fetal Surgery Reigstry

From 1982 to 1985, the International Fetal Surgery Registry contained 39 reported cases of fetal hydrocephalus treated by in utero decompression.[46] Thirty-seven of the 39 cases were treated with indwelling shunts for a mean duration of 2.1 ± 1.3 weeks (range less than 1 to 7 weeks). The average gestational age at diagnosis was 25 ± 2.7 weeks, while the mean age at treatment was 27 ± 2.6 weeks. The survival rate was 82.1 percent, with a procedure-related death rate of 10.25 percent. One fetus died at the time of shunt placement from brain trauma, while three others died from premature delivery related to the surgical procedure. Three deaths occurred that were not procedure related: two with severe associated anomalies, one unexplained.

Neonatal diagnoses were aqueductal stenosis (32 cases) and one case each of Dandy-Walker syndrome, holoprosencephaly, Arnold-Chiari syndrome, and porencephalic cyst. In three cases, the cause of hydrocephalus was unknown. Associated anomalies in other organ systems were found in 15.4 percent of fetuses: diaphragmatic hernia, arthrogryposis multiplex congenita, myelomeningocele, trisomy 21, massive facial cleft, pulmonary hypoplasia, and multiple anomalies.

Follow-up of the survivors for a mean of 8.2 ± 6 months showed the majority to be abnormal (65.6 percent). Eighteen of 39 treated fetuses (56.25 percent) have severe handicap, and all tested exhibited developmental quotients of less than 50. Five of these infants have cortical blindness, two have severe seizure disorders, and two have spastic dysplegia. The only neurologically normal fetuses in the series were those with aqueductal stenosis. Of the 32 cases with this diagnosis, 34 percent are normal, 50 percent have a severe handicap, and 12.5 percent died of procedure-related complications.

It is difficult to compare the outcomes in groups of untreated and treated fetuses with hydrocephalus, as both groups suffer from selection bias; however, a prospective randomized controlled trial does not exist. Preliminary analysis of treated fetuses with isolated hydrocephalus compared with historical controls indicates that in utero treatment may increase survival by allowing severely handicapped fetuses to survive. Manning et al.[46] compared the above Registry statistics for aqueductal stenosis with published reports of the outcome of fetal aqueductal stenosis managed expectantly. Only 40 percent of the 20 reported cases that were not shunted in utero survived, but six of the eight survivors (75 percent) were normal at follow-up. In the Registry's treated group, 87.5 percent survived, but only 37.5 percent of these were normal.

CONCLUSION

In utero shunting for hydrocephalus has offered no clear benefit to the fetus. While intrauterine therapy may improve outcome for a small group of fetuses, accurate antenatal selection of that group has not yet been demonstrated. Improvements are needed in our ability to determine etiology, document increased intracranial pressure, and rule out irreversible brain damage. More information on the natural history and long-term outcome of fetal hydrocephalus is essential before the role of in utero treatment can be properly evaluated. At the same time, experimental studies are necessary in order to develop a model that closely parallels isolated human hydrocephalus. Experimental models can also help in refining shunt procedures in order to lower the morbidity of shunt placement and decrease the need for repeated procedures.

While some conditions are better left untreated until after delivery, in utero therapy of severe erythroblastosis fetalis and obstructive uropathy can prevent progressive disease leading to fetal or neonatal death. Other potentially correctable disorders currently under investigation include diaphragmatic hernia, severe combined immune-deficiency disease, and spina bifida. Fetal invasive therapy is only in its infancy and will continue to develop as the natural history of disorders is elucidated and strategies to overcome technical difficulties perfected.

REFERENCES

1. Liley AW: Liquor amnii analysis in the management of the pregnancy complicated by Rhesus sensitization. Am J Obstet Gynecol 82:1359, 1961
2. Nicolaides KH, Rodeck CH, Millar DS, et al: Fetal hematology in rhesus isoimmunization. Br Med J 290:661, 1985
3. Chitkara V, Wilkins I, Lynch L, et al: The role of sonography in assessing severity of fetal anemia in Rh and Kell isoimmunized pregnancies Obstet Gynecol 71:393, 1988
4. Benacerraf BR, Frigoletto FD: Sonographic sign for the detection of early fetal ascites in the management of severe isoimmune devise without intrauterine transfusion. Am J Obstet Gynecol 152:1039, 1985
5. Barss VA, Benacerraf BR, Green MF, Frigoletto FD: Use of a small gauge needle for intrauterine fetal transfusion. Am J Obstet Gynecol 155:1057, 1986
6. Bowman JM: Rh erythroblastosis 1975. Semin Hematol 12:189, 1975
7. Bowman JM: The management of Rh-isoimmunization. Obstet Gynecol 52:1, 1978
7a. Bowman JM, Manning FA: Intrauterine Fetal Transfusions: Winnipeg 1982. Obstet Gynecol 61:203, 1983
8. Berkowitz RL: Intrauterine transfusion, 1980: An update. Clin Perinatol 7:285, 1980
9. Jeanty P, Rodesch F, Romero R, et al: How to improve your amniocentesis technique. Am J Obstet Gynecol 1983:146, 593
10. Rodeck CH, Nicolaides KH: Ultrasound guided invasive procedured in obstetrics. Clin Obstet Gynecol 10:515, 1983
10a. Rodeck CH, Nicolaides KH, Warsof SL, et al: The management of severe rhesus isoimmunization by fetoscopic intravascular transfusion. Am J Obstet Gynecol 150:769, 1984

10b. Grannum PA, Copel JA, Plaxe SC, et al: In utero exchange transfusion by direct intravascular injection in severe erythroblastosis fetalis. N Engl J Med 314:1431, 1986

11. Berkowitz RL, Chitkara U, Goldberg JD, et al: Intravascular intravascular transfusion for severe red blood cell isoimmunization: Ultrasound-guided percutaneous approach. Am J Obstet Gynecol 155:574, 1986

12. Harrison MR, Filly RA, Golbus MS, et al: Fetal treatment 1982. N Engl J Med 306:1651, 1982

13. Kurjak A, Latin V, Mandruzzto B, et al: Ultrasound diagnosis and perinatal management of fetal genito-urinary abnormalites. J Perinat Med 12:291, 1984

14. Hobbins JC, Romero R, Grannum P, et al: Antenatal diagnosis of renal anomalies with ultrasound. I. Obstructive uropathy. Am J Obstet Gynecol 148:868, 1984

15. Potter EL, Craig JM: Pathology of the Fetus and Infant. Year Book, Chicago, 1975

16. Quinlan RW, Cruz AC, Huddleston JF: Sonographic detection of fetal urinary tract anomalies. Obstet Gynecol 67:558, 1986

17. Reuss A, Wladimiroff JW, Scholtmeijer RJ, et al: Antenatal evaluation and outcome of fetal obstructive uropathies. Prenatal Diagnosis 8:93, 1988

18. Frydman M, Magenis RE, Mohandas TK, et al: Chromosomal abnormalities in infants with prune belly anomaly: Association with trisomy 18. Am J Med Genetics 15:145, 1983

19. Nevin NC, Nevin J, Dunlop JM, et al: Antenatel detection of grossly distended bladder owing to absence of the urethra in a fetus with trisomy 18. J Med Genetics 20:132, 1983

20. Manning FA, Harrison MR, Rodeck C, et al: Catheter shunts for fetal hydronephrosis and hydrocephalus. Report of the International Fetal Surgery Registry. N Engl J Med 315:336, 1986

21. Harrison MR, Golbus MS, Filly RA, et al: Management of the fetus with congenital hydronephrosis. J Pediatr Surg 17:728, 1982

22. Fitzsimmons RB, Keohane C, Galvin J: Prune belly syndrome with ultrasound demonstration of reduction of megacystis in utero. Br J Radiol 58:374, 1985

23. Avni EF, Rodesch F, Schulman CC: Fetal uropathies: Diagnostic pitfalls and management. J Urol 134:921, 1985

23a. Nakayama DK, Harrison MR, deLorimer AA: Prognosis of posterior urethral valves presenting at birth. J Pediatr Sur 21:43, 1986

24. Nakayama DK, Glick PL, Villa RL, et al: Experimental pulmonary hyperplasia due to oligohydramnios and its reversal by relieving thoracic compression. J Pediatr Surg 18:347, 1983

25. Grupe WE: Hydronephrosis. p. 431. In Avery ME, Taeusch HW (eds): Schaffer's Diseases of the Newborn. WB Saunders, Philadelphia, 1984

26. Berkowitz RL, Glickman MG, Smith GJW, et al: Fetal urinary tract obstruction: What is the role of surgical intervention in utero? Am J Obstet Gynecol 144:367, 1982

27. Harrison MR, Golbus MS, Filly RA, et al: Fetal surgery for congenital hydronephrosis. N Engl J Med 306:591, 1982

28. Manning FA, Harman CR, Lange IR, et al: Antepartum chronic fetal vesicoamniotic shunts for obstructive uropathy: A report of two cases. Am J Obstet Gynecol 145:819, 1983

29. Golbus MS, Harrison MR, Filly RA, et al: In utero treatment of urinary tract obstruction. Am J Obstet Gynecol 142:383, 1982

30. Mahoney BS, Filly RA, Callen PW, et al: Sonographic evaluation of renal dysplasia. Radiology 152:143, 1984

31. Golbus MS, Filly RA, Callen P, et al: Fetal urinary tract obstruction: Management and selection for treatment. Semin Perinatol 9(2):91, 1985

32. Nicolaides KH, Rodeck CH: Fetal therapy. p. 40. In Studd J (ed): Progress in Obstetrics and Gynecology. Vol. 5. Churchill Livingstone, 1985

33. Wilkins I, Chitkara U, Lynch L, et al: The nonpredictive value of fetal urinary electrolytes: Preliminary report of outcomes and correlations with pathologic diagnosis. Am J Obstet Gynecol 157:694, 1987

34. Johnson ML, Dunne MG, Mack LA, et al: Evaluation of fetal intracranial anatomy by statis and realtime ultrasound. J Clin Ultrasound 8:311, 1980

34a. Jeanty P, Dramaix-Wilmet M, Delbeke D: Ultrasonic evaluation of fetal ventricular growth. Neuroradiology 21:123, 1981

35. Chervenak FA, Berkowitz RL, Romero R, et al: The diagnosis of fetal hydrocephalus. Am J Obstet Gynecol 147:703, 1983

36. Chervenak FA, Berkowitz RL, Tortora M, et al: Diagnosis of ventriculomegaly before fetal viability. Obstet Gynecol 64:652, 1984

37. Clewell WH, Meier PR, Manchester DK, et al: Ventriculomegaly: Evaluation and management. Semin Perinatol 9(2):98, 1985

38. Burton BK: Recurrence risk for congenital hydrocephalus. Clin Genet 16:47, 1979

39. Ricardi VM, Marcus ES: Congenital hydrocephalus and cerebellar agenesis. Clin Genet 13:443, 1978

40. Chervenak FA, Berkowitz RL Tortota M, et al: The management of fetal hydocephalus. Am J Obstet Gynecol 151:933, 1985

41. Glick PL, Harrison RM, Nakayama DK, et al: Management of ventriculomegaly in the fetus. J Pediatr 105:97, 1984

42. Pretorius DH, Davis K, Manco-Johnson ML, et al: Clinical course of fetal hydrocephalus: 40 cases. Am J Radiol 144:827, 1985

43. Chervenak FA, Duncan C, Ment LR, et al: Outcome of fetal ventriculomegaly. Lancet 2:179, 1984

44. Vintzileos AM, Campbell WA, Weinbaum PJ, et al: Perinatal management and outcome of fetal ventriculomegaly. Obstet Gynecol 69:5, 1987

45. Clewell WH, Johnson ML, Meier PR, et al: A surgical approach to the treatment of fetal hydrocephalus. N Engl J Med 306:1320, 1982

46. Manning FA: International Fetal Surgery Registry: 1985 update. Clin Obstet Gynecol 29:551, 1986

12 Hydrops Fetalis

ARTHUR C. FLEISCHER
DINESH M. SHAH
PHILIPPE JEANTY
GLYNIS A. SACKS
FRANK H. BOEHM

Hydrops fetalis refers to a variety of conditions associated with a markedly swollen and edematous fetus. The severely affected fetus usually has effusions into the peritoneal, pleural, and/or pericardial spaces.

Hydrops fetalis is divided into those causes that are associated with isoimmunization to an erythrocyte antigen (isoimmune hydrops; IIH) and those that are not (nonimmune hydrops; NIH). Each type has a relatively specific cause and predictable prognosis. With the more widespread use of Rh immune globulin (RhIG) prophylaxis over the past several years, the relative incidence of nonimmune to isoimmune hydrops has changed significantly. Although the actual incidence of NIH to IIH varies depending on the screened population, at most medical centers the incidence of NIH is far greater than that of IIH.

Isoimmunization to a particular erythrocyte antigen usually results in severe hemolytic anemia of the fetus. With the advent of RhIG prophylaxis, the incidence of hemolytic disease in newborns declined from 40.5 births to 14.3 per 10,000 live births between 1970 and 1979.[1] Despite the widespread use of RhIG prophylaxis for nonsensitized Rh mothers, approximately 1.5 percent of all pregnancies are complicated by isoimmunization. The use of both ante- and postpartum RhIG has further reduced the incidence of isoimmunization to 0.1 to 0.3 percent. Despite its low incidence, IIH is associated with a perinatal mortality rate of 25 to 30 percent.[2]

As opposed to IIH, NIH results from a variety of anatomic and/or functional disorders not related to an immunologic cause.[3] It has been estimated that 3 percent of all fetal mortality is related to NIH.[1] Unfortunately, anywhere from 70 to 90 percent of fetuses affected by NIH die during the perinatal period.[1]

This review discusses the new developments in sonographic detection and evaluation and sonographically guided procedures of the hydropic fetus, in particular, the role of percutaneous umbilical cord blood sampling for fetal karyotyping, hematocrit determination, blood analysis, and transfusions. The importance of a detailed sonographic evaluation of the fetus for determining the specific cause and severity of nonimmune hydrops is emphasized. The expanded role of real-time observations concerning the assessment of the fetal condition by sonography is also discussed.

NONIMMUNE HYDROPS

The sonographic findings common to both severe nonimmune and immune hydrops include peritoneal, pleural, or pericardial effusions and/or skin thickening (anasarca).[4] The specific anomalies that can be associated with NIH are related to the underlying structural and functional defect. Table 12.1 lists the various etiologies of NIH. These are classified as fetal, placental, and maternal abnormalities.

Even though NIH is associated with specific fetal structural and functional anomalies, in approximately 30 to 40 percent of cases, the precise etiology cannot be found.[1] Depending on the population studied, probably one of

TABLE 12.1. Conditions associated with nonimmune hydrops

Fetal
    Cranial
        Hydrocephalus
        Vein of Galen aneurysm
    Cardiovascular
    Severe congenital heart disease (i.e., ASD, VSD, hypoplastic left heart, pulmonary valve insufficiency, Ebstein anomaly, subaortic stenosis)
    Premature closure of foramen ovale
    Myocarditis
    Large arteriovenous malformation
    Tachyarrhythmias (i.e., atrial flutter, supraventricular tachycardia)
    Bradyarrhythmias (i.e., especially those associated with heart block)
    Fibroelastosis
    Pulmonary
        Cystic adenomatoid malformation of lung
        Pulmonary lymphangiectasia
        Pulmonary hypoplasia
        Congenital chylothorax
        Mediastinal teratoma
        Extralobar pulmonary sequestration

(Table continues)

TABLE 12.1 (*Continued*)

Fetal (*Continued*)
  Renal/Retroperitoneal
    Congenital nephrosis
    Renal vein thrombosis
    Neuroblastomatosis
  Multisystem disorders
    Chromosomal
      Trisomy 21
      Turner syndrome 45,XO
      Other trisomies
      Triploidy
      Mosaicism
    Intrauterine infections
      Syphilis
      Toxoplasmosis
      Cytomegalovirus
      Leptospirosis
      Chagas disease
      Congenital hepatitis
      Herpes simplex
    Hematologic
      Homozygous α-thalassemia
      Chronic fetomaternal transfusion
  Miscellaneous congenital anomalies
    Meconium peritonitis
    Tuberous sclerosis
    Small bowel volvulus
    Twin-to-twin transfusion
    Cystic hygroma

Placental/umbilical cord
  Umbilical vein thrombosis
  Chorioangioma
  Umbilical cord knots

Maternal disease
  Diabetes mellitus
  Toxemia
  Severe anemia

Idiopathic

the most common disorders associated with NIH is congenital heart disease or arrhythmias. The second most common cause of NIH is most likely chromosomal abnormalities. Hematologic abnormalities probably account for the third most common cause of NIH. As in cases of IIH, these disorders have in common a cardiovascular derangement, since structural abnormalities of the heart are common in fetuses with a chromosomal disorder.

Although it is extremely rare, there have been reports of spontaneous resolution of fetal ascites.[5] We have documented a case of spontaneous resolution of a left-sided pleural effusion, and there have been reports of resolution of a chylothorax after repeated sonographically guided thorocenteses at 20 to 23 weeks.[6]

Sonographic evaluation for evidence of hydrops should initially focus on the presence or absence of peritoneal, pleural, or pericardial fluid. Since the fetus does not remain stationary in utero, the precise location of these collections will vary. Small intraperitoneal collections usually begin to collect within the peritoneum surrounding the liver or spleen. One should be aware that the abdominal wall musculature usually appears as a hypoechoic band near the umbilical cord insertion on the ventral abdominal wall. One way of determining whether a hypoechoic area represents fluid is by close examination of the area of the abdomen near where the umbilical cord enters the body. If both sides of the umbilical vein can be seen clearly as it traverses the anterior abdominal wall, intraperitoneal fluid is probably present.[7] Abnormal thickening of the skin is usually first recognized around the calvaria. One should not mistake excessive fat in the subcutaneous layer of a fetus of a diabetic (macrosomia) mother with anascara seen in the hydropic fetus.

Once the hydropic fetus is identified, the sonographer should systematically examine the fetus for anatomic and/or functional abnormalities that may be associated with NIH. In the head, one can detect a dilated lateral ventricle secondary to a viral encephalopathy or associated with a chromosomal anomaly. Rarely, a vein of Galen aneurysm may produce sufficient arteriovenous shunting to result in a hydropic fetus.

Cardiac arrhythmias and malformations are among the most common causes of NIH.[8] The heart should be closely examined for any structural malformations, such as hypoplastic left ventricle, and the cardiac rate and rhythm evaluated by M mode (Fig. 12.1). Supraventricular tachyarrhythmias can be treated in utero and are some of the more common arrhythmias associated with hydrops.[8]

Thoracic lesions that result in obstruction to venous return, such as a mediastinal teratoma or cystic adenomatoid malformation, should be excluded by detailed sonographic evaluation of the thorax and its contents (Fig. 12.2A).

Renal disorders associated with NIH include congenital nephrosis that results in NIH probably due to urinary protein loss. To date, no definite sonographic anatomic abnormalities of the kidney have been reported with this disorder. Neuroblastomatosis may result in NIH secondary to obstruction of venous return in the inferior vena cava.

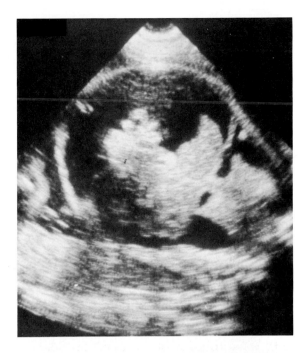

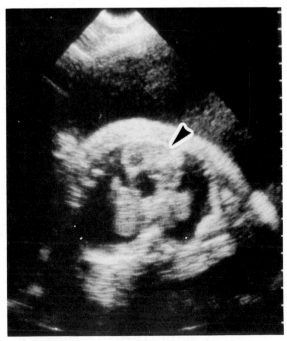

FIG. 12.1. Nonimmune hydrops associated with severe bradycardia and multiple cardiac defects. (A) Massive ascites and pleural effusions. (B) Short-axis view of heart showing its midline location and thickened myocardium (arrowhead).

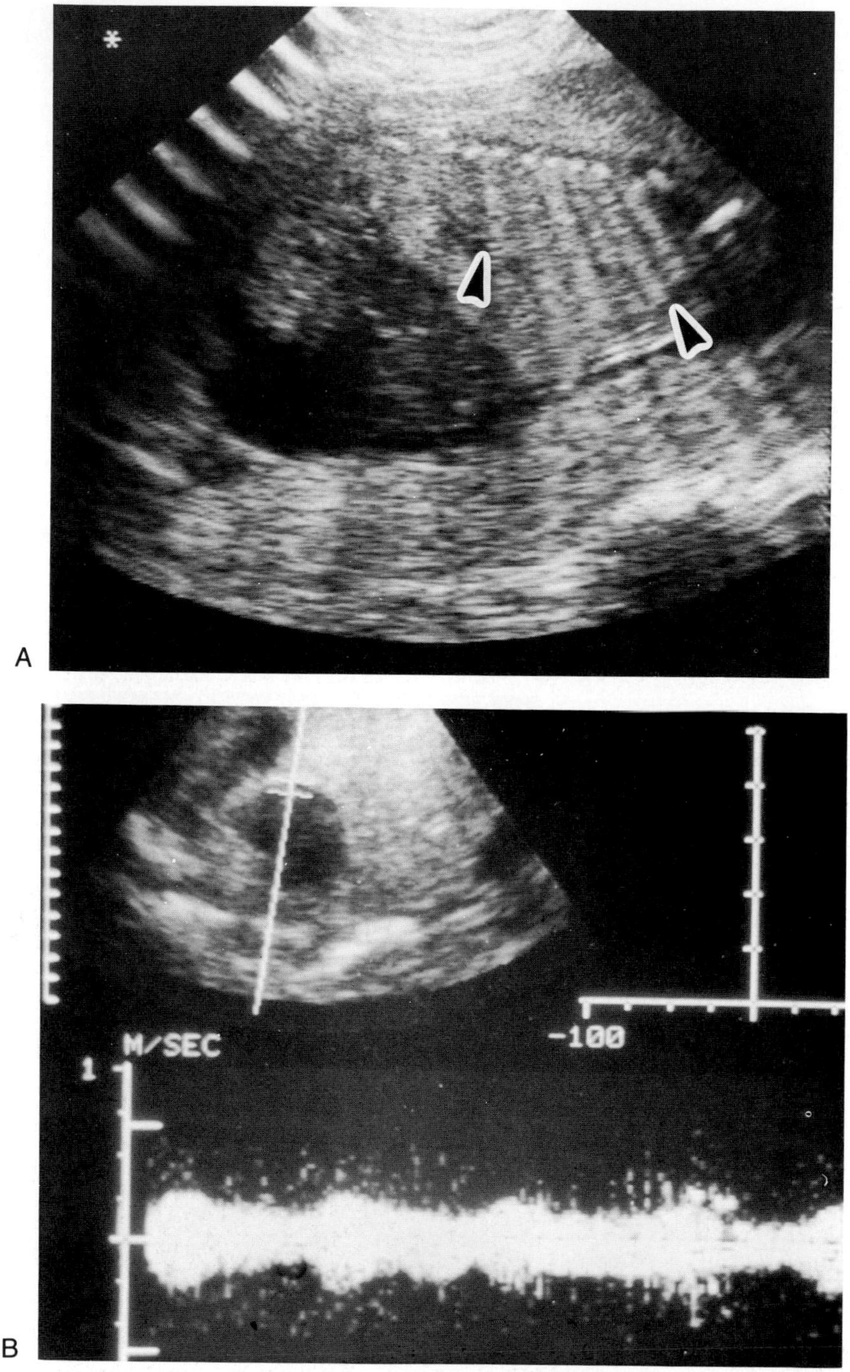

FIG. 12.2.   Miscellaneous causes of nonimmune hydrops. (A) Cystic adenomatoid malformation (microcystic type) appearing as solid mass (arrowhead) enlarging the right lung. (B) Chorioangioma appearing as hypoechoic mass near cord origin. Turbulent arterial and venous flow was detected on duplex Doppler examination. (*Figure continues.*)

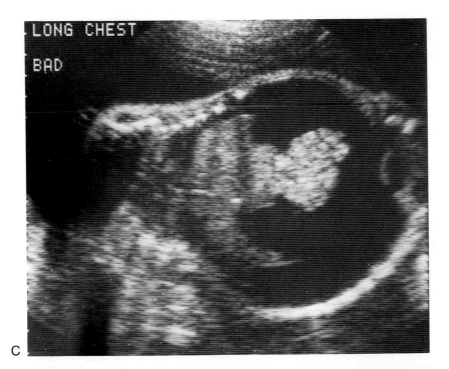

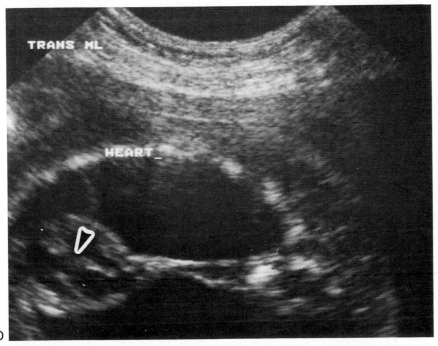

Fig. 12.2 (*Continued*).   (C) Massive hydrops secondary to cytomegalovirus infection in a 27-week fetus. No liver or brain calcifications were seen. (D) Massively hydropic 22-week fetus with a large ventricular septal defect and an overriding aorta. (*Figure continues.*)

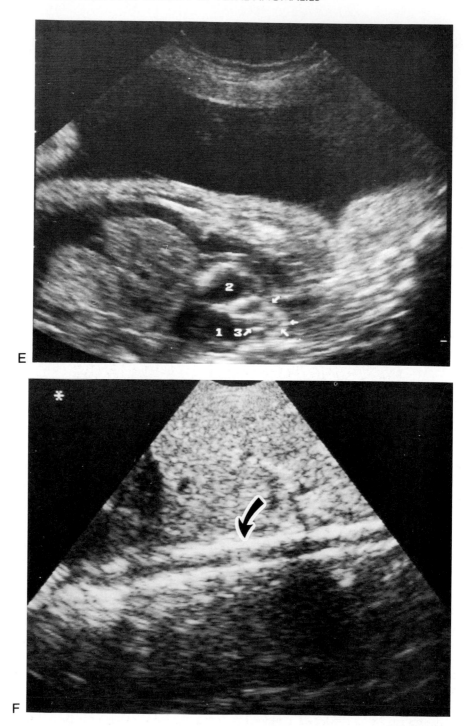

Fig. 12.2 *(Continued)*.   (E) Hydrops associated with arterial calcinosis. The aortic arch (arrows) is calcified. 1 = left ventricle, 2 = right ventricle, 3 = mitral valve. (F) Long-axis view of calcified aorta (arrow) in neonate. *(Figure continues.)*

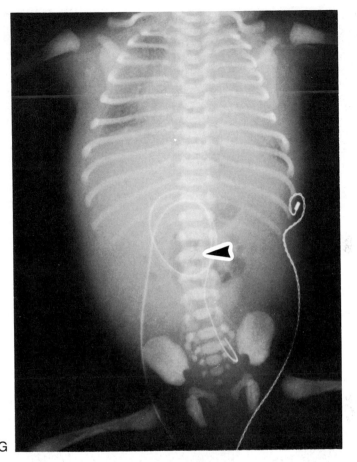

G

Fig. 12.2 (*Continued*).   (G) Radiograph of neonate shown in E and F showing calcified distal abdominal aorta and common iliac a (arrow).

Several multisystem disorders may result in NIH. These include conditions associated with systemic infections, hematologic abnormalities, and syndromes associated with abnormal chromosomal composition. Percutaneous umbilical vein sampling is useful in detecting the hematologic disorders such as α-thalassemia, which may result in NIH. Rarely, NIH is associated with placental or umbilical cord abnormalities (Fig. 12.2B). Hydrops fetalis associated with a placental chorioangioma can be attributed to excessive arteriovenous shunting that occurs within the tumor. This may result in reduced blood flow to the fetus. The plethoric twin affected by twin–twin transfusions can also become hydropic related to high-output failure (Fig. 12.3).

Thus, a variety of disorders may result in NIH. In general, the hydropic fetus should be considered a severely compromised fetus, one that may be agonal (near death). Serial biophysical profile testing and non-stress testing should be used to assess the condition of the hydropic fetus. In fact, these two tests were successfully used to follow some affected fetuses who would

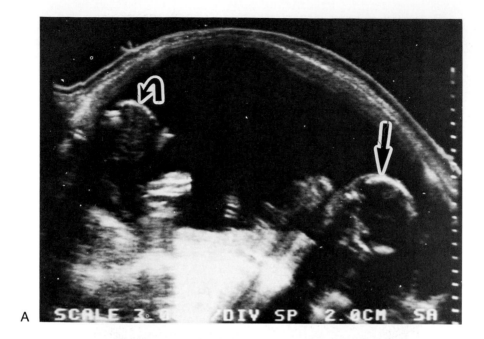

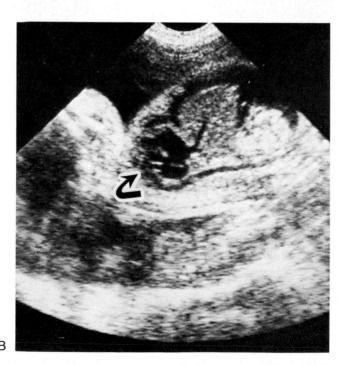

FIG. 12.3. Nonimmune hydrops associated with a twin–twin transfusion. (A) Static sonogram showing twins (arrows) and hydramnios. (B) Long-axis view of hydropic twin showing enlarged heart and liver floating within ascites. (*Figure continues.*)

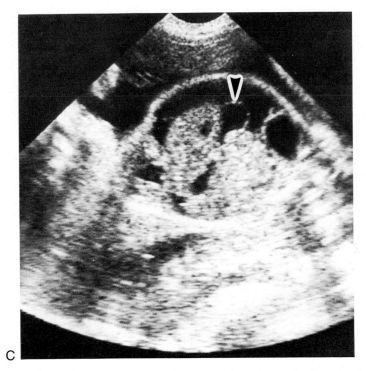

C

Fig. 12.3 (*Continued*).   (C) Long-axis view of abdomen showing omentum (arrowhead) floating within ascites.

previously have been treated by multiple intrauterine transfusions or early delivery.[9]

Other abnormalities that may be encountered with a hydropic fetus include hydramnios, oligohydramnios, and an abnormally thickened placenta. Hydramnios may be secondary to a lack of fetal swallowing due to a compromised fetal condition. Oligohydramnios usually portends a poor prognosis and may indicate poor fetal renal function. A thickened placenta may result from vascular engorgement secondary to increased resistance to forward flow to the fetus. It is postulated that this condition might be detected with continuous-wave Doppler as a high systolic peak of umbilical artery flow.

Sonography has an important role in the management of NIH that is not associated with a specific anatomic or functional abnormality. Because of the high incidence of chromosomal abnormalities associated with NIH, amniocentesis or percutaneous cordocentesis is indicated to determine whether the condition is related to an abnormal karyotype[10] (Fig. 12.4 and 12.5). Amniocentesis can be performed if hydrops is detected prior to 20 to 22 weeks, since 2 to 4 weeks is required for all culture. The technique of percutaneous cordocentesis has been described in detail in several papers.[11,12] As reported by Daffos et al.,[10] the complication of this procedure is low, with a fetal death rate of 1.1 percent and a spontaneous abortion rate of 0.8 percent.

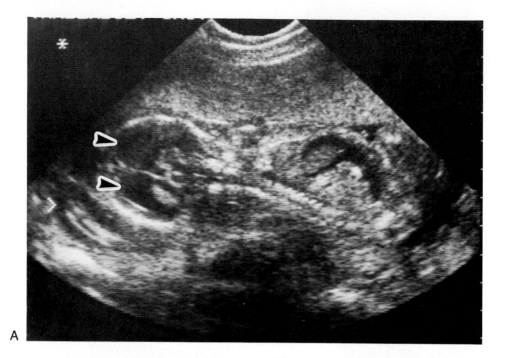

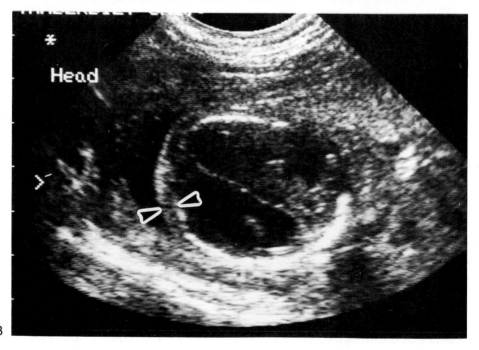

FIG. 12.4. Nonimmune hydrops associated with trisomy in 17-week fetus. (A) Long-axis view of 16-week fetus showing ascites and dilated lateral ventricles (arrowheads). (B) Axial sonogram through head showing dilated lateral ventricles and skin edema (arrowheads). (*Figure continues.*)

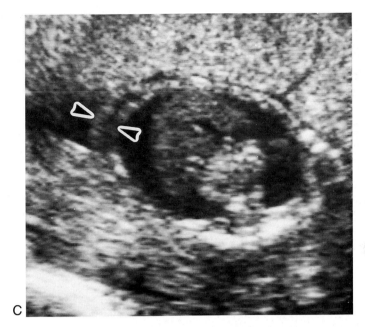

FIG. 12.4. (*Continued*)   (C) Anasarca of abdominal wall (arrowheads).

The data obtained from this procedure concerning the karyotype of the fetus permit coherent and coordinated management of the IIH fetus, especially one who does not exhibit a recognizable structural anomaly.

ISOIMMUNE HYDROPS

Isoimmune hydrops occurs when there is a maternal IgG antibody response to fetal red blood cell (RBC) antigen, leading to hemolysis and anemia. This is most frequently seen, but is not limited to, anti-D. RhIG treatment is unable to prevent incompatibility with some erythrocyte antigens, such as the K antigen in the Kell system, FY antigen in the W system, and C and E antigens in the Rhesus system.

Before the routine and widespread use of sonography, the amount of breakdown of bilirubinoid pigments in the amniotic fluid (ΔOD_{450}) was one of the only means of serially following the severity of hemolysis and determining the prognosis of the affected fetus. However, it should be noted that the Liley curves were first developed from data in fetuses from 27 weeks of age to term; these curves were only derived from linear extrapolation back to the second trimester.[1] Thus, their accuracy in determining the severity of hemolysis can be questioned. Data from pre-27-week fetuses suggested a lower ΔOD_{450} cutoff for intervention than was inferred from the Liley curve.[13]

Serial sonograms of the fetus combined with nonstress testing results are currently used to monitor the affected fetus (Fig. 12.6). This requires testing every third or other day. Special attention is directed toward detecting any

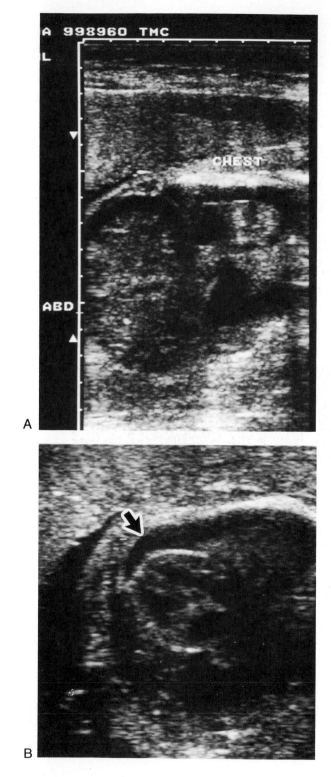

FIG. 12.5. Nonimmune hydrops associated with trisomy 21 in 26-week fetus. (A) Massive ascites and pleural effusions. (B) Long axis of the heart showing pericardial effusion (arrow).

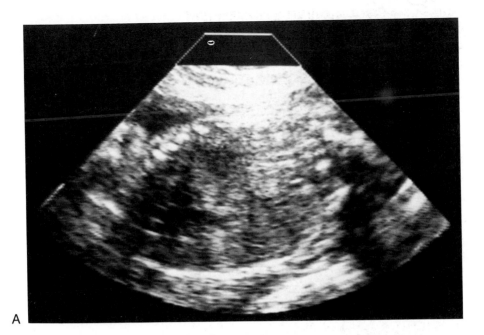

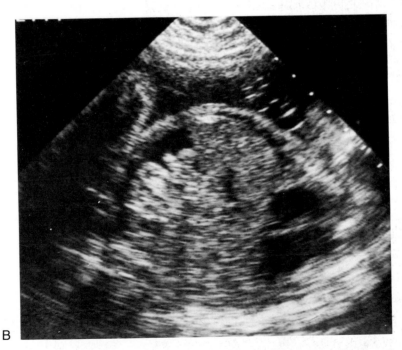

FIG. 12.6.   Serial sonography documenting the development of immune hydrops. (A) Long-axis view of isoimmunized fetus at 21 weeks showing no ascites. (B) At 26 weeks, the hemolysis became severe, and intraperitoneal fluid was detected.

changes in the fetal condition (breathing, movements) or interval development of skin edema or effusions as well as placental thickening.[9]

Although the precise pathophysiology in the development of IIH remains unclear, severe chronic anemia acting through tissue hypoxia is thought to be the most likely initiating factor.[1] Data from fetoscopic studies have indicated that fetal hydrops usually does not occur until hemoglobin levels drop below 4 g/dl.[14] Clearly, hydrops is worsened by hypoproteinemia and hypoalbuminemia. The diffuse extramedullary hematopoiesis that occurs in the liver and spleen may increase the resistance to forward flow through these organs, causing portal and umbilical vein hypertension. Combined with high-output failure, these disorders result in the loss of vascular competency, which is probably a major factor contributing to the production of hydrops.

SONOGRAPHY IN MANAGEMENT OF IIH

Sonography has an important role in several aspects of the management of the fetus affected by IIH, including serially guided amniocentesis for determination of the severity and/or progression of hemolysis and guidance of transfusions. With sonographically guided amniocentesis, there is less likelihood that the needle will traverse the placenta (which could further the extent of isoimmunization).

Over the past 10 years, sonography has replaced fluoroscopy as a means of accomplishing intraperitoneal instillation of blood. In addition to continuously monitoring the location of the needle, the real-time capability of sonography affords monitoring of heart rate during the procedure, since a significant (less than 60 beats/min) bradycardia may indicate fluid overload.[7] This technique of blood instillation into the peritoneum of the fetus depends on resorption of blood via the mesenteric and/or diaphragmatic lymphatics. This process is slow and occurs at an unpredictable rate, especially in the hydropic fetus.

The primary aim of treatment of the IIH fetus in whom delivery is contraindicated involves correction of the severe fetal anemia secondary to hemolysis. Over the past 5 years, direct puncture of the umbilical vein under fetoscopic visualization has been used to transfuse the affected fetus.[15,16] Percutaneous cordocentesis has replaced fetoscopically guided cord aspirations to determine the severity of fetal anemia and for direct intravascular transfusions.[11,12] Normal values for fetal hemoglobin levels average 12 ± 1.2 g/dl. A major disadvantage of fetoscopic transfusions included a fetal loss rate of approximately 2 to 5 percent, probably related to the relatively large (1.7-mm-diameter) endoscope needed to introduce the needle.[1] Using the fetoscopic approach for the management of 50 severely isoimmunized pregnancies, Warsof et al.[1] have achieved an overall survival rate of 84 percent, 92 percent in the nonhydropic and 71 percent hydropic fetuses. Reversal of hydrops was seen in successful transfusions.[1]

A major improvement in the techniques used for fetal transfusions has recently come about with the use of percutaneous cordocentesis for direct-exchange transfusions of the IIH fetus[11,12] (Fig. 12.7). The advantage of this technique includes the ability to monitor the hematocrit of the fetus during the transfusion such that the amount of blood infused is appropriate to the severity of the hemolytic anemia, the ability to withdraw and transfuse blood directly with the fetal circulation, and the relatively low complication rate.[11]

Percutaneous cordocentesis is preferred over direct introduction of the needle into umbilical vein within the fetal liver. This technique probably poses a higher threat of trauma to the fetus than cordocentesis; it also requires transient paralysis of the fetus with an intramuscular injection of curare in the thigh of the fetus.[17]

The technical and clinical sophistication required for direct transfusion into the fetus mandates that it be performed in tertiary care centers that are well equipped and experienced in the management of such cases.[18] Intraperitoneal instillation should be considered as an alternate when it is not possible to perform direct intravascular transfusion.[11] The blood transfused directly into the intraperitoneal cavity takes approximately 8 to 12 days (up to 50 ml and more than 50 ml, respectively) to resorb, depending on the amount instilled.[19]

Since the use of direct intravascular intrauterine transfusions is relatively new, the clinical efficacy of this approach cannot be determined at this time.

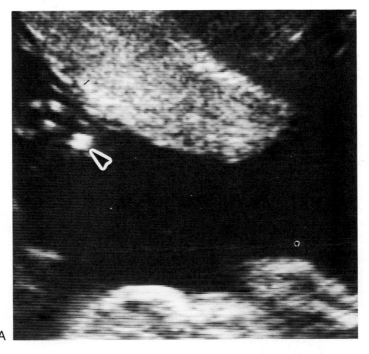

A

FIG. 12.7. Sonographically guided procedures. (A) Percutaneous umbilical vein transfusion. The tip of the needle (arrowhead) is lodged within the umbilical vein. (*Figure continues.*)

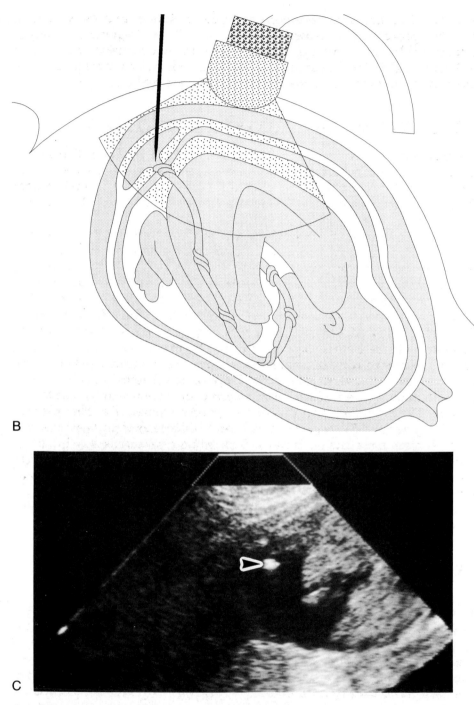

Fig. 12.7 (*Continued*).   (B) Diagram of umbilical vein transfusion shown in A. (C) Intraperitoneal instillation of blood. The tip of the needle (arrow) is within the ascites surrounding the liver.

Thus far, 38 procedures have been reported, indicating that the technique can be performed successfully, with or without significant complications.[11,12,15] Additional experience is needed to determine the optimal technique and timing for serial transfusions. Earlier and more frequent treatments may improve the chances of avoiding severe hydrops.

SONOGRAPHIC MIMICS OF FETAL HYDROPS

Certain conditions may be associated with sonographic findings that mimic those of the hydropic fetus. In most cases, these disorders involve excess fluid in a particular body cavity, such as the peritoneum or pleural spaces. Rarely, excessively thick skin of a macrosomic fetus may mimic the anasarca seen in the severely hydropic fetus.

Specifically, conditions that may mimic the findings of hydrops include urinary ascites secondary to bladder or renal collecting system rupture, intraperitoneal fluid resulting from a rupture of a viscus, chylothorax resulting in an accumulation of chylous fluid secondary to thoracic duct rupture, and intraperitoneal and pleural effusions seen with cystic hygromas (Fig. 12.8). Although it may not be possible to differentiate these disorders from those associated with true hydrops using sonography, certain features may be suggestive. These include distention of the bladder and/or renal collecting systems associated with urinary ascites secondary to posterior urethral valves in a male fetus, abnormally distended loops of bowel associated with meconium peritonitis, and unilateral hydrothorax on the left with thoracic duct rupture. The redundant skin covering a shrunken thorax of a thantotrophic dwarf may mimic a hydropic fetus, but the fetal limbs are significantly shortened. A cystic mass arising from the back of the neck can usually be recognized in a fetus with cystic hygroma. The intraperitoneal and pleural effusions occasionally seen with cystic hygromas are associated with disruption in lymphatic return. Thickening of the skin secondary to lymphangiectasia can also be seen. Cystic hygromas in females are frequently associated with Turner syndrome.

PROGNOSIS FOR THE HYDROPIC FETUS

Even with accurate sonographic diagnoses and aggressive treatment, the hydropic fetus has, in general, a poor prognosis. In NIH, the prognosis is related to the underlying anatomic, chromosomal, or structural abnormalities. In one series of severely hydropic fetuses with NIH, only 32 percent of diagnosed NIH fetuses survived the neonatal period, with five of the nine survivors having an uncertain or poor prognosis.[8,20] The best prognosis in the NIH group usually involves the fetus that has a potentially correctable arrhythmia. The prognosis for the IIH fetus is usually better than that for the NIH fetus; it is hoped that the prognosis will improve with more extensive experience in sonographically assisted cord transfusions. Interventional ther-

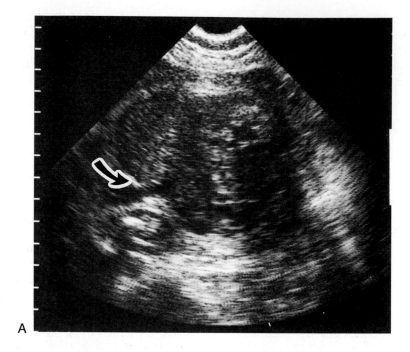

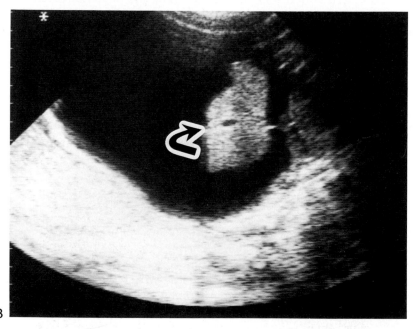

FIG. 12.8. Sonographic mimics of hydrops. (A) "Pseudoascites" appearing as a hype-choic band (arrow) along the anterior abdominal wall. (B) Massive urinary ascites secondary to ruptured renal collecting systems associated with posterior urethral valves. (*Figure continues.*)

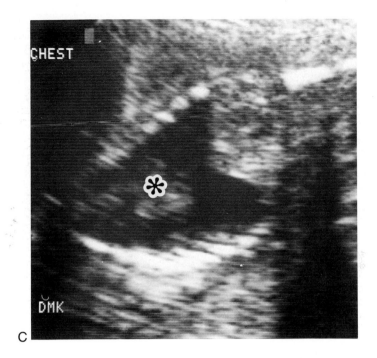

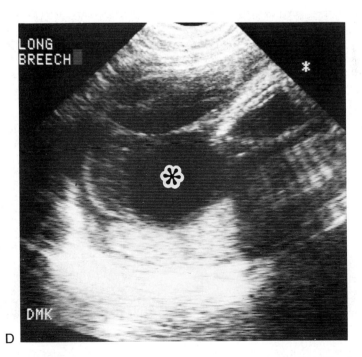

Fig. 12.8 (*Continued*).   (C) Bilateral pleural effusions surrounding the lung (*) in a 16-week fetus. (D) Same patient as in C showing cystic hygroma (8). (*Figure continues.*)

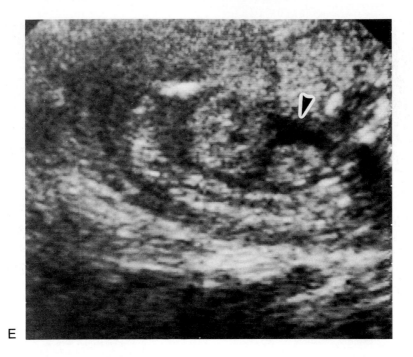

FIG. 12.8 (*Continued*).   (E) Left-sided hydrothorax (arrowhead) in a 16-week fetus. (F) One month later, the left-sided effusion has spontaneously resolved (arrowhead).

(*Figure continues.*)

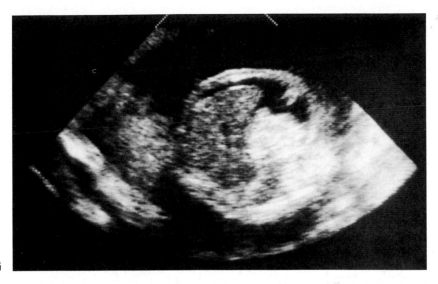

G

FIG. 12.8 (*Continued*). (G) Intraperitoneal fluid secondary to bowel perforation from meconium obstruction.

apy of the IIH fetus is potentially gratifying for the fetus, parents, and physicians.

In rare cases, hydrops has resolved spontaneously. We observed a left-sided effusion detected at 16 weeks resolve before 21 weeks (Fig. 12.8E,F). Several isolated case reports have documented transitory fetal ascites. One case of transitory fetal ascites was attributed to the sequelae of twin–twin transfusion.[21] In general, cases of spontaneous regression are extremely rare; once hydrops is present, it rarely resolves except after successful therapeutic intervention.[6]

SUMMARY

Sonography has a major role in the identification, evaluation, and treatment of the hydropic fetus. Although the prognosis of the NIH fetus is generally poor, the IIH fetus can frequently be treated effectively by transfusions performed by percutaneous needling of the umbilical vein. In addition, sonographic guidance of percutaneous umbilical vein sampling affords an accurate assessment of the etiology of NIH by facilitating karyotyping of the fetal blood.

ACKNOWLEDGMENTS

We thank Joan Johnson and John Bobbitt for their assistance in preparation of the manuscript.

REFERENCES

1. Warsof SL, Nicolaides KH, Rodeck C: Immune and nonimmune hydrops. Clin Obstet Gynecol 29:533, 1986

2. Freda VJ: Hemolytic disease of the newborn. p. 359. In Danforth DN (ed): Obstetrics and Gynecology. Harper & Row, Hagerstown, MD, 1977

3. Etches PC, Lemons JA: Nonimmune hydrops fetalis: Report of 22 cases including three siblings. Pediatrics 64:326, 1979

4. Fleischer AC, Killam AP, Boehm FH, et al: Hydrops fetalis: Sonographic evaluation and clinical implications. Radiology 141:163, 1981

5. Platt LD, Collea JV, Joseph DM: Transitory fetal ascites: An ultrasound diagnosis. Am J Obstet Gynecol 132:906, 1978

6. Benacerraf B, Frigoletto F, Wilson M: Successful mid-trimester thorocentesis with analysis of the lymphocyte population in pleural effusion. Am J Obstet Gynecol 155:398, 1986

7. Hashimoto BE, Filly RA, Callen PW: Fetal pseudoascites: Further anatomic observations. J Ultrasound Med 5:151, 1986

8. Kleinman CS, Donnerstein RL, DeVore GR, et al: Fetal echocardiography for evaluation of in utero congestive heart failure. N Engl J Med 306:568, 1982

9. Frigoletto FD, Greene MF, Benacerraf BR, et al: Ultrasonographic fetal surveillance in the management of the isoimmunized pregnancy. N Engl J Med 315:430, 1986

10. Daffos F, Capella-Pavlovsky M, Forestier F: Fetal blood sampling during pregnancy with use of a needle guided by ultrasound: A study of 606 consecutive cases. Am J Obstet Gynecol 153:655, 1985

11. Berkowitz RL, Chitkara U, Goldberg JD, et al: Intrauterine intravascular transfusions for severe red blood cell isoimmunization: Ultrasound-guided percutaneous approach. Am J Obstet Gynecol 155:574, 1986

12. Berkowitz RL, Chitkara U, Isabelle W, et al: Technical aspects of intravascular intrauterine transfusions: Lessons learned from thirty-three procedures. Am J Obstet Gynecol 157:4, 1987

13. Nicolaides KH, Rodeck CH, Mibashan RS, Kemp JR: Have Liley charts outlived their usefulness? Am J Obstet Gynecol 155:90, 1986

14. Rodeck CH, Nicolaides KH, Warsof SL, et al: The management of severe rhesus isoimmuniacation by fetoscopic intravascular transfusions. Am J Obstet Gynecol 150:769, 1984

15. Grannum PA, Copel JA, Plaxe SC, et al: In utero exchange transfusion by direct intravascular injection in severe erythroblastosis fetalis. N Engl J Med 314:1431, 1986

16. Nicolaides KH, Rodeck CH, Lange I, et al: Fetoscopy in the assessment of unexplained fetal hydrops. Br J Obstet Gynecol 92:671, 1985

17. de Crepigny LC, Robinson HP, Quinn M, et al: Ultrasound-guided fetal blood transfusion for severe Rhesus Isimmunization. Obstet Gynecol 66:529, 1985

18. Queenan JT: Erythroblastosis fetalis: Closing the circle. N Engl J Med 314:1448, 1986

19. Hashimoto B, Filly RA, Callen PW, Parer JT: Absorption of fetal intraperitoneal blood after intrauterine transfusion. J Ultrasound Med 6:421, 1987

20. Mahony BS, Filly RA, Callen PW, et al: Severe nonimmune hydrops fetalis: Sonographic evaluation. Radiology 151:757, 1984

21. Lubinsky M, Rapoport P: Transient fetal hydrops and "prune belly" in one identical female twin. N Engl J Med 308:256, 1983

Index

Page numbers followed by an f indicate figures; those followed by a t indicate tables.